Neurobiology and Mental Health Clinical Practice

This book illustrates the current findings of interpersonal neurobiology from leading mental health clinician-scholars that inform knowledge building and clinical practice. Representing the fields of social work, psychology and psychiatry, these authors creatively apply research findings from the ongoing revolution in social and behavior neuroscience to a diverse array of clinical issues. Contributions include elaborations of theory (the evolving social brain; new directions in attachment, affect regulation and trauma studies); practice (neurobiologically informed work with children, adults, couples and in the conduct of supervision); and emerging neuroscientific perspectives on broader mental health issues and concerns (substance abuse; psychotropic medications; secondary traumatic stress in clinicians; the neurodynamics of racial prejudice; the dangers of forfeiting humanism to our current romance with the biological). Together, these chapters equip readers with state-of-the-art knowledge of the manner in which new understandings of the brain inform and shape today's professional efforts to heal the troubled mind.

This book was originally published as a special issue of *Smith College Studies in Social Work*.

Dennis Miehls, PhD, LICSW, is a professor at Smith College School for Social Work, Northampton, Massachusetts, USA. He is chair of the Human Behavior Sequence of the School. He has published extensively in the areas of trauma, couple therapy, neurobiology and supervision. He maintains a private psychotherapy practice in Northampton, Massachusetts, USA.

Jeffrey Applegate, PhD, is professor emeritus at the Graduate School of Social Work and Social Research, Bryn Mawr College, Pennsylvania, USA. Currently he is adjunct professor at the School of Social Policy and Practice, University of Pennsylvania, USA. His scholarly work focuses on the application of psychoanalytic theory to social work research, practice and education.

Neurobiology and Mental Health Clinical Practice

New Directions, New Challenges

Edited by
Dennis Miehls and Jeffrey Applegate

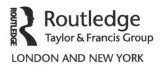

Routledge
Taylor & Francis Group

LONDON AND NEW YORK

First published 2015 by Routledge

2 Park Square, Milton Park, Abingdon, Oxon OX14 4RN
711 Third Avenue, New York, NY 10017, USA

Routledge is an imprint of the Taylor & Francis Group, an informa business

First issued in paperback 2017

British Library Cataloguing in Publication Data
A catalogue record for this book is available from the British Library

ISBN 13: 978-1-138-86075-9 (hbk)
ISBN 13: 978-1-138-05956-6 (pbk)

Typeset in ITC Garamond
by RefineCatch Limited, Bungay, Suffolk

Publisher's Note
The publisher accepts responsibility for any inconsistencies that may have
arisen during the conversion of this book from journal articles to book chapters,
namely the possible inclusion of journal terminology.

Disclaimer
Every effort has been made to contact copyright holders for their permission to
reprint material in this book. The publishers would be grateful to hear from any
copyright holder who is not here acknowledged and will undertake to rectify
any errors or omissions in future editions of this book.

Contents

CONTENTS

Citation Information

The chapters in this book were originally published in the journal *Smith College Studies in Social Work*, volume 84, issues 2–3 (2014). When citing this material, please use the original page numbering for each article, as follows:

Chapter 1
Introduction to Neurobiology and Clinical Work
Dennis Miehls and Jeffrey Applegate
Smith College Studies in Social Work, volume 84, issues 2–3 (2014) pp. 145–156

Chapter 2
Why We Need Therapy—and Why It Works: A Neuroscientific Perspective
Louis J. Cozolino and Erin N. Santos
Smith College Studies in Social Work, volume 84, issues 2–3 (2014) pp. 157–177

Chapter 3
Regulation Theory and Affect Regulation Psychotherapy: A Clinical Primer
Judith R. Schore and Allan N. Schore
Smith College Studies in Social Work, volume 84, issues 2–3 (2014) pp. 178–195

Chapter 4
Selected Neurobiological Arousal Issues as Manifested in a Clinical Case Illustration
Arlene Montgomery
Smith College Studies in Social Work, volume 84, issues 2–3 (2014) pp. 196–218

Chapter 5
The Interpersonal Neurobiology of Clinical Intuition
Terry Marks-Tarlow
Smith College Studies in Social Work, volume 84, issues 2–3 (2014) pp. 219–236

Chapter 6
Working Implicitly in Couples Therapy: Improving Right Hemisphere Affect-Regulating Capabilities
Francine Lapides
Smith College Studies in Social Work, volume 84, issues 2–3 (2014) pp. 237–254

Please direct any queries you may have about the citations to
clsuk.permissions@cengage.com

Notes on Contributors

Jon G. Allen, PhD, is a senior staff psychologist and Helen Malsin Palley chair in Mental Health Research at The Menninger Clinic, and professor of Psychiatry at the Menninger Department of Psychiatry and Behavioral Sciences at the Baylor College of Medicine.

Jeffrey Applegate, PhD, is professor emeritus, the Graduate School of Social Work and Social Research, Bryn Mawr College, Pennsylvania, USA. Currently he is adjunct professor at the School of Social Policy and Practice, University of Pennsylvania, USA. His scholarly work focuses on the application of psychoanalytic theory to social work research, practice and education.

Susanne Bennett, PhD, LICSW, is an associate professor at the National Catholic School of Social Service, The Catholic University of America in Washington, DC, where she teaches theory, practice and research in the master's and doctoral programs and has a scholarship focus on attachment theory and neurobiology.

Susan Bliss, PhD, LCSW, is an associate professor of social work at Molloy College and teaches in the Fordham University/Molloy College MSW Program.

Louis J. Cozolino, PhD, is a clinical psychologist with a consulting practice in Los Angeles, California, and a professor of psychology at Pepperdine University.

Yvette M. Esprey is a clinical psychologist (BA Hons, MA) working in private practice in Johannesburg, South Africa. She has a particular interest in the inter-subjectivity of race in the clinical setting.

Rosemary L. Farmer, PhD, LCSW, is an associate professor at the School of Social Work, Virginia Commonwealth University, where she teaches clinical social work practice, psychopathology and social work practice and the neurosciences.

Francine Lapides, MFT, is a founding member of the Santa Cruz Psychoanalytic Psychotherapy Society and writes and teaches in the area of attachment and psychoneurobiological theories and their applications to relational, psycho-dynamic psychotherapy. She has trained extensively with Daniel Siegel and is a member of Allan Schore's Berkeley study group. She has taught workshops and conferences across the United States. She offers small, personal monthly study groups online and in her office in Felton, CA, for clinicians wishing to learn more about applying neuroscience findings to their practices. She has online courses at www.PsyBC.com and at https://www.psychsem.com.

Terry Marks-Tarlow, PhD, is a clinical psychologist in private practice in Santa Monica, California, who teaches affective neuroscience at Reiss Davis Child Study Center and is author most recently of *Clinical Intuition in Psychotherapy* (2012, Norton) and *Awakening Clinical Intuition* (2014, Norton).

Dennis Miehls, PhD, LICSW, is a professor at Smith College School for Social Work. He is chair of the Human Behavior Sequence of the School. Dr. Miehls earned his BA from the University of Western Ontario in London, Ontario; his MSW from Wilfrid Laurier University in Waterloo, Ontario; and his PhD from Smith College School for Social Work in Northampton, MA. Dr. Miehls has published extensively in the areas of trauma work, couple therapy, neurobiology and supervision. In 2006, Dr. Miehls was named a Distinguished Practitioner by the National Academies of Practice in Social Work. He maintains a private psychotherapy practice in Northampton, MA. Dr. Miehls specializes in longterm psychotherapy with individuals and couples.

Arlene Montgomery, PhD, LCSW, is a clinical social worker with a private practice specializing in trauma issues and clinical supervision. She is an adjunct faculty member at The University of Texas School of Social Work, and Smith College School for Social Work.

Patricia Petrash, MSW, LICSW, is a psychotherapist and psychoanalyst in private practice and chair of the Institute of Contemporary Psychotherapy and Psychoanalysis (ICP+P) Psychotherapy Training Program in Washington, DC.

Brian Rasmussen, PhD, is an associate professor in the School of Social Work at the University of British Columbia, Okanagan Campus, and an adjunct associate professor at Smith College School for Social Work.

Erin N. Santos is a graduate student in psychology at Pepperdine University.

Allan N. Schore, PhD, is on the clinical faculty of the UCLA David Geffen School of Medicine, editor of the *Norton Series on Interpersonal Neurobiology*, and the recipient of a number of awards from the American Psychological Association and the American Psychoanalytic Association. He is the co-chair of the child section of the upcoming *Psychodynamic Diagnostic Manual* (2nd edition).

Judith R. Schore, PhD, is a clinical social worker in private practice, dean of students and core faculty at the Sanville Institute, associate director of Clinical Training and Curriculum Development at Reiss-Davis Child Study Center, and faculty at The Graduate Center for Child Development and Psychotherapy.

Jacqueline R. Strait, DSW, is a clinical social worker in private practice in Philadelphia, PA. She is also a lecturer at the University of Pennsylvania School of Social Policy and Practice.

Karen Zilberstein, MSW, is a child and family therapist and clinical director of the Northampton, MA, chapter of A Home Within, a national non-profit devoted to providing pro bono psychotherapy to foster care youth and alumni.

Introduction to Neurobiology and Clinical Work

The purpose of this article[1] is to familiarize the readers of this Special Issue of *Smith College Studies in Social Work* with fundamental theoretical concepts that are elaborated and deepened in the following articles in the journal. We informed our authors that we would provide the introductory framework to neurobiology so as to give them the flexibility to focus with more specificity on their respective topic areas. The dizzying pace of development and advancing literature in a number of converging fields makes the study of neurobiology and clinical work an exciting and daunting task. We recognize that literature from the broad fields of attachment theory, infant research, trauma theory, cognitive neuroscience, relational theory, relational analytic trauma theory, and nonlinear dynamic systems theory (to name a few) are converging in a synergistic and interesting manner. These theories underscore that human beings are resilient and that change is possible across the life cycle, even if individuals have experienced unfortunate traumatic beginnings. We use the term *neurobiology* to discuss current research findings on brain structure and function(s). We agree with Louis Cozolino (2006) when he suggested that there is no such thing as a "single brain" and that an individual's brain and mind functions, which effect a multitude of intrapsychic and interpersonal factors, are fundamentally shaped in interaction with other people. There are many implications to this statement—this article illuminates some of these implications, especially as they inform clinical work based on the understanding that the treatment relationship is a central component of change in brain functioning that leads to therapeutic change with a diverse range of clients. The purpose of this article is twofold. First, we outline some "brain basics" that give the reader foundational knowledge of neurobiology. Second, we briefly discuss the importance of "relationship" as the foundation for change in brain function.

BRAIN BASICS

At the outset, it is important to recognize that our study and knowledge of how the brain functions is rapidly expanding. Current technology such as functional magnetic resonance imaging (fMRI) and positron emission tomography (PET) facilitates research that illuminates where particular brain activity

1

is occurring under various conditions (Applegate & Shapiro, 2005; Basham & Miehls, 2004). Researchers are able to trace the parts of the brain that are activated during different (interpersonal) experiences, and we can hypothesize how mental processes affect one's subjective experiences. The work of Schore (2003a, 2003b) and other infant and trauma researchers (Cozolino, 2006; Siegel, 1999, 2007) has extended our working knowledge of brain functions related to affect regulation, normative development, and interrupted development. Studying the effects of disrupted attachment on the developing emotional security of infants and children has been particularly useful in understanding the essential components of brain physiology that contribute to overall positive mental health.

Generally, we understand that individuals develop symptoms of mental distress as a result of a combination of genetic vulnerabilities and environmental factors that lead to alterations in the way in which neurotransmitters and hormones are produced. These alterations lead to changes in brain functions that may result in the development of disorders. Consider the interactive effects on brain physiology for individuals who experience depression. Feelings of hopelessness in depressed individuals likely interact with neurological vulnerabilities that result in potential impairment of body–brain functions. In other words, there is a reciprocal effect of genetic vulnerability interacting with the emotional world of depressed individuals that leads to actual changes in brain physiology and certain brain functions.

Three parts of the brain, composing what's referred to as the "triune brain," are intricately connected (Levine, 1997). At its most basic, the triune brain is a combination of the reptilian brain, the limbic system, and the neocortex. The reptilian brain, or brain stem, is that part of our brain that is instinctual and promotes basic survival by regulating basic physiological processes like respiration, body temperature, and sleep cycles. Regions of the limbic system integrate and regulate key mental and emotional processes, including attachment. The neocortex is that part of our brain that is the thinking, cognitive, and perceptual processing center. A vertical integration of reptilian, limbic, and neocortex functions promotes the capacity to sense the ebb and flow of empathic connection in our own bodies (Badenoch, 2008). However, if the natural integration of our triune brain is interrupted (e.g., as a result of trauma), the capacity to experience and hold complex affective states is compromised. Compromised individuals develop a range of symptoms and responses to stimuli that fundamentally shape their interactions with the world around them, including their relationships with others.

Various parts of the brain have a sophisticated way of communicating with each other. The brain is estimated to have one hundred billion cells called "neurons" that facilitate communication among brain areas. Applegate and Shapiro (2005) suggest that neurons "maintain an electrical charge and are composed of three parts: the *cell body*, which contain the substances that govern its metabolism; hundreds of branding appendages, called *dendrites*;

and a single appendage called an *axon*" (p. 4). Neural systems are formed through a process called "synaptogenesis"—in this process, the axon of one neuron connects with the dendrite of another. A minute gap (synapse) allows the transmission of chemical molecules (neurotransmitters) from one neuron to another. Those neurons that electrically fire together form connections that influence enduring patterns of behavior in individuals. That is, neurons that fire together repeatedly form connections that enable them to survive. Those neurons not connected to others in this manner die off in a process of parcellation, or "neural pruning." This use-it-or-lose-it principle ultimately determines the manner in which the brain achieves its ultimate differentiation into various functional neural networks (Applegate & Shapiro, 2005).

With these beginning understandings of how the brain organizes the complexity of interactions among its various parts, we now summarize brain physiology in terms of, the different functions of the right- and left-brain hemispheres, the systems of memory, and the role that attachment experiences play in the development of neural networks and associated brain functions. We also discuss how these brain functions are activated and used in the clinical relationship toward repair of earlier disrupted attachments and/or the sequelae of trauma.

Right- and Left-Brain Hemisphere Development and Functions

The brain is divided into right and left hemispheres that are connected by filaments of white matter called the "corpus collosum." Briefly, the right hemisphere registers the global aspects, or the "big picture" of incoming information. It processes emotional experience, aspects of nonverbal communication such as gestures, prosody, tone of voice, and somatic sensations such as touch and body positioning. The left hemisphere, in contrast, "specializes in identifying and processing the details of a situation and is therefore superior in processing the semantic aspects of language, making causal connections between phenomena, and coordinating fine motor movements" (Applegate & Shapiro, 2005, p. 8). These hemispheric differences give rise to common parlance that refers to individuals as either "right brained" (feeling/artistic) or "left brained" (intellectual/rational). These characterizations do have some foundation in the neurobiology of brain hemispheric characteristics and functions; but increasingly we are able to understand how the brain integrates information and experiences on multiple levels (Badenoch, 2008; Cozolino, 2006; Siegel, 2007).

Because of its leading role in language development the left hemisphere was considered the dominant hemisphere for understanding emotions for most of the 20th century. New technologies, however, have enabled neuroscientists to learn more about the crucial role of the right hemisphere in emotional life. Right hemispheric activity is experienced in a holistic and nonlinear manner. It is "specialized for perceiving and processing visual and spatial information – such as sending and receiving nonverbal signals, the centerpiece of social understanding" (Badenoch, 2008, p. 19). Nonverbal interactions such as observing the facial expression of another and sensing danger from another are processed in the right hemisphere. These reactions develop early in infants who can sense safety or danger from the nonverbal behaviors of parental/caregiver figures. From these experiences, babies begin to develop intrapsychic mental representations of themselves and others. It is important to note that most right-brain functions occur outside conscious awareness. We develop a template of responses that are beyond our awareness and, as Cozolino (2006) noted, "because the right brain develops first, it organizes and stores many emotional experiences that can emerge in later relationships, especially when we are under stress" (p. 68).

Innumerable interactions with attachment figures during the first 18 months of life shape right-brain circuitry. This development is directly related to the infant's burgeoning abilities to regulate emotions. Such regulation is a joint endeavor—the infant develops its right-brain circuitry while in connection with the right brain of the attachment figure. In other words, the "linking of right hemispheres is accomplished through eye contact, facial expressions, soothing vocalizations, caresses, and exciting exchanges" (Cozolino, 2006, p. 72). The attuned parent knows when to engage and/or disengage with the infant so that the infant can begin self-regulating emotions without becoming overwhelmed. As described below, disrupted attachment and traumatic events can wreak havoc with right-brain development and the achievement of emotional regulation.

The left hemisphere develops somewhat later than the right and is often characterized as serving the executive functions of logic, language, and linearity. In other words, the left hemisphere takes the lead in consciously processing information that is accessible to the individual's memory. The left brain potentiates language to explain, order, and characterize experiences.

When there has been healthy and synchronized attunement with an attachment figure the infant/toddler begins to integrate the functions of the two hemispheres. Badenoch (2008) referred to this synchronization of the two hemispheres as "horizontal integration." Individuals with adaptive horizontal integration have the capacity to move fluidly between the functions of the two hemispheres. This ability leads to the capacity to verbalize affective states while in the midst of experiencing states of nonconscious activation of bodily sensations. Recall that the right-brain responses are activated through a range of nonverbal activities and that these activities are often encoded on an unconscious basis. The left brain, then, begins to register conscious ideas that help explain the autonomic responses of the right brain. For example, an adult who experiences panic when he sees a barking German Shepherd will be able to calm himself when the left brain accurately registers and brings into conscious thought a childhood experience of being terribly frightened by a large dog. This individual has achieved horizontal integration of the two hemispheres. However, if the child had been unable to feel safe in the childhood experience, the right-brain response will dominate the current experience, and the logic and calming messages of the left brain will be mute. In other words, the emotions that the individual experiences are altered dependent on the intensity of the childhood experiences and dependent on the ability of an attachment figure to help the frightened child process and mediate them.

Information Processing and Memory

As noted above, well-integrated right- and left-brain hemispheres function collaboratively to ensure healthy adaptation to internal and external stimuli. When working well together, the left brain is able to organize experiences in such a way that the individual does not feel threatened and is able to continue to explore novel situations and enjoy the positive emotions associated with growth and development. However, if a child feels overtly threatened and is not in the presence of a calming, affectively balanced attachment figure, less adaptive templates of responses become more powerfully ingrained. As noted above, resulting templates influence the response and the meaning system of individuals. Cozolino (2006) noted that "states of stress, anxiety, fear, trauma, and pain all result in heightened activation in right-sided structures" (p. 74). We tend to use the defense strategies of fight, flight, or freeze when experiencing such powerful negative emotions. Right-brain activation tends to be biased toward negative emotions whereas left-brain activation tends to be biased toward positive emotions. Citing Keenan et al., Cozolino (2006) suggested that

> an unfortunate artifact of the evolution of laterality may be that the right hemisphere, biased toward negative emotions and pessimism, develops first and serves as the core of self-awareness and self-identity. To be human may be to have vulnerability towards shame, guilt, and depression. (p. 75)

This vulnerability is particularly heightened if the individual has experienced disrupted attachment and/or traumatic events in her early development.

Memory is the means by which the brain responds to experiences, and neural connections are formed that potentiate implicit or explicit memory. Implicit, or nondeclarative, memory is operable at birth and is dominant until about age 18 months. Siegel and Hartzell (2003) noted that it "results in the creation of the particular circuits of the brain that are responsible for generating emotions, behavioral responses, perception, and probably the encoding of bodily sensations" (p. 22). Implicit memories are nonverbal and become activated on an unconscious basis. What is encoded in infancy in certain situations may become restimulated when an adult experiences similar circumstances. Badenoch (2008) explained: "When implicit memories are activated in our day-to-day experience, they have no time stamp, so we interpret the emotional, visceral, perceptual, behavioral surge as being entirely *caused by something occurring in the present moment*" (p. 25). An essential goal of clinical intervention is to assist individuals to transform implicit memories into explicit memories.

Explicit memory, in contrast, becomes possible with the development of the hippocampus, a part of the brain promotes the capacity to recall consciously and articulate experiences and related emotional responses. "There are two components of explicit memory: *semantic, or factual*, memory, which becomes available at around a year and a half of age, and *autobiographical* memory, which begins to develop sometime after the second birthday" (Siegel & Hartzell, 2003, p. 23). The later development of the hippocampus explains why individuals universally experience childhood amnesia and explains why humans are not able to remember details of experiences of their first 2 years of life. Autobiographical memory allows children to begin to narrate their stories and to make sense or meaning of their experiences. Badenoch (2008) emphasized that this type of remembering is related to empathic connections to caregivers. As she noted, *"Empathic attunement is the key factor that fosters this all-important integrative step in children*, and it is also part of the reason that solid therapy can rewire the brain so efficiently" (p. 28).

Autobiographical memory links the hippocampus and the front part of the brain called the "prefrontal cortex." Siegel and Hartzell (2003) suggested that "the prefrontal cortex is extremely important for a wide range of processes, including autobiographical memory, self-awareness, response flexibility, mindsight, and the regulation of emotions" (pp. 24–25). Research demonstrates that the development of the prefrontal cortex is profoundly influenced by interpersonal relationships. Secure attachment relationships contribute to sound development of the functions associated with the prefrontal cortex. Siegel (2007) drew together research findings and lists nine integrative functions of the middle prefrontal cortex.[2] These functions are (1) regulation of the body, (2) attuned communication, (3) emotional regulation, (4) response flexibility, (5) empathy, (6) insight, (7) fear modulation, (8) intuition, and (9) morality.

Studying the brains of depressed individuals offers some interesting data suggesting that certain brain functions are altered in conjunction with certain mental health vulnerabilities. The functions of the prefrontal cortex, for example, are significantly altered in the depressed individual. Citing Bremner et al., Badenoch (2008) noted that "recent neuroimaging studies have revealed that the *medial orbitofrontal cortex* of people who suffer from *major depression* is 32% smaller than in nondepressed people" (p. 122). This suggests that these individuals have less capacity to integrate cognitive and emotional processes and are also more challenged than nondepressed individuals in regulating their bodily functions and emotions. Badenoch (2008) also suggested that the volume of the hippocampi of depressed individuals is 19% less than individuals without depression. Recalling that the hippocampus is that part of our brain that aids the individual to have explicit memories, it follows that depressed individuals have a neurophysiological reason for experiencing memory and cognitive deficits during depressive episodes.

Depressed individuals also experience heightened arousal of the amygdala, an almond shaped part of the limbic system that generates feelings of fear and anxiety. In addition to experiencing waking periods of anxious depression, their overactive amygdala can lead to sleeping difficulties as they remain "on alert" to danger and associated anxiety even during sleep periods (Badenoch, 2008).

The Influence of Trauma on Brain Development

Humans are resilient beings. However, certain traumatic events will shape the response of individuals in particular ways. It is important to recognize that trauma is a relative concept and that there will be variability in individual responses to certain types of disrupted attachment, neglect, abuse, and other extreme stressors. We discuss how these sorts of traumatic events influence one's ability to remember and process these events in an adaptive manner. When individuals experience symptoms of post-traumatic stress disorder, including dissociation, their capacities to work through aspects of trauma are compromised.

The adult brain regresses to an infantile state when experiencing stressors and/or traumatic events. Van der Kolk (1996) pointed out that traumatic memories are not encoded in narratives—rather, individuals store unprocessed traumatic events in somatic, bodily sensations. Basham and Miehls (2004) noted:

> First, the psychophysiological effects following trauma include extreme autonomic responses that are reminiscent of the actual trauma. Alternating patterns of hyperarousal and numbness plague trauma survivors, who are disturbed regularly by startle responses, lowered thresholds to sound intensities, and a reduced electrical pattern in cortical events. (p. 76)

The amygdala of the trauma survivor is aroused by the sympathetic regulatory system when there is a familiar traumatic stimulus coming toward the individual. Citing Cahill and McGaugh, Cozolino (2002) wrote that the "activation of the amygdala (and the related physiological and biological changes) is at the heart of the modulation of emotional and traumatic memory" (p. 271). The heightened arousal of the amygdala disrupts the ability of the hippocampus to facilitate explicit memory of the event. In other words, the functions of the hippocampus that are related to understanding, attaching language to and consciously remembering the event may be hijacked by the trauma survivor's amygdala.

An individual processes the relative danger and/or safety of situations in rapid fashion. Any new stimulus is quickly appraised by right-brain functions by reading facial expressions, body language, and posture of the other participant. If the behavior/stimulus is familiar to the individual and has previously been experienced as benign, then she can move forward with the interaction with increasing complexity. If the hippocampus is unfamiliar with the situation then a message is picked up by the brain essentially saying "be alert" or "wake up"—something is going on that needs to be tended to and controlled. Then, the amygdala takes over and the implicit memories are predominant and the individual experiences sensoriomotor or bodily responses to the stimuli. Explicit or declarative memory functions may cease to function.

This process explains why trauma memories are often encoded outside of conscious awareness of the survivor. A current situation reminds the individual of a previous traumatic event that was neither processed nor encoded as explicit memory. Rather, the event was "remembered" through sensoriomotor memory. In clinical social work, then, the therapeutic process aids the individual in translating these implicit memories into more readily accessible conscious explicit memories. Often trauma survivors will try to make sense of their sensorimotor memories by talking to family (to confirm history, for example), to friends or to clinicians. An individual will suffer less and will become less likely to repeat traumatic patterns when she attaches words to these experiences. Making meaning of, categorizing, schematizing, and articulating previous traumatic events diminish their strength.

These understandings of brain function aid our understanding of certain clinical phenomena that many trauma survivors exhibit in treatment. Amygdalar fear networks are activated when a trauma survivor experiences flashbacks during sessions. Flashbacks are powerful and intrusive images of previous traumatic events. Cozolino (2002) suggested that

> traumatic flashbacks are memories of a quite different nature than are those of nontraumatic events. To begin with, they are stored in more primitive circuits with less cortical and left-hemisphere involvement. Because of this, they are strong somatic, sensory, and emotional, as well as inherently nonverbal. (p. 272)

Clinical interventions aid the trauma survivor to begin to modulate the intensity of the flashback experience.

Dissociation is a commonly used defense by trauma survivors. Here too, the client is affected by implicit communication that reminds her of painful earlier traumatic events. This unconscious process can trigger a dissociative response. Understood as an adaptation to stressors related to traumatic events, the dissociated individual client needs therapeutic assistance to regulate more adaptively the powerful affect that is being triggered by the implicit memory.

Finally, it is important to note that the functions of the part of the brain that is related to the development of speech and language (Broca's area) are also compromised for many trauma survivors. Some appear frozen or are rendered silent due to speechless terror and a sense of numbness. Cozolino (2002) suggested that

> this inhibitory effect on Broca's area will impair the encoding of conscious memory for traumatic events at the time they occur. It will then naturally interfere with the development of narratives that serve to process the experience and lead to neural network integration and psychological healing. (p. 274)

Here too, clinical work can assist trauma survivors in attaching words and meaning to their potentially paralyzing experiences.

The Treatment Relationship: The Cornerstone of Clinical Work Informed by Neurobiology

The last trimester of pregnancy and the first 3 years of an infant's life are crucial time periods for the development of a number of brain functions that have been described above. The primary relationship between the child and caregiver(s) influences the relative strengths, health, and/or deficits in brain functions. Secure attachment contributes to optimal brain development; however, unpredictable or otherwise "traumatic" parenting leads to the development of self-protective behaviors in the child that impair certain mental functions of the developing brain. A secure attachment relationship between caregiver and child leads to the child's ability to manage highly charged affective states (Schore, 2003b). Infant researchers (Beebe & Lachmann, 2002; Stern, 1985) have demonstrated that parents need to help modulate children's primitive affective states for optimal development to occur. Caregivers who experience difficulties with their own affect regulation often have a difficult time in assisting their children to deal adaptively with their emotional development, often resulting in anxious and insecure attachment patterns which affect their abilities to form satisfying relationships. Parents convey information to their children in implicit (right brain) and explicit (left brain) communication patterns. Clinicians and clients also form their treatment relationship by attunement with each other in implicit and explicit interactions. A client receives and understands the clinician's implicit messages by observing nonverbal responses of the clinician (facial expression, tone of voice, posture, etc.). Language, interpretation, and insight promote the client's developing capacities for left-brain activities. This movement between implicit and explicit communication mirrors the development between caregiver and child during early phases of emotional development.

The sensitively attuned treatment relationship is a highly empathic one—and one that holds the promise of corrective experiences for adult clients. Crucial for the development of trust in the treatment relationship, the clinician's understanding that her nonverbal right-brain attunement with her client's right-brain activity leads to satisfying and healing affect synchronizing possibilities. The functions of the clinician change over the course of the treatment relationship. More active in the early phase of treatment, the clinician attends to left-brain processes by assisting the client to recognize, feel, and manage affective states. With increasing capacity to be aware of her own affective states, the client becomes more able to self-regulate emotions while in the presence of the clinician and others in her relational environment. Responding to this shift, the clinician can focus more directly on right-brain processes that promote conscious insight and the creation of new patterns of interactions with others. Clients can then alter their internal representations of relationships and redesign their views of self and others in interpersonal exchanges—all while altering associated brain structures.

It is important for the clinician to appreciate the inevitability that her clients are tuning into her complex internal world via observations of her facial expressions, tone of voice, and postural changes. In addition, the clinician's own affective response to a client may serve as information about powerful unconscious aspects of the client that remain unverbalized. Most clinicians have been trained to conduct clinical work as predominantly a left-brain activity. They have been taught to encourage clients to verbalize, seek insight, and to update memories. Although acknowledging these necessary therapeutic activities, Badenoch (2008) suggested that there are risks to staying focused solely on left-brain activities when working with a client. One drawback may be that the client does not utilize bodily sensations as important diagnostic indicators of anxiety and other mental health vulnerabilities. Ignoring such implicit communication may lead the client/clinician dyad to miss opportunities to lessen the client's "typical" defensive postures of interaction with others. Second, a clinician who ignores her own right-brain responses may reduce her abilities to receive crucial information about her clients' right-brain processes and dynamics.

The Power and Promise of Neural Plasticity

As documented above, trauma can change the brain in ways that compromise its key structures and functions. Fortunately, evidence mounts that neurologically informed clinical intervention can facilitate reparative and growthful change in these structures and functions (Badenoch, 2008; Baylis,

2006; Cozolino, 2002; Schwartz & Begley, 2002). The capacity for this sort of brain modification is referred to as "neural plasticity." Simply put, *neural plasticity* refers to the brain's capacity to reshape itself in response to new experience. Although brain cells and pathways are most plastic during the rapid developmental transformations of the first 3 years of life, recent findings suggest that adult relational experience, including psychotherapy, can alter the architecture of neural networks and foster the growth of new neurons in a process called "neurogenesis" (Badenoch, 2008). Areas of the brain that appear most able to generate new neurons include the hippocampus, the amygdala, and the cerebral cortex (Cozolino, 2002)—areas crucial to the capacity to retrieve and modify the affective intensity of memories and foster adaptive affect regulation.

CONCLUSION

Cozolino (2002) asserted that all forms of psychotherapy "will be successful to the degree to which they foster neural growth and integration" (p. 27). From its inception, social workers have asserted that human distress results from a combination of biological, psychological, and social factors. Progress in interpersonal neurobiology over the last two decades now offers the field the opportunity to strengthen the biological dimension of this biopsychosocial perspective and its implications for effective intervention. The following articles in this special issue give voice to the dynamic and creative manner in which today's scholars are exploring and documenting the vast potential of this new direction in clinical knowledge building and practice.

Dennis Miehls
Professor, Smith College School for Social Work
Guest Coeditor
and
Jeffrey Applegate
Adjunct Professor, School of Social Policy and Practice,
University of Pennsylvania
Guest Coeditor

NOTES

1. This article is an updated version of a previously published chapter by Dennis Miehls (2011). Some material is duplicated in its exact form with copyright permission from SAGE Publications.

2. For a more detailed description of Siegel's work, the reader is encouraged to see Siegel (2007).

REFERENCES

Applegate, J., & Shapiro, J. (2005). *Neurobiology for clinical social work: Theory and practice*. New York, NY: W.W. Norton.

Badenoch, B. (2008). *Being a brain-wise therapist: A practical guide to interpersonal neurobiology*. New York, NY: W.W. Norton.

Basham, K., & Miehls, D. (2004). *Transforming the legacy: Couple therapy with survivors of childhood trauma*. New York, NY: Columbia University Press.

Baylis, P. (2006). The neurobiology of affective interventions: A cross-theoretical model. *Clinical Social Work Journal*, *34*(1), 61–81.

Beebe, B., & Lachman, F. M. (2002). *Infant research and adult treatment: Co-constructing interactions*. Hillsdale, NJ: Analytic Press.

Cozolino, L. (2002). *The neuroscience of psychotherapy: Building & re-building the human brain*. New York, NY: W.W. Norton.

Cozolino, L. (2006). *The neuroscience of human relationships: Attachment and the developing social brain*. New York, NY: W.W. Norton.

Levine, P. (1997). *Waking the tiger: Healing trauma*. Berkeley, CA: North Atlantic Books.

Miehls, D. (2011). Neurobiology and clinical social work. In J. Brandell (Ed.), *Theory and practice in clinical social work* (2nd ed., pp. 81–99). Thousand Oaks, CA: Sage.

Schore, A. (2003a). *Affect dysregulation & disorders of the self*. New York, NY: W.W. Norton.

Schore, A. (2003b). *Affect regulation & the repair of the self*. New York, NY: W.W. Norton.

Schwartz, J. M., & Begley, S. (2002). *The mind and the brain: Neuroplasticity and the power of mental force*. New York, NY: Regan Books.

Siegel, D. (1999). *The developing mind*. New York, NY: Guilford Press.

Siegel, D. (2007). *The mindful brain: Reflection and attunement in the cultivation of well-being*. New York, NY: W.W. Norton.

Siegel, D., & Hartzell, M. (2003). *Parenting from the inside out*. New York, NY: Penguin Publishers.

Stern, D. N. (1985). *The interpersonal world of the infant: A view from psychoanalysis and developmental psychology*. New York, NY: Basic Books.

van der Kolk, B. (1996). The body keeps score: Approaches to psychobiology of posttraumatic stress disorder. In B. van der Kolk, A. McFarlane, & L. Weisaeth (Eds.), *Traumatic stress: The effects of overwhelming experience on mind, body and society* (pp. 214–241). New York, NY: Guilford Press.

Why We Need Therapy—and Why It Works: A Neuroscientific Perspective

LOUIS J. COZOLINO and ERIN N. SANTOS

Pepperdine University, Los Angeles, California, USA

Evolution has woven together genetics, biology, and relationships with minds, tribes, and culture over a vast expanse of time to create a remarkable social organ. This deep history accounts for the profound connections among our bodies, minds, and attachment to others. Due to their very complexity, our brains are extremely vulnerable to dysregulation, dissociation, and emotional distress. Fortunately for us, we possess the tools to heal one another—communication, trusting relationships, and empathy. In this article, the authors explore the brain's evolutionary history with two concerns in mind: why we need therapy and why therapy works.

Evolution is a problem-creating as well as a problem-solving process. (Jonas Salk, 1983)

WHY WE NEED THERAPY

Anatomically, modern humans evolved from our primate ancestors around 100,000 years ago. It took another 50,000 years for our brains and culture to evolve sufficient complexity to make us capable of language, planning, and creativity. But alas, this very complexity has a downside. The more recently emergent aspects of our brains, which give us such astonishing powers of thought, logic, imagination, empathy, and morality, are interdependent with much older circuitry that we share with our mammalian and reptilian fore-bears. So, even today, one of the most basic human challenges is integrating and coordinating the complex and very different systems that make up our brains.

For example, the neo-cortex, the part of the brain that organizes our powers of conscious thought and imagination, must coexist and cooperate with ancient survival networks conserved by natural selection through hun-dreds of thousands of generations. Beneath our newer equipment, capable of writing sonnets and dreaming of a utopian future, are structures driven by instincts, unconscious impulses, and primitive anxieties. Related to the difficulties of coordinating systems from different stages of evolution are a number of challenges that result in psychological suffering.

Five Artifacts of Evolution: Vulnerabilities to Emotional Distress

Through a million years of conservation, innovation, and mutation, our brains have become a government of old and new systems, many with opposing goals, different languages, and operating at vastly different speeds. Below are five of those artifacts that make us vulnerable to the mental distress that brings us and our clients to psychotherapy. Although we have divided them for definitional purposes, you will see that they are all interdependent and mutually reinforcing.

#1 THE VITAL HALF-SECOND

> Man is an over-complicated organism who may die out for want of simplicity. (Ezra Pound, 1938)

As Freud and many before him recognized, our brains have at least two major tracks of information processing: a very fast primitive system that pro-cesses sensory, motor, and emotional data that we share with most other animals and a modern, slower system that processes conscious information. The primitive system, which is nonverbal and inaccessible to conscious con-sideration, is referred to as implicit memory, the unconscious, or somatic memory. The slow system, which has given rise to consciousness experi-ence, self-awareness, and the capacity to self-reflect, gave rise to narratives, stories, and imagination; our newer, complex system is dependent on a well-developed and fully integrated cerebral cortex.

Similar to computers, a half second is an eternity for neural connections within the fast system. Evidence of this fast neural activity reveals itself every day. If we touch a hot stove or are cut off while driving, our body reacts faster than our conscious awareness. We discover ourselves having avoided a collision or having lifted our hand off of the stove, but we experience it as a choice we made. In stark contrast, consciousness is the result of broad and complex neural activity; in other words, it's a complicated accomplishment. Although our brains process sensory, motor, and emotional information in 10 to 50 milliseconds, it takes 500 to 600 milliseconds (a half second) for brain activity to register in conscious awareness.

Although a half second is a long time in terms of neural communication, it is barely noticeable within our normal stream of conscious awareness. During this vital half-second, our brains work like search engines unconsciously scanning our memories, bodies, and emotions for relevant information. In fact, 90% of the input to the cortex comes from this internal neural processing. This half second gives our brains the opportunity to construct present experience based on a template from the past that our minds interpret as current objective reality. The result is that we feel we are living in the present moment when in reality we live a half second behind. These neural mechanisms also help us to understand why so many of us continue in old and ineffective patterns of behavior despite repeated failure.

By the time we become consciously aware of an experience, it has already been processed many times, activated memories, and set in motion complex patterns of behavior. An example of this process is transference, where the brain signals the mind to use past relationships to shape perceptions of our motivations, thoughts, feelings, and intentions in the absence of external information. This projective process can damage a lifetime of relationships without us ever being aware that it is taking place.

#2 THE PRIMACY OF EARLY LEARNING

Limits, like fears, are often just an illusion. (Michael Jordan, 2009)

The conceptual and abstract learning controlled by our neocortex evolved and develops last. The early years of life are dominated by more primitive systems dedicated to sensory-motor, emotional, and relational abilities.

The parents are the primary environment to which a baby's brain adapts, and their unconscious minds are a child's first reality. Their nonverbal communications and patterns of responding to the infant's basic needs shape the baby's brain and how he or she perceives the world. Because the first few years of life are a period of exuberant brain development, early experience has a disproportionate impact on the development of neural systems, with lifelong consequences. Because the cortical systems of conscious learning and awareness take years to develop, all of our early sensory, motor, social, and emotional learning is stored in fast, unconscious systems. This means that childhood has a powerful and lifelong influence on the way the brain constructs reality.

Even before birth, primitive regions of our brains begin to learn, and they are deeply affected by our social and emotional experiences. The amygdala, for example, which serves as the executive center of fear processing, is fully mature by 8 months of gestation. On the other hand, the cortical networks that will come to regulate and inhibit the amygdala will take two decades or more to mature. As a result, we can experience intense fear for years before we can regulate it. The amygdala also happens to be a central component in the development of our attachment schema, our ability to regulate our emotions, and our sense of self-worth.

Misattuned parents, brutal social systems, war, and prejudice can have a tremendous impact on early brain development, thus creating severe conflicts. For most of us, these memories remain forever inaccessible to conscious consideration or modification. We mature into self-awareness years later, having been programmed by early experiences that we automatically assume to be true. As adolescents and adults, we seek therapy because we find ourselves unable to form meaningful relationships, to manage our emotions, or to feel worthy of love.

The fact that so much learning occurs early in life is one of nature's standard operating procedures for mammals like ourselves. In the womb, the child's biology is shaped by the mother's day-to-day experience. After birth, a child is shaped by its interactions with the environment and its interactions with his mother and other caretakers. All of this flexibility is good and bad news. The good news is that each brain is shaped to adapt to a particular environment. This is adaptive from an evolutionary point of view because, unlike most animals, every human baby can learn to "fit in" to whatever physical and social environment he or she is born into—which might change radically from culture to culture, generation to generation, climate to climate.

Our parents' attitudes and behaviors serve as the models that shape our brains. In good times and with good enough parents, this early brain building will serve the child well throughout life. The bad news comes when factors are not so favorable, such as in the case of parental psychopathology where the brain may be sculpted in ways that become maladaptive later in life. Abused and neglected children often enter adolescence and adulthood with little awareness of their early experiences, but with a variety of symptoms. Explosive anger, eating disorders, drug and alcohol problems, and promiscuity are quite common. They also have identity disturbances and poor self-images, which are exacerbated by their negative emotions and behaviors.

In the absence of an ability to consciously connect these feelings and thoughts with past experiences, negative feelings and behaviors seem to arise without cause from within. Victims are then left to make sense of their internal chaos and negative behavior, which they perceive as their own faulty character. Psychotherapy guides us in an exploration of our early experiences and helps us to create a healthier narrative that connects these early experiences to the ways in which our brains and minds distort our current lives. In the process, our symptoms come to be understood as forms of implicit memory for consciously forgotten events instead of signs of insanity or character pathology. This process can open the door to greater empathy and compassion for oneself and for the possibility of healing.

#3 Core Shame

> Nothing you have done is wrong, and nothing you can do can make up for it. (Gershen Kaufman, 1974)

Although core shame is clearly an aspect of the primacy of early learning, its prevalence in society and its power to create suffering warrants it special attention. Core shame describes the process wherein some children come to experience themselves as fundamentally defective, worthless, and unlovable—the polar opposite of self-esteem. Core shame needs to be differentiated from the appropriate kinds of shame and guilt that emerge later in childhood. Appropriate shame is about behavior that violates social rules, and it requires an ability to judge one's behaviors in a social context and the cortical development required to inhibit impulses. Core shame is about the self, a sense of worthlessness, a fear of being "found out," and a desperate attempt to be perfect to avoid detection. In essence, core shame is tied to our primitive survival need; we need to be part of the tribe for survival, yet core shame feels like we are always on the bubble and at risk for exile.

During the first year of life, parent–child interactions are mainly positive, affectionate, and playful. Infants' limited mobility keeps them close to caretakers who provide for their physical and emotional needs. As infants grow into toddlers, their increasing motor abilities, impulsivity, and exploratory urges cause them to plunge head-first into danger. The unconditional affection of the first year gives way to loud and abrupt inhibitions designed to stop a child in his or her tracks. A chorus of "no's" replaces the smiles and soft tones. "Don't," "stop!," and a shift in the use of the child's name from a term of affection to a command or warning, often with the addition of middle and last names, characterizes this period.

Differences in temperament and personality between parent and child can contribute to the development of core shame because they can result in so much misattunement. A parallel to these experiences may occur in early attachment relationships when a child's excited expectation of connection is met with indifference, disapproval, or anger from a parent or caretaker. This misattunement in the attachment relationship likely triggers the same rapid shift from sympathetic to parasympathetic control and is translated by the developing psyche as shame, rejection, and abandonment. These experiences are stored as visceral, sensory, motor, and emotional memories, creating an overall expectation of positive or negative feelings and outcomes during future social interactions.

What began as a survival strategy to protect our young has unfortunately become part of the biological infrastructure of later evolving psychological processes related to attachment, safety, and self-worth. For social animals like ourselves, the fundamental question of "Am I safe?" has become woven together with the question "Am I loveable?" And with core shame, the answer is usually a painful and resounding "No!"

Because shame is a powerful, preverbal, and physiologically based organizing principle, the overuse of shame as a disciplinary tool predisposes children to long-standing difficulties with emotional regulation and self-esteem. Chronically shaming parents have children who spend much of their time anxious, afraid, and at risk for depression and anxiety. On the other hand, attentive parents rescue children from shame states by reattuning with them as soon as possible after a break in their connection. It is thought that repeated and rapid returns from shame states to attunement states result in the rebalance of autonomic functioning while contributing to the gradual development of self-regulation.

Applying this to psychotherapy, the reparenting that takes place taps into this attuned-misattuned-reattuned pattern in an attempt to modify the experience of insecure to secure attachment. In one of the author's experience (LC), it has become clear that core shame is very difficult to cure—it is difficult to tell if he has ever had complete success either with his clients or himself. In fact, he has come to think of core shame as a chronic illness, like diabetes, that needs to be managed instead of cured. Core shame distorts thoughts and feelings that have to be vigilantly monitored for accuracy and checked with others.

#4 THE ANXIETY BIAS AND THE SUPPRESSION OF LANGUAGE UNDER STRESS

Evolution favors an anxious gene. (Beck, Emery, & Greenberg, 1990)

The prime directive of survival for every living thing, from single-cell organisms to human beings, is to approach what sustains life while avoiding what puts us at risk. The better and faster a species is at discerning between the two, the more likely it is to survive. Originally, reptiles evolved a structure called the amygdala that has been conserved during the evolution of mammals and primates. The primary job of the amygdala is to appraise the desirability or danger of things in our world and to motivate us toward or away depending on its decision.

When our amygdala becomes aware of danger, it sends signals to the autonomic nervous system to become aroused and to prepare to fight or flee. A half second later, we consciously experience anything from anxiety to panic. Some things that trigger fear signals in the amygdala, such as snakes and heights, appear to be hard wired, genetic memories that harken back to our tree-dwelling ancestors. Others are learned associations that are triggered during the vital half-second that can make us avoid dogs, public speaking, or intimacy.

Because vigilance and approach-avoidance reactions are central mechanisms of the process of natural selection, Aaron Beck postulated that evolution favors an anxious gene. In other words, natural selection weeds out those of us who are too laid back. This idea has been supported by research that has shown that once the neurons in the amygdala create an association between a stimulus and danger, it is difficult to impossible to change the connection. Our best guess is that when we get over a fear or phobia, the connection still remains within our amygdala, but we have built new connections to inhibit the activation of a fight–flight reaction.

It appears that evolution has shaped our brains to err on the side of caution whenever it might be remotely useful—not such a bad idea for animals of prey in the wild, but a really bad idea for us. Humans have really big brains that create large societies filled with complexity and stress. These societies are created by our extensive imaginations, which can also, unfortunately, create nightmares. As we said before, the amygdala reacts to traffic jams, the thought of asteroids hitting the earth, and being shamed by others as threats to life and limb. This design flaw provides psychotherapists with an abundance of job security.

Fear inhibits executive function, problem-solving abilities, and emotional regulation. In other words, fear makes us rigid, inflexible, and dumb. We become afraid of taking risks and learning new things, leading us to remain in dysfunctional patterns of behavior, hold on to failed strategies, and remain in destructive relationships. The amygdala seems to use survival as vindication of its strategy, leading the agoraphobic to assume: "I haven't set foot outside my house in ten years and I'm still alive, which *must* be because I haven't set foot outside my house in ten years." The amygdala's job is to keep us alive, and it has the neural authority to veto happiness and well-being for survival. Psychotherapy has to break into this closed logic and interrupt the cycle of dysfunction and reinforcement.

During high states of arousal, brain areas responsible for speech (Broca's area) become inhibited. This may explain a variety of human phenomena, such as becoming tongue tied when talking to the boss or the speechless terror of trauma. For us, shutting down sound means losing the language we need to connect with others and organize our conscious experience. In humans, language serves the integration of neural networks of emotion and cognition, which supports emotional regulation and attachment. Putting feelings into words and constructing narratives of our experiences make an invaluable contribution to a coherent sense of self.

Central tenants of psychotherapy include expressing the unexpressed, making the unconscious conscious, and integrating thoughts and feelings. Experiences that occur before we develop speech or that occur in the context of trauma remain unintegrated and isolated in dissociated neural networks. By stimulating Broca's area, connecting words with feelings, and helping clients to construct a coherent narrative of their experience, we help restore a sense of perspective, agency, and an ability to edit dysfunctional life stories. Language has evolved to connect us to each other and to ourselves, a primary reason why Freud called psychotherapy "the talking cure."

#5 ILLUSION

Beware of Maya. (George Harrison, 1970)

In case you haven't heard, our minds are masters of illusion. Highly dedicated men and women—from psychoanalysts to neuroscientists to Zen Buddhists—have spent their lives trying to penetrate these illusions to discern the nature of reality. Much like using gasoline to put out a fire, using an illusion generator to see beyond illusion has its limitations. Although much still remains a mystery, one thing is clear—conscious experience distorts reality in endless ways. Although many of these distortions are designed to enhance survival, they also make us vulnerable to the kind of suffering that brings people to psychotherapy.

Our minds construct conscious experience based on three misperceptions: (1) we are experiencing the present moment, (2) we possess unlimited free will, and (3) we have access to accurate information about ourselves and the world. As you might imagine, the combination of these three illusions allows us to act with confidence and without hesitation. Of course, all you need to do is read the front page of any newspaper to see that, as a species, we still have a lot to learn. Let's look at these three beliefs.

Primates, including humans, possess brains with complex neural networks that become activated as we observe and interact with those around us. Neurons called mirror neurons in the premotor regions of our frontal lobes fire when we observe someone engaging in a specific behavior, such as saying a specific word or grasping an object. Some mirror neurons are so specific that they only fire when an object is grasped in a certain way by particular fingers. These same neurons fire when we perform the action itself. Mirror neurons link observation and action, allowing us to (1) learn from others through observation; (2) anticipate and predict the actions of others, which supports group coordination and self-defense; and (3) activate emotional states supportive of emotional resonance and empathy.

We also have circuits that analyze the actions and gestures of others to develop a theory of mind—what others know, what their motivations may be, and what they might do next. This ability to intuit what's on someone else's mind helps us predict their behavior. The existence of these mirror neurons and theory of mind systems reflects the fact that millions of years of evolution have been dedicated to refining systems for reading the emotions, thoughts, and intentions of others. We are quick to think we know others because these processes, and the attributions and emotions they trigger, are preconscious, automatic, and obligatory. All of this dedicated circuitry makes us very good at coming up with ideas about the motives and intentions of other people. It also allows us to learn through observation and practice new behaviors in our minds.

Of course, there is an obvious down side to this ability—we are also fairly prone to misreading other people. One reason is that though evolution has equipped us with awareness of others, it has not as yet seen fit to invest much circuitry into self-awareness and personal insight. It is easy to see what is wrong with someone else, but it can be an elaborate process before we can see what is wrong with our perception or our behavior. In fact, the capacity to challenge our own perceptions of ourselves may have even been selected against because it can lead to self-doubt, hesitation, and demoralization. This may be why humans have so many ways of distorting reality in their favor.

In fact, we often project our own thoughts and feelings (which we may not recognize as our own) onto others and assume it is their truth, not our own. Although Freud saw these projective processes as defensive, they may in part be a natural by-product of how our brains have evolved to process social information. Projection is automatic and lessens anxiety whereas self-awareness can generate anxiety and requires sustained effort. Self-analysis is difficult because our inner logic is so interwoven with our natural reflex to impute motives to others and our need to avoid anxiety.

Freud's defense mechanisms and all of the attribution biases of social psychology point to the ways in which we distort experiences in self-favorable ways. In fact, it has often been suggested that depression results from too accurate a perception of reality—a sort of denial deficit disorder. Repression, denial, and humor certainly grease the social wheels and lead us to put a positive spin on the behavior of those around us. Defenses also help us to regulate our internal states by decreasing anxiety and shame.

Although self-deception decreases anxiety, it also increases the likelihood of our successfully deceiving others. If we believe our self-deceptions, we are less likely to give away our real thoughts and intentions via nonverbal signs and behaviors. Reaction formations, or behaviors and feelings that are opposite of our true desires, are often quite effective in deceiving others. The most naive observer can see many things about us more clearly than we can see them ourselves.

Attachment schemas are another example of implicit memory patterns that shape our experience of others during the vital half-second. Given that most of us are unaware of transference and attachment schemas, we believe that our distortions are an accurate interpretation of external realities. These and other distortions give us far more confidence in our judgments than we should have, and they lead us to repeatedly make maladaptive decisions.

In short, distortions of conscious awareness are not character flaws but by-products of having a human brain. Our illusions, distortions, and misperceptions create the need for reality testing in psychotherapy. These illusions have evolved as part of our brains because they have had survival value. They help us to be strong, assertive, and without self-doubt in the face of threat. Our distortions allow us all to believe that we are above average and for two warring nations to believe that god is on their side.

The downside of these distortions comes when we have so much confidence in our point of view that we repeat the same dysfunctional behaviors for decades, filtering reality through character flaws, anxiety disorders, and depression. The questioning of one's assumptions, internalizing interpretations, and learning about how the brain mismanages information are all potential avenues for positive change. The following four topics are ways in which information is biased during the first half-second between sensation and perception.

In psychotherapy, we provide our clients with an alternative perspective and add new information to a closed, dysfunctional system. When therapy is at its most useful, clients are sometimes able to internalize perceptions and insights from others that improve their ability to test the reality of their experience beyond the habitual, self-serving distortions created by their brains.

WHY THERAPY WORKS

Let's begin with the take home message. Psychotherapy is a specialized learning situation that relies on three fundamental mechanisms. The first is that the brain is a social organ of adaptation, shaped by evolution to connect with and change in response to others. The second is that this change occurs via neuroplastic processes. The third mechanism is the co-creation of narratives between client and therapist that support neural and psychic integration. This intimate interaction between human connection and learning has been forged over the eons in the crucible of the social brain's evolution. Psychotherapy leverages the ability of brains to connect, attune, join together, and trigger neuroplasticity in the service of positive change.

As social and neural complexity played evolutionary leap-frog with one another over thousands of generations, they slowly became inextricably interwoven. Successful social behavior required increasingly complex brains whereas complex brains required more help from other brains to stay organized and on track. Eventually, this double helix of complexity and sociality wove families and tribes into superorganisms—a word used to describe larger organisms made up of many smaller organisms that serve a collective survival. The more social our brains became, the more important the role of relationships became as sociostatic regulators of our minds, bodies, and emotions. For those of you familiar with systems therapy, this is nothing new; studies from evolution, to psychoneuroimmunology, to neuroscience all support what people like Murray Bowen, Virginia Satir, and Carl Whittaker taught us decades ago.

Two consequences of human evolution seem particularly relevant to the birth and success of psychotherapy. The first is that we evolved into social animals who are highly attuned to one another's inner experiences. This sympathetic attunement allows us to influence each other's thoughts, feelings, and behaviors. The second is that our brains remain plastic throughout life, especially those circuits dedicated to attachment. If you have any doubts about this, just ask grandparents how they feel about their grandchildren. Thus, the fact that our brains are so social and overly complex provides both the need for therapy and the tools for its success—secure human attachments. Through the new science of epigenetics, we now know that we participate in the way each other's brains are built, how they develop, and how they function.

As social animals, we possess strong instincts to connect to other humans, and our brains are wired to love and work. In modern terms, we want to love and be loved, have successful careers, and be thought of well by others. So if we have healthy relationships, make babies, be creative, feel fulfilled, and live up to our potential, we most likely lack the need for psychotherapy. These people are linked to the group mind and can use their social connections to process and heal life's traumas naturally, much as a cut naturally forms a scab and heals over time. The need for psychotherapy arises when the social connections are absent, distorted, or damaging due to trauma, depression, or any number of causes.

Five Artifacts of Evolution: Tools for Healing

Fortunately for us, the same brain that gave rise to all of these difficulties also provides us with the tools to heal. Now it is time to review five evolutionary artifacts that are our tools for healing and succeeding in psychotherapy.

#1 NEUROPLASTICITY

> Plasticity . . . means the possession of a structure weak enough to yield to an influence, but strong enough not to yield all at once. (William James, 1890)

What does neuroplasticity mean? The birth, growth, development, and connectivity of neurons are the basic mechanisms of all adaptation and learning. All of these changes are expressions of neuroplasticity, or the ability of the brain to change in response to experience. Existing neurons grow through the expansion and branching of the dendrites that they project to other neurons in reaction to new experiences and learning. Neurons interconnect to form neural networks, and neural networks, in turn, integrate with one another to perform increasingly complex tasks.

When one or more neural networks necessary for optimal functioning remain underdeveloped, under-regulated, or underintegrated with others, we experience the complaints and symptoms for which people seek therapy. Because a brain is such a complicated government of systems, the possibilities of disconnections, misconnections, and failures of adaptations are almost endless. The real miracle is how we function as well as we do! Because our brains depend so much on experience to help them develop properly, a lot can go wrong in the normal course of day-to-day life, something Freud loved to refer to as the "vicissitudes" of experience.

We now assume that when psychotherapy results in symptom reduction or experiential change, the brain has, in some way, been altered. New connections have been made; dysfunctional systems are altered or inhibited; disconnected networks are reintegrated. This suggests that as we are engaged in the talking cure, all psychotherapists are neuroscientists in the business of changing the human brain.

Safe and attuned connections create internal biological states conducive to neuroplastic and epigenetic modifications of the brain. Through the therapeutic relationship, something new is offered into a previously closed and dysfunctional system. This is how relatives, friends, and tribal members are molded into units that enhance survival and lead to the emergence of group mind and culture. This is also why relationships are the most challenging aspects of life. Although there is endless debate about the relative merits of different forms of therapy, they all depend on the same underlying biopsychosocial mechanisms.

#2 THE SOCIAL BRAIN

> Everything can be acquired in solitude, except sanity. (Friedrich Nietzsche, 1951)

An interesting thing happened during the evolution of our social brains. The primitive processes of neuroplasticity became interwoven with the more recently evolved aspects of sociality. This means that the quality of attachment relationships influences learning—secure relationships support flexible, adaptive learning, and insecure attachments support rigid trauma-based learning. This is why establishing a therapeutic relationship—a secure attachment—is the alpha and omega of psychotherapy. We use the leverage of evolution via secure attachment, attunement, and empathy to stimulate plasticity in neural circuits of social and emotional processing.

Like neurons, we send and receive messages from one another across a synapse—the social synapse. Although we may be a bit more complicated, the basic strategy remains the same. As therapists, we connect with our clients and exchange energy and information with them. Let's look at this first in terms of the direction of flow across the social synapse—input and output—and the resulting interconnection.

Input: Listen, understand, attune, sympathize, empathize, support, cheer-lead, and champion. The goals of input are to establish emotional and cognitive connection, to link hearts and minds.

Output: Question, clarify, suggest, interpret, educate, assign homework, share our own experiences, and sometimes even give advice. The over-all goal of our output is to offer new information to our clients' minds and brains. We try to help them gain clarity, make the unconscious conscious, and expand emotional, physical, and cognitive awareness while encouraging appropriate risk taking.

Interconnection: What can be called the therapeutic alliance, attunement, or intersubjectivity is the joining together in an attempt to be of a common mind. Interconnection allows for mutual sociostatic regulation and provides us with the leverage to trigger neuroplasticity in the service of positive change. Establish a bridge of emotional attunement and empathy that allows your clients to use your brain as a set of external neural circuits until they are able to reshape their own in a more adaptive and productive way.

To accomplish this empathic bridge, we rely on many neural systems that process social and emotional information. We gather huge amounts of information from clients across the social synapse, consciously and unconsciously—facial expressions, body posture, blushing, pupil dilation, eye gaze, and many still-to-be-discovered channels. We create hypotheses about the unconscious internal states of others, all in the service of attempting to articulate experiences that they are unable to articulate themselves. We utilize our own mirror neurons to establish internal representations of what is happening within them by simulating their internal states within us. We rely on attachment circuitry to establish bonds and to know how to apply the optimal balance of challenge and support to help our clients grow.

Openness and trust are fragile creatures even with the people we love most. The training of the therapist and the therapeutic context itself are designed to increase neuroplasticity in networks of the social brain to enhance support, trust, and availability. It turns out that a secure and positive therapeutic alliance generates a double neuroplastic punch. A positive emotional connection stimulates rewarding metabolic processes that activate neuroplasticity, and secure relationships protect against stress, which inhibits protein synthesis and other biological processes necessary for brain growth.

An important remnant of our evolutionary past, the amygdala, rests at the core of each of our brains. This ancient executive center has retained veto power over our modern brains when it detects a threat. Also, like an elephant; it never forgets. Fear becomes reinforced through avoidance, and it is only inhibited by confrontation. This is also why a decrease in "avoidance behavior" is highly correlated with therapeutic success.

In other words, approaching danger and surviving inhibits the amygdala's triggering of the fight–flight system. These situations can be as far-reaching as picking up a spider, finishing the last class to get a degree, or going out on a first date. Risking new and seemingly dangerous experiments in the service of positive change requires a combination of courage, emotional support, and a good plan for success. Thus, successful therapists learn to be "amygdala whisperers" to help our clients face their fears in the safe environment that we co-create during sessions.

#3 LANGUAGE, STORYTELLING, AND CO-CONSTRUCTED NARRATIVES

There is no greater agony than bearing an untold story inside you. (Maya Angelou, 2009)

Human beings are natural storytellers. Through countless generations, we have gathered to listen to stories of the hunt, the exploits of our ancestors, and morality tales of good and evil. The urge to tell and listen to stories is embedded in our psyches, wired into our brains, and woven into our DNA. The success of the talking cure harkens back to gatherings around ancient campfires. For most of human history, oral communication and verbal memory constituted the repository of our collective knowledge.

Although stories may appear imprecise and unscientific, they serve as powerful tools for neural network integration. The combination of a linear storyline and visual imagery, woven together with verbal and nonverbal expressions of emotion, activates circuitry of both hemispheres, cortical and subcortical networks, the various regions of the frontal lobes, the hippocampus, and the amygdala. This integrative process may also account for the positive correlations between coherent speech and secure attachment. These coherent narratives provide for the integration of sensations, feelings, and behaviors within conscious awareness. Further, shared stories link individual brains to the group mind.

An engaging story, containing conflicts, resolutions, gestures, expressions, and thoughts flavored with emotion, connects people and integrates neural networks. In listening to our clients tell their stories, we are analyzing their narratives for missing elements and a lack of balance that correlates with their emotional distress. We then attempt to edit the narrative in some manner. With clients who are preverbal or nonverbal, we still create a narrative that guides our interventions, allows us to assess our progress, and judge success.

Narratives are so powerful because they allow us to have an objective distance on direct experience, creating the possibility of alternate points of view. We can escape the emotions and influences of the moment to some degree to reflect on the experience. Through stories, we have the opportunity to ponder ourselves in an objective way across an infinite number of contexts. We can share versions of possible selves and receive input from others about our thoughts and perspectives. Finally, we can experiment with new emotions, actions, and language as we edit the scripts of our lives.

As children we are told by others, and we gradually begin to tell others, who we are, what is important to us, and what we are capable of. These self-stories are co-constructed with parents and peers. Although it sometimes seems that children are little scientists discovering the world, what we often miss is that they are primarily engaged in discovering what the rest of us already know, especially about them. This serves the continuity of culture from one generation to the next as we reflexively strive to re-create ourselves. Often, narratives are maladaptive and need to be rewritten. But first, they need to be made conscious and understood so that they can be edited and emotionally retooled.

The role of language and narratives in neural integration, memory formation, and self-identity makes them powerful tools in the creation and maintenance of the self. Stories are powerful organizing forces that serve to perpetuate healthy and unhealthy forms of self-identity. There is evidence that positive self-narratives aid in emotional security while minimizing the need for elaborate psychological defenses. In the same way, anxious and traumatized parents pass along their negative experiences in the stories they tell. The recognition of the negative power of personal narrations containing negative self-statements stimulated the development of rational and cognitive based therapies.

Putting feelings into words (affect labeling) has long served a positive function for many individuals suffering from stress or trauma. Labeling emotions correlates with decreased amygdala response and an increase in right prefrontal activation. It has also been found that amygdala and right frontal activation are inversely correlated and that this homeostatic balance is mediated by the orbital medial prefrontal cortex. This suggests that the labeling process may require the lateral and medial prefrontal regions for cognitive processes to have a modulatory impact on our emotional activation. The narrative, which simultaneously activates an array of networks, enhances metabolic activity and neural balance.

Even writing about your experiences supports top-down modulation of emotion and bodily responses. Journaling about important emotional issues, especially related to close personal relationships, serves the same function.

Journaling has been shown to reduce physical symptoms, physician visits, and work absenteeism; it also increases immunological health. Our ability to tame the amygdala in this way results in a cascade of positive physiological, behavioral, and emotional effects.

#4 SELF-REFLECTIVE CAPACITY

> The key to growth is the introduction of higher dimensions of conscious-
> ness into our awareness. (Lao Tzu [as cited in Henderson, 2010])

Self-reflective capacity correlates with secure attachment and successful psychotherapy. This same ability is called "psychological mindednesss" by psychoanalysts and "mindfulness" in most blue states. The central idea is metacognition, the ability to reflect on one's own thinking. Self-awareness is expanded and reinforced through the creation of a narrative that includes language for this possibility. This is what happens in therapy when we ask clients the questions they never think to ask themselves. Through these more inclusive narratives and a deeper awareness of inner experience, we learn that we are capable of evaluating and choosing whether to follow the expectations of others or the mandates of our childhoods.

Therapy attempts to create this meta-cognitive vantage point from which the shifting states of mind that emerge during day-to-day life can be thought about. We accomplish this by interweaving the narratives of client and therapist, hopefully leading them in a more healthful direction. You begin by making a client aware of one or more of the narrative arcs of their life story and then help them understand that change is possible by offering alternative story lines. As the editing process proceeds, new narrative arcs emerge, as do the possibilities to experiment with new ways of thinking, feeling, and acting. The importance of the unconscious processes of parent and therapist is highlighted by their active participation in the co-construction of the new narratives of their children and patients. This underscores the importance of the proper training and adequate personal therapy for therapists who will be putting their imprint on the hearts, minds, and brains of their clients. In essence, therapists hope to teach their clients that they are more than their present story; they can also be editors and authors of new stories.

#5 ABSTRACT THOUGHT AND IMAGINATION

> Imagination is more important than knowledge. (Albert Einstein [as cited
> in Viereck, 1929])

As the size of primate groups expanded, the grooming, grunts, and hand gestures that worked fine within a small group became inadequate, and they were gradually shaped into spoken language. Language made possible far more disparate, precise, multilayered, and subtle communications among a much larger group of individuals than a relatively small, early hominid tribe. As social groups grew larger and language became more complex, more cortical landscape was required to process a greater amount of social information.

The transition to the human brain is also characterized by the growth of a small area near the back of the brain called the inferior parietal cortex. This area, in collaboration with the prefrontal cortex, appears to have allowed us to do three things that border on the miraculous. The first is that our brains allow us to construct three dimensional models of external objects inside our heads.

Second, we are able to manipulate objects in our imagination. And third, we can transform them into new objects that we can use as templates for what we create in the external world. In other words, we have imagination and the ability to apply it in the world. And we can apply our imagination, not only to objects in the environment, but to ourselves.

Thus, humans are capable of imagining an alternative self, creating narratives of how to become this self, and then using these narratives as blueprints for the journey. Countless blueprints are created and discarded during development; children and adolescents try out different identities. As we progress, we naturally outgrow old self stories like a snake outgrows its skin, and we need to write new stories. People often forget this and become symptomatic when they are contained by a life that no longer fits them. This is the hero's journey of every culture—with shamans, medicine women, wise elders, and psychotherapists serving as guides. Our imaginations allow us to escape the present moment, create alternative realities, and then begin our journey to find them.

PULLING IT TOGETHER

Shift happens. (Candace Perth, 2009)

As Dr. Salk observed decades ago, evolution solves old problems and creates new ones. The very processes that created the need for psychotherapy have also provided us with the tools to heal. Thus, the interwoven processes of brain, mind, and relationship that create the distortions of the vital half-second have also supplied the tools for change. The first is the power of secure relationships to stimulate neuroplasticity and brain growth. The second is the ability of the body and the conscious mind to use self-awareness, stories, emotions, and bodily awareness to reshape neural circuitry in the service of improved adaptation.

Thus, our brains are inescapably social, their structure and function deeply embedded in connections with other brains. Because our brains have evolved in this social context, we have individually developed the ability to link with other brains—attuning with each other, regulating each other's emotional systems, and helping to grow each other's neural networks. The good news is that this capacity to integrate our brains with other brains allows us to counterbalance some of evolution's less than stellar decisions. This ability of one brain to influence another brain is at the heart of psychotherapy.

WHY SCIENCE MATTERS TO PSYCHOTHERAPY

Science is more than a body of knowledge. It's a way of thinking. (Carl Sagan [as cited in Head, 2006])

Many therapists protest the integration of neuroscience and psychotherapy, calling it irrelevant or reductionistic. Would Rogers, Kohut, or Beck have been better therapists if they had been trained as neuroscientists? Probably not. On the other hand, it's hard for us to grasp how the brain could be irrelevant to changing the mind. And though we dislike reductionism as much as the next person, doesn't a tendency toward reductionism say more about the thinker than the nature of natural phenomena? Our knowledge of neuroscience highlights the fact that we primates have complex and imperfect brains, and we should remain skeptical about what we think we know. In other words, primates would be wise to doubt their beliefs and remain open to new ideas.

The psychotherapist as healer exists within a long tradition of rabbis, priests, medicine women, and shamans. At the same time, findings in social neuroscience make it clear that we are also in the current scientific mainstream. In contrast to technological medicine, we understand our profound personal role in the healing relationship while simultaneously respecting the subjective experience of our clients. In the absence of a brain-based model of change, the leaders of our fields have learned to stimulate and guide neuroplastic processes to help build, integrate, and regulate our clients' brains. But why does an academic understanding of neuroscience make any difference to our work?

Knowing about neuroscience is valuable for therapists not only because it will give rise to new theories and techniques, but also because it provides us with a deeper understanding of the mechanisms of the talking cure. As a social organ, the brain has evolved to link to and be changed by other brains; psychotherapy relies upon the power of relationships to trigger neuroplastic processes necessary for new learning and growth. In our daily work, psychotherapists are in effect "applied neuroscientists," altering the functioning and structures of our clients' brains. Findings from neuroscientific research are making it increasingly clear that psychotherapists operate well within the scientific mainstream.

On a practical level, adding a neuroscientific perspective to our clinical thinking allows us to talk with clients about the shortcomings of our brains instead of the problems with theirs. Information about the brain and how it evolved helps us communicate with clients about their problems in a more objective and nonshaming manner. The truth appears to be that many human struggles, from phobias to obesity, are consequences of brain evolution, not deficiencies of character. Identifying problems that we hold in common and developing methods to circumvent or correct them is a solid foundation upon which to base a therapeutic alliance.

Learning about what is happening in their brains and how these billions of neural events have shaped their emotional lives and behavior is more likely to inspire interest and curiosity in clients rather than defensiveness or feelings of shame. One of the authors (LC) has experienced increased buy-in by skeptical clients after they have a scientific explanation for what happens in therapy—especially if it contains an acceptable rationale for why it is sometimes necessary to feel worse before you can feel better.

As the value of interdisciplinary care becomes increasingly recognized, a neuroscientific perspective provides a common language for us to communicate with professionals from other fields. We can at least all agree that we are working with the same brain! Our hope is that a brain-based model of treatment may someday lead us to a more evidence-based rationale for eclectic treatment approaches and provide us with more practical, valid, and measurable means of evaluating treatment outcome.

CONCLUSION

It is humbling and more than a little frightening to realize that we rely on what may be the most complex structure in the universe with little knowledge of how it works. But despite the fact that we are only at the dawn of understanding the brain, an appreciation of its evolutionary history, developmental sculpting, and peculiarities of design can surely encourage us to begin to use it more wisely. Practical things—like understanding the neural damage resulting from drugs, stress, and early deprivation—should influence everything from personal decision making to public policy. The neural network dissociation that often results from exposure to combat should make us pay closer attention to those whom we put in harm's way. Even our tendencies to distort reality in the direction of personal experience and egocentric needs should lead us to examine our beliefs and opinions more carefully.

Our brains are inescapably social, their structures and functioning deeply embedded in the family, tribe, and society. And though the brain has many shortcomings and vulnerabilities, our ability to link with, attune to, and regulate each other's brains provides us with a way of healing. This is why the power of human relationships is at the heart of psychotherapy. From our perspective, the value of neuroscience for psychotherapists is not to explain away the mind or generate new forms of therapy, but to help us grasp the neurobiological substrates of the talking cure in an optimistic and enthusiastic continuation of Freud's "Project for a Scientific Psychology" (1895).

We carry within our brains the entire history of biological evolution from its primitive origins to the vastly complex organ we possess today. Evolution is still underway as we adapt to everything from space travel and the Internet to the ever expanding demands of child rearing. One thing we can be sure of is that the individual brain and the social dynamics of the entire human race are becoming increasingly intertwined. And, perhaps for the first time in history, we can truly begin to get some sense of the vast, interconnected web that connects every human brain on earth. This is a cause for awe and humility—awe at the potential of our collective cerebral tapestry and humility about how much unnecessary suffering a bunch of primates can create as we struggle with the shadows of our collective histories.

REFERENCES

Angelou, M. (2009). *I know why the caged bird sings*. New York, NY: Ballantine Books.

Beck, A. T., Emery, G., & Greenberg, R. L. (1990). *Anxiety disorders and phobias: A cognitive perspective*. New York, NY: Basic Books.

Freud, S. (1895). Project for a scientific psychology. In J. Strachey (Ed.), *The Standard edition of the complete psychological works of Sigmund Freud* (Vol. 1, pp. 3–182). London, UK: Hogarth Press.

Harrison, G. (1970). Beware of darkness. On *All Things Must Pass* [Record]. United States: Harrisongs Ltd.

Head, T. (2006). *Conversations with Carl Sagan*. Jackson, MS: University Press of Mississippi.

Henderson, J. (2010). *Multi-dimensional perception*. Cape Town, South Africa: Kima Global Publishers.

James, W. (1890). *The principles of psychology* (Vol. I). New York, NY: Henry Holt and Company.

Jordan, M. (2009, September 11). *Michael Jordan's acceptance to the Basketball Hall of Fame*. Lecture conducted from Naismith Memorial Basketball Hall of Fame, Springfield, MA. Retrieved from https://www.youtube.com/watch?v=XLzBMGXfK4c

Kaufman, G. (1974). The meaning of shame: Towards a self-affirming identity. *Journal of Counseling Psychology, 21*(6), 568–574.

Nietzsche, F. (1951). *My sister and I*. New York, NY: Boar's Head Books.

Perth, C. (2009). *Molecules of emotion: The science behind mind-body medicine*. New York, NY: Simon and Schuster.

Pound, E. (1938). *Guide to Kulchur*. New York, NY: New Directions Publishing.

Salk, J. (1983). *Anatomy of reality*. New York, NY: Columbia University Press.

Viereck, G. S. (1929, October 26). What life means to Einstein. *The Saturday Evening Post*, pp. 17, 110, 113–114, 117.

Regulation Theory and Affect Regulation Psychotherapy: A Clinical Primer

JUDITH R. SCHORE

Sanville Institute and Reiss-Davis Child Study Center, Los Angeles, California, USA

ALLAN N. SCHORE

David Geffen School of Medicine, University of California, Los Angeles, Los Angeles, California, USA

This article offers an essay on the influence of advances in developmental neuroscience and neuropsychoanalysis for our understanding of the interpersonal neurobiological change mechanisms embedded in the mother–infant and client–therapist relationship. Regulation theory and affect regulation therapy are reviewed, along with attachment, affect regulation, and the development of the right brain. Right-brain communications within the therapeutic alliance are described, leading to the conclusion that the right brain is dominant in psychotherapy. Changes in not only the client's but also the clinician's brain over long-term clinical experiences are discussed.

We want to thank Dennis Miehls and Jeffrey Applegate for inviting us to contribute to this important edition of the Smith College Studies in Clinical Social Work. It is a privilege to be a part of this distinguished group of clinicians who have incorporated neurobiology in their theory and practice. As one of us (J. Schore, 2012) has recently written in this journal, interpersonal neurobiological models mesh nicely with the biopsychosocial-cultural perspective of clinical social work, perhaps more than any other area of the social work profession. Psychodynamic social workers are now actively integrating recent scientific and theoretical advances into more complex yet highly pragmatic models of individual and social change that translate into more effective and profound therapeutic approaches.

For more than two decades our own contributions toward that effort have focused on two essential questions of human development. First, how do relational experiences structuralize the early maturation of the right lateralized "emotional brain," and thereby indelibly affect its essential role in all later social-emotional, intersubjective, and stress-regulating functioning, including those operating in the therapeutic relationship? And the parallel question, how do object relational experiences at the beginning of life fundamentally influence the growth of the unconscious mind, especially in intimate contexts? (see A. N. Schore, 1994, 2003, 2012; J. R. Schore & Schore, 2008, 2010).

Grounded in Freud's (1895/1966) "Project for a Scientific Psychology," his primordial attempt to construct a model of the mind in terms of its underlying neurobiological mechanisms, and in *The Interpretation of Dreams* (1900/1953), his seminal description of the central role of the unconscious in everyday life, the body of our neuropsychoanalytic work has offered an evidence-based, clinically relevant model of the right hemisphere as the biological substratum of the human unconscious mind. Extending the pioneering work of developmental psychoanalysts such as Winnicott, Bowlby, Stern, and others, our ongoing studies of the early relational, interpersonal neurobiological origins of the subjective implicit self-represent a coherent theory of the development of the unconscious mind, over the course of the life span (for recent updates, see A. N. Schore, 2013b; J. R. Schore, 2012).

Indeed a considerable amount of interdisciplinary research now supports the assertion that early relational, bodily based experiences, much of it operating at nonconscious levels and occurring before the maturation of the verbal conscious mind, indelibly influences all future development (see A. N. Schore, 1994, 2003, 2012). Mirroring this research, a large body of clinical studies also indicates that the development of adaptive nonverbal social-emotional functions and not verbal cognitions lie at the core of the unconscious right lateralized brain/mind/body, the "subjective self." As a result, updated models of psychotherapy are focusing on emotion and changes in intersubjective affective processes that operate beneath conscious awareness. We have therefore emphasized the relevance of developmental, affective, and social neuroscience (more so than cognitive neuroscience) for the theory and practice of psychotherapy.

Essentially, the contributions of regulation theory (A. N. Schore, 1994) to the field of interpersonal neurobiology attempt to explain how these early experiences indelibly affect and alter the developing right brain, which for the rest of the life span is centrally involved in the innate psychobiological need for affiliation and social connection, and thereby for emotion regulation and personal growth. The work continues to describe, in some detail, the psychoneurobiological mechanisms by which the early attachment relationship cocreates the organization of the developing personality, expressed in the individual's adaptive or maladaptive abilities to cope with later stress, especially relational stress. In other words, the emotional environment provided by the primary caregiver shapes, for better or worse, the experience-dependent maturation of the brain systems involved in attachment affect communicating and affect regulating functions that are accessed throughout the life span (see A. N. Schore, 2013b, for a recent application of the theory for the early assessment of attachment and autistic spectrum disorders).

In this article, we offer the reader not so much a documentation of scientific evidence for regulation theory as an essay on the influence of advances in developmental neuroscience and neuropsychoanalysis for our understanding of the interpersonal neurobiological change mechanisms embedded in the mother–infant and client–therapist relationship.

REGULATION THEORY AND AFFECT REGULATION THERAPY (ART)

Regulation theory specifically models how relational experiences affect the development of what has previously been termed "psychic structure," which we identify with more complex right-brain bodily based systems that operate beneath conscious awareness. We contend that neuroscience can do more than confirm or disconfirm existing clinical theories. Rather it can expand our clinical interventions and allow us to work more deeply and more broadly, at conscious and especially unconscious levels, with a wider array of psychopathologies.

Knowledge of brain ontogeny teaches us that the right hemisphere (the unconscious mind) evolves earlier than the left (the conscious mind), thus emphasizing its unique properties of nonverbal, intuitive, holistic processing of emotional information and social interactions (see Decety & Lamm, 2007; Hecht, 2014; McGilchrist, 2009; A. N. Schore, 2012; and Semrud-Clikeman, Fine, & Zhu, 2011, for recent comprehensive descriptions of right hemispheric functions).

Updated brain–mind–body models that integrate biology and psychology can thus serve as a source for more effective treatment interventions for a wide range of disorders. As opposed to past trends that compared and contrasted one form of psychotherapy with another, we believe that we can now finally move toward a deeper understanding of the common psychoneurobiological mechanisms that underlie the change processes common to infants, children, adolescents, and adults. It is important to have theories that don't need to invent concepts and assume or project meaning into the infant's unconscious mind. The arcane, convoluted early psychoanalytic constructs were used because they didn't understand how the biological development of the brain–mind–body really worked. We now have simpler yet more comprehensive and understandable models with which to more accurately describe the rapid attachment communications of the relational unconscious that occur within any emotionally intimate dyad.

Indeed, in the last 10 years, the rapid growth in attachment theory has allowed it to become the most complex theory of the development of the brain–mind–body available to science. We think the reason for this is that attachment theory, as opposed to other developmental theories, from its origins has always been an integration of psychology and biology. In his classic 1969 volume, *Attachment*, Bowlby used the perspectives of Freud and Darwin to understand the instinctive mother–infant bond in terms of psychoanalysis and behavioral biology, and even speculated about the brain systems involved in the evolutionary mechanism of attachment. Today it is clear that framing attachment solely in terms of psychological constructs is limited and inadequate. This principle applies to the expression of attachment dynamics in the early developmental and later psychotherapeutic contexts. At present researchers and clinicians are exploring the essential neurological and biological mechanisms that underlie all psychological functions. Neuroscience allows us to know in greater detail and in real time the mechanisms of early attachment relationships and how they shape the formation of deep, internal psychic structures across the life span, especially within "in depth psychotherapy."

Classical chroniclers of child development such as Spitz, Winnicott, Erikson, Mahler, and Bowlby (all psychotherapists), coupled with the modern "up close," intimate, intersubjective infant research of Beebe, Tronick, and Lyons-Ruth (also psychotherapists) provide a solid developmental psychoanalytic base for regulation theory, including a modeling of the changes in the core of the personality that can result from optimal and less-than-optimal intersubjective, psychosocial contexts. What we have clinically, intuitively known about how humans change, about how character is formed is now mirrored, confirmed, and expanded by science—biological development occurs in a psychosocial context. It is not an isolated unfolding of a self in a psychological vacuum, without an intimate other. Human infants are dependent on the physical, relational, emotional environment not only for their actual survival, but also for the social matrix out of which they will emerge as individuals with their own psychic structure. Each individual "hatches" and grows in a relational context, for better or worse. It is the business of social work to pay attention to this on a micro- and macrolevel.

A major theme of our ongoing studies has been to integrate an interpersonal neurobiological perspective into a developmentally informed, affectively focused model of psychotherapy. Our work on regulation theory, on the centrality of affect regulation for attachment, right-brain maturation, and social emotional development lies at the core of our clinical model of treatment, affect regulation therapy (ART). This understanding of the therapeutic change process focuses on strengths and limitations in affect regulation and social intersubjective functions across a wide variety of self-pathologies and personality disorders.

In the following sections we offer a primer on regulation theory, beginning with a condensed explication of the right-brain interpersonal neurobiology of the early mother–child relationship, and then the reactivation of the same unconscious mechanisms in the therapist patient relationship. The clinical model, ART, is thus anchored in the developmental model of regulation theory, which we term modern attachment theory (J. R. Schore & Schore, 2008).

ATTACHMENT, AFFECT REGULATION, AND DEVELOPMENT OF THE RIGHT BRAIN

In the last two decades two major trends of research have converged to confirm the basic tenets of regulation theory. Number one, from psychology: as opposed to earlier models that posited the beginnings of personality between the 3rd and 4th year, we now have good evidence that the prenatal and postnatal stages of human infancy represent the critical period for the organization of the central dimensions of the personality. Number two, from neuroscience: the peak interval of attachment formation overlaps the most rapid period of massive human brain growth that takes place from the last trimester of pregnancy through the end of the 3rd year.

We now know that the evolutionary mechanism of attachment does more than just provide the baby with a sense of safety and security (A. N. Schore, 2013a). Rather, attachment drives brain development, five sixths of which happens postnatally. In fact the brain grows more extensively and more rapidly in infancy than at any other stage of life. Forty thousand new synapses are formed every second in the infant's brain (Lagercrantz & Ringstedt, 2001), and cortical and especially subcortical brain volume doubles in the first year (Knickmeyer et al., 2008). Importantly, this brain growth is influenced by "social forces" and therefore is "experience-dependent." It requires not only nutrients, but also the emotional experiences embedded in the relationship it cocreates with the primary caregiver.

According to neurobiologically informed modern attachment theory (J. R. Schore & Schore, 2008) the essential task of the first year of human life is the cocreation of a secure attachment bond of emotional communication between the infant and his or her primary caregiver. The baby communicates its burgeoning positive emotional states (e.g., joy, excitement) and negative emotional states (e.g., fear, anger) to the caregiver so that she can then regulate them. The attachment relationship shapes the ability of the baby to communicate with not just the mother, but ultimately with other human beings. This survival function—the capacity to communicate one's own subjective internal states to other human beings and to receive their resonant responses—is the basis of all later social relations.

Thus, the major developmental accomplishments of human infancy are the capacity to communicate emotional states, and subsequently the capacity for self-regulation, that is, the ability to auto-regulate emotional states. At the most fundamental level, the attachment relationship represents more than mental communications—rather, they are psychobiological, and bodily based. We repeat—the essential nonverbal communication involved in attachment formation in the first year is fundamentally nonverbal and emotional, more so than verbal and cognitive. It is not until the middle of the 2nd year that the left hemisphere and the speech centers in Broca's and Wernicke's language areas come online. The baby's ability to communicate his or her emotional states is thus essential, and nature has made sure that emotion circuits come online before the verbal language circuits.

Bowlby (1969) originally stated that mother–infant attachment communications are "accompanied by the strongest of feelings and emotions" (p. 242). We think in some ways our psychotherapy fields have lost sight of this, with such a heavy emphasis on cognition, and even mind *over* body. Developmental neuroscience research demonstrates that the limbic system processes emotional information, and the autonomic nervous system is responsible for the bodily based/somatic aspects of emotion. Studies show that both are in a critical period of growth in the first and much of the 2nd year, and that the maturation of these emotional brain circuits is significantly influenced by early socioemotional experience. We also know that the right hemisphere is more connected into the limbic and autonomic systems, and that it develops pre- and postnatally, before the left hemisphere. The bodily based brain systems involved in attachment and emotion are thus located in the right hemisphere (for recent neuroscience research, see A. N. Schore, 2012, 2013a, 2013b).

Attachment forms through communications that occur essentially between the right brain of the baby and the right brain of the primary caregiver. They are not transmitted through language, or semantics (a finding that is significant to our understanding of attachment at all points of the life span including attachment dynamics in psychotherapy). Rather, from the beginning of human development, these are nonverbal, social-emotional communications. Specifically, attachment communication is expressed in (1) visual, face-to-face transactions; (2) auditory expressions of the emotional tone of the voice; and (3) tactile-gestural cues of the body. All of these are performed very rapidly by the right brains of the infant and mother. For the rest of the life span, we use these nonverbal communication skills in all of our interpersonal relationships.

Here is another new insight about attachment, informed by neuroscience. Bowlby thought that the key to the attachment bond was that the mother was soothing, or regulating the baby's negative fear states. There is now strong evidence that the secure primary attachment figure not only down-regulates negative fear states, but also up-regulates positive emotions in loving and play states. When we are evaluating an attachment relationship, we should be looking at not only the ability to calm and soothe, but also the ability to stimulate the baby into states of joy, interest, and excitement. These positive emotions are important for brain development. So what we have in the attachment relationship is the developing ability of the child to communicate and to regulate positive and negative emotional states, which are components of healthy self-esteem.

Right-brain development is not just genetically encoded; it is shaped by "epigenetic" social forces and requires these human intimate experiences for its optimal growth. What the child is looking for, and what the child is gaining from the attachment relationship and imprinting into the circuits of its maturing right brain, are these critical emotional, right brain-to-right brain experiences. How those experiences are provided or not provided by the primary caregiver is going to affect the wiring of the circuits of that right brain. The mother's history of her own secure or insecure emotional experiences, including when she was an infant with her own mother, are stored in her right brain, creating what we call the epigenetic transmission of attachment patterns across generations.

Regulation theory also offers a model of psychopathogenesis—early social-emotional experiences may be either predominantly regulated or dysregulated, imprinting secure or insecure attachments. Developmental neuroscience clearly demonstrates that all children are not "resilient" but rather are "malleable," for better or worse (A. N. Schore, 2012). In marked contrast to the earlier described optimal growth-facilitating attachment scenario, in a relational growth-inhibiting early environment of attachment trauma (abuse and/or neglect) the primary caregiver of an insecure disorganized-disoriented infant induces traumatic states of enduring negative affect in the child (A. N. Schore, 2003). This caregiver is too frequently emotionally inaccessible and reacts to her infant's expressions of stressful affects inconsistently and inappropriately (intrusiveness or disengagement) and therefore shows minimal or unpredictable participation in the relational arousal regulating processes. Instead of modulating she induces extreme levels of stressful stimulation and arousal levels, very high in abuse and/or very low in neglect. Because she provides little interactive repair, the infant's intense negative affective states are long lasting. Over the last few years neurobiological research is now exploring not just disorganized insecure attachments, but organized "insecures," looking at the impact of maternal dismissive attachments on the infant's brain (see Ammaniti & Gallese, 2014).

A large body of research now highlights the central role of insecure attachments in the psychoneuropathogenesis of all psychiatric disorders (A. N. Schore, 2003, 2012, 2013b). Watt observed, "If children grow up with dominant experiences of separation, distress, fear and rage, then they will go down a bad pathogenic developmental pathway, and it's not just a bad psychological pathway but a bad neurological pathway" (2003, p. 109). More specifically, during early critical periods, frequent dysregulated and unrepaired, organized, and disorganized-disoriented insecure attachment histories are "affectively burnt in" the infant's early developing right brain. Not only traumatic experiences but also the defense against overwhelming trauma, dissociation, is stored in implicit-procedural memory as well.

In this manner attachment trauma ("relational trauma"; A. N. Schore, 2001) is imprinted into right cortical-subcortical systems, encoding disorganized-disoriented insecure internal working models that are nonconsciously accessed at later points of interpersonal emotional stress. These insecure working models are of central interest in affectively focused psychotherapy of early forming self-pathologies and personality disorders. Such deficits in right-brain relational processes and resulting affect dysregulation underlie all psychological and psychiatric disorders. All models of therapeutic intervention across a span of psychopathologies now share a common goal of attempting to improve emotional auto-regulatory and interactive regulatory processes (see A. N. Schore, 2003, for a discussion of these dual regulatory processes).

ATTACHMENT, AFFECT DYSREGULATION, AND RIGHT-BRAIN COMMUNICATIONS WITHIN THE THERAPEUTIC ALLIANCE

Bowlby (1988), a psychoanalyst, asserted that the reassessment of nonconscious internal working models of attachment is a primary goal of any psychotherapy. These interactive representations of early attachments encode strategies of affect regulation and contain coping mechanisms for maintaining basic regulation and positive affect in the face of stressful environmental challenge. Acting at levels beneath conscious awareness this internal working model is accessed to perceive, appraise, and regulate social-emotional information and guide action in familiar and especially novel interpersonal environments. Regulation theory dictates that in "heightened affective moments" the patient's unconscious internal working model of attachment, whether secure or insecure, is reactivated in right-lateralized implicit-procedural memory and reenacted in the psychotherapeutic relationship (A. N. Schore, 2003, 2012).

In light of the commonality of nonverbal, intersubjective, implicit right brain-to-right brain emotion transacting and regulating mechanisms in the caregiver–infant and the therapist–client relationship, developmental attachment studies have direct relevance to the treatment process. The early responding right brain, which is more "physiological" than the later responding left, is involved in rapid bodily based intersubjective communications of dysregulated affect within the therapeutic alliance. At all life stages the right hemisphere holistically and nonverbally processes threats and mediates states of fear and vulnerability (A. N. Schore, 1994; Hecht, 2014). From the first point of intersubjective contact the psychobiologically attuned clinician tracks not just the verbal content but the nonverbal moment-to-moment rhythmic structures of the patient's internal states and is flexibly and fluidly modifying his or her own behavior to synchronize with that structure, thereby cocreating with the patient a growth-facilitating context for the organization of the therapeutic alliance.

Decety and Chaminade's (2003) characterization of higher functions of the right brain is directly applicable to the psychotherapeutic relational context:

> Mental states that are in essence private to the self may be shared between individuals . . . self-awareness, empathy, identification with others, and more generally intersubjective processes, (and) are largely dependent upon . . . right hemisphere resources, which are the first to develop. (p. 591)

As the right hemisphere is dominant for subjective emotional experiences (Wittling & Roschmann, 1993), the communication of affective states between the right brains of the client–therapist dyad is thus best described as "intersubjectivity."

In accord with a relational model of psychotherapy, right-brain processes that are reciprocally activated on both sides of the therapeutic alliance lie at the core of the psychotherapeutic change process. These implicit clinical dialogues convey much more essential organismic information than left-brain explicit, verbal information. Rather, right-brain interactions "beneath the words" nonverbally communicate essential nonconscious bodily based affective relational information about the inner world of the client (and therapist). Rapid communications between the right-lateralized "emotional brain" of each member of the therapeutic alliance allow for moment-to-moment "self-state sharing," a cocreated, organized, dynamically changing dialogue of mutual influence. Bromberg (2011) noted, "Self-states are highly individualized modules of being, each configured by its own organization of cognitions, beliefs, dominant affect, and mood, access to memory, skills, behaviors, values, action, and regulatory physiology" (p. 73). In this relational matrix both partners match the dynamic contours of different emotional-motivational self-states and simultaneously adjust their social attention, stimulation, and accelerating/decelerating arousal in response to the other's signals.

Regulation theory models the mutual psychobiological mechanisms that underlie any clinical encounter, whatever the verbal content. Lyons-Ruth (2000) described the affective exchanges that communicate "implicit relational knowledge" within the therapeutic alliance. Neuroscience characterizes the role of the right brain in these nonverbal communications. At all stages of the life span, "The neural substrates of the perception of voices, faces, gestures, smells and pheromones, as evidenced by modern neuroimaging techniques, are characterized by a general pattern of right-hemispheric functional asymmetry" (Brancucci, Lucci, Mazzatenta, & Tommasi, 2009, p. 895). More so than conscious left-brain verbalizations, right brain-to-right brain visual-facial, auditory-prosodic, and tactile-gestural subliminal communications reveal the deeper aspects of the personality of the client, as well as the personality of the therapist (see A. N. Schore, 2003, for a right brain-to-right brain model of projective identification, a fundamental process of implicit communication between the relational unconscious systems of client and therapist).

To receive and monitor the client's nonverbal bodily based attachment communications the affectively attuned clinician must shift from constricted left hemispheric attention that focuses on local detail to more widely expanded right hemispheric attention that focuses on global input (Derryberry & Tucker, 1994), a characterization that fits with Freud's (1912/1958) description of the importance of the clinician's "evenly suspended attention." In the session, the empathic therapist is consciously, explicitly attending to the client's verbalizations to objectively diagnose the patient's dysregulating symptomatology. However, she is also listening and interacting at another level, an experience-near subjective level, one that implicitly processes moment-to-moment attachment communications and self-states at levels beneath awareness. Bucci (2002) observed, "We recognize changes in emotional states of others based on perception of subtle shifts in their facial expression or posture, and recognize changes in our own states based on somatic or kinesthetic experience" (p. 194). In this manner the empathic clinician is able to resonate with the client's unconscious communications, so he or she can feel at an implicit level how this person experiences the world "from the inside out" (Bromberg, 2011). This enables the therapist to find ways of relating with this specific client that allows the patient's right brain to shift toward more integration and vitality.

Writing on therapeutic "nonverbal implicit communications," Chused (2007) asserted,

> It is not that the information they contain cannot be verbalized, only that sometimes only a nonverbal approach can deliver the information in a way it can be used, particularly when there is no conscious awareness of the underlying concerns involved. (p. 879)

These nonverbal communications are examples of "primary process communication." According to Dorpat (2001), "The primary process system analyzes, regulates, and communicates an individual's relations with the environment" (p. 449). He proposed,

> Affective and object-relational information is transmitted predominantly by primary process communication. Nonverbal communication includes body movements (kinesics), posture, gesture, facial expression, voice inflection, and the sequence, rhythm, and pitch of the spoken words. (Dorpat, 2001, p. 451)

The right brain thus processes "the music behind the words."

The organizing principle for working with unconscious primary process communications dictates that just as the left brain communicates its states to other left brains via conscious linguistic behaviors, so the right nonverbally communicates its other states to other right brains that are tuned to receive these communications. Bromberg (2011) observed,

> Allan Schore writes about a right brain-to-right brain channel of affective communication – a channel that he sees as "an organized dialogue" comprised of "dynamically fluctuating moment-to-moment state sharing." I believe it to be this process of state sharing that . . . allows . . . "a good psychoanalytic match." (p. 169)

Writing in the psychiatry literature, Meares (2012) described "a form of therapeutic conversation that can be conceived . . . as a dynamic interplay between two right hemispheres" (for other clinical examples of right brain-to-right brain tracking, see Chapman, 2014; Marks-Tarlow, 2012; Montgomery, 2013; A. N. Schore, 2012).

THE RIGHT BRAIN IS DOMINANT IN PSYCHOTHERAPY

On the matter of the verbal content, the words in psychotherapy—it has long been assumed in the psychotherapeutic literature that all forms of language reflect left hemispheric functioning of the conscious mind. Current neuroscience now indicates this is incorrect. In an overarching review Ross and Monnot (2008) concluded, "Thus, the traditional concept that language is a dominant and lateralized function of the left hemisphere is no longer tenable" (p. 51). These authors pointed out that

> the right hemisphere is essential for language and communication competency and psychological well-being through its ability to modulate affective prosody and gestural behavior, decode connotative (non-standard) word meanings, make thematic inferences, and process metaphor, complex linguistic relationships and non-literal (idiomatic) types of expressions. (p. 51)

Other studies reveal that the right hemisphere is dominant for the processing of, specifically, emotional words (Kuchinke et al., 2006). These data strongly suggest that the use of language in emotional and relational contexts such as intimate moments of the therapy involves right- and not left-brain language functions.

Left-brain interactions, that is, interpretations and rational explanations, are not the essential work of intersubjective psychotherapy, especially in heightened affective moments of the treatment. In fact, left-brain analyses will only contain and manage temporarily in a specific context. Insight will not solve long-standing emotional and interpersonal problems in relating. Right-brain-challenged clients will look to psychotherapy for left-brain solutions—conscious, willed changes in thoughts, intentions, and strategies, when what they need for lasting change is someone to emotionally engage with them right brain to right brain. What should this look like? In essence right-brain communications are experience-near in a reliable and consistent manner. For the therapist, "The key mechanism is *how to be with the patient*, especially during affectively stressful moments when the patient's implicit core self is dis-integrating in real time (right brain focus)" (A. N. Schore, 2012, p. 103, italics added).

We maintain that the core skills of any effective psychotherapist are right-brain implicit capacities which include empathy, the regulation of one's own affect, the ability to receive and express nonverbal communication, the sensitivity to register very slight changes in another's expression and emotion, and an immediate awareness of one's own subjective and intersubjective experience. All other techniques and skills sit atop this essential relational substratum. As Valentine and Gabbard (2014) eloquently stated, "Technique, in general, should be invisible. The therapist should be viewed by the patient as engaging in a natural conversational dialog growing out of the patient's concerns; the therapist should not be perceived as applying a stilted, formal technique" (p. 60).

The most important part of the therapist's trying to understand the client's "attachment emotional narrative" (much of which is nonverbal) is thus a spontaneous affective resonance that echoes the moment-to-moment shifts in client's affective and bodily states. The therapist tracks the intensity and direction of the affective charge, providing interactive affect regulation that allows for a safe holding of this interpersonally shared moment as it emerges without interpretation. The safety created by this new experience of being felt and regulated by another is repeated many times, so that the client will eventually be able to stay with this amplified affective state as it emerges in the interpersonal context of the therapeutic alliance, and ultimately even begin to talk about it or reflect on its meaning to her. In this process, unconscious affect becomes experienced, sustained, regulated affect, which can then become organized as a subjectively experienced emotional state and integrated into an expanding right-lateralized autobiographical self. The interactively regulated relationship with the therapist begins to provide an alternative to the defensive auto-regulatory withdrawal from others to protect the vulnerable self. The client learns to be with himself differently as well, within this safe connection with the attuned, engaged therapist.

As the client is able to contact, describe, and regulate his own emotional experience within the relational field, right-brain insight comes organically, building upon the emotional experience. The client develops a more complex ability to feel the connections between remembered history, sense of self, and working models of relationships. This right-brain insight includes a deeper awareness as a feeling/thinking/choosing person, and the creation of a more meaningful and authentic personal narrative. In terms of neuroscience, this change reflects more interconnectivity in his right brain, horizontally and laterally, more brain systems involved in the processing, communication, and regulation of emotion, thereby increasing the neuroplasticity of the emotional brain. Resultingly, the client becomes increasingly able to experience a broader range of and more complexity in emotions, as well as less rigidity in defenses. This more developed way of being, of self-regulation, will prove to be more flexible and useful than the previous characterological reliance on defensive affect-deadening dissociation. The client's bodily-based affective states, rather than being experienced as threats to self-cohesion, will now promote the development and unification of her sense of self. This emotional growth, in turn, allows her to be in a better position to intersubjectively communicate positive and negative affective states, to solve relationship problems with more resilient right-brain strategies, and to find emotional connection and satisfaction in interpersonal relationships (A. N. Schore, 2012).

Intersubjectivity is more than a communication or match of explicit verbal cognitions or overt behaviors. Regulated and dysregulated bodily based affects are communicated within an energy-transmitting intersubjective field coconstructed by two individuals that includes not just two minds but two bodies. At the psychobiological core of the coconstructed intersubjective field is the attachment bond of emotional communication and interactive regulation. Implicit intersubjective communications express bodily based emotional self-states, not just conscious cognitive "mental" states. The essential biological function of attachment communications in all human interactions, including those embedded in the therapeutic alliance, is the regulation of right brain–mind–body states. Intersubjective, relational, affect-focused psychotherapy is not the "talking cure," but the "affect-communicating cure." Neurobiologically informed relational infant, child, adolescent, and adult psychotherapy can thus potentially facilitate the intrinsic plasticity of the right brain, the biological substrate of the human unconscious.

The experience of being known and held in the understanding and affirming gaze of the therapist is what heals a broken or underdeveloped self and enables the client to grow emotionally: not insight, catharsis, or strategies to change behaviors and thoughts. Any lasting change in the deeper subjective sense of self can only emerge in the emotional presence of the therapists' empathy, authenticity, and unconditional positive regard. This has been written about since the middle of the last century, when Carl Rogers (1951) placed it at the core of client-centered therapy. Within psychoanalysis Heinz Kohut (1971) continued this central focus on empathic attunement. More recently the Boston Change Process Study Group (2010) highlighted what they call "now moments" that occur between therapist and client that have the power to alter and expand "implicit relational knowledge," what a client implicitly or unconsciously knows about how relationships really work and who he is in them. In earlier writings we identified the right hemisphere as the processor of implicit relational knowledge (J. Schore & Schore, 2010). Furthering this idea, we now propose that the shared social-emotional experiences of the intimate psychotherapeutic context can affect brain plasticity and expand the client's "social intelligence," a right-brain capacity for "identifying social stimuli, understanding the intentions of other people, awareness of the dynamics in social relationships, and successful handling of social interactions" (Hecht, 2014, p. 1).

CODA: LONG-TERM CLINICAL EXPERIENCE AND CHANGES IN THE CLINICIAN'S BRAIN

Regulation theory models changes in not only the client, but also in the clinical social worker. With clinical experience (the proverbial "10,000 hours" needed for the development of "expertise") psychotherapists of all schools can become expert in nonverbal intersubjective processes and implicit relational knowledge that enhance therapeutic effectiveness. The professional growth of clinicians reflects progressions in right-brain relational processes that underlie clinical skills. These right-brain expert functions of the emotionally sensitive therapist are expressed implicitly in an expanded ability to intuitively communicate with the bodily based unconscious minds across a wide variety of different client populations. The clinical experiences of psychodynamic psychotherapists also cultivate an implicit ability to regulate unconscious affect.

On this matter—the neuropsychoanalytic perspective of ART focuses attention on the increasing complexity of therapist's right-brain clinical intuition, more so than left-brain analytic reasoning, and on an expanding ability to process right brain-to-right brain dynamics within the coconstructed therapeutic alliance. The source of the most complex professional learning is what we learn from our clients, if we are open to this knowledge. Some of this knowledge can only be gained by exposing oneself to the darker side of the human experience. Other forms of this self-knowledge come from the intense intimacy and relational play that one encounters in deep psychotherapy. Our work leads us to believe that certain parts of our personalities can only grow in the presence of a receptive, emotionally communicating "other."

There is a limit to what we can learn by moving into a space apart from others, and self-reflecting. Mindfulness is often a left-brain attempt to auto-regulate and is thus self-limiting in terms of more efficient interactively regulated emotional experiences. Reflective consciousness ("mentalization") can only get one so far in terms of "understanding" oneself, especially the relational implicit self that interacts with another implicit self. We need trusted, empathic, resonant others who can mirror and amplify our deepest unconscious self-states and thereby bring them into working memory and awareness (see J. R. Schore, 2012, for a discussion of implicit and explicit memory systems).

The clinical model of regulation theory, ART, is a blend of classic attachment theory, internal object relations theory, self-psychology, and contemporary relational theory, all informed by neuroscience and infant research. The practice of psychotherapy is fundamentally relational: the therapeutic alliance, the major vector of change, is, in essence, a two-person system for (implicit) self-exploration and relational healing. At all points in the life span, this emotional growth of the self that supports emotional well-being is facilitated in relational contexts. The importance of "context" is currently highlighted by all scientific and clinical disciplines. For most of the last century science equated context with the organism's physical surround; this has now shifted to the social, relational environment. All human interactions, including those between therapist and client as well as researcher and experimental subject, occur within a relational context, in which essential nonverbal communications are transmitted and regulated at levels beneath conscious awareness, thereby activating/deactivating basic homeostatic processes in both members of an intersubjective dyad. We suggest that the inclusion of right-brain neuroscience and neuropsychoanalysis into a developmentally oriented, affectively focused treatment model can offer us more complex understandings of the science and the art of psychotherapy.

REFERENCES

Ammanitti, M., & Gallese, V. (2014). *The birth of intersubjectivity. Psychodynamics, neurobiology, and the self.* New York, NY: Norton.

Boston Change Process Study Group. (2010). *Change in psychotherapy: A unifying paradigm.* New York, NY: Norton.

Bowlby, J. (1969). *Attachment and loss. Vol. 1: Attachment.* New York, NY: Basic Books.

Bowlby, J. (1988). *A secure base* (2nd ed.). New York, NY: Basic Books.

Brancucci, A., Lucci, G., Mazzatenta, A., & Tommasi, L. (2009). Asymmetries of the human social brain in the visual, auditory and chemical modalities. *Philosophical Transactions of the Royal Society of London Biological Sciences*, *364*, 895–914.

Bromberg, P. M. (2011). *The shadow of the tsunami and the growth of the relational mind*. New York, NY: Routledge.

Bucci, W. (2002). The referential process, consciousness, and the sense of self. *Psychoanalytic Inquiry*, *5*, 766–793.

Chapman, L. (2014). *Neurobiologically informed trauma therapy with children and adolescents. Understanding mechanisms of change*. New York, NY: Norton.

Chused, J. F. (2007). Nonverbal communication in psychoanalysis: Commentary on Harrison and Tronick. *Journal of the American Psychoanalytic Association*, *55*, 875–882.

Decety, J., & Chaminade, T. (2003). When the self represents the other: A new cognitive neuroscience view on psychological identification. *Consciousness and Cognition*, *12*, 577–596.

Decety, J., & Lamm, C. (2007). The role of the right temporoparietal junction in social interaction: How low-level computational processes contribute to meta-cognition. *The Neuroscientist*, *13*, 580–593.

Derryberry, D., & Tucker, D. M. (1994). Motivating the focus of attention. In P. M. Niedentahl & S. Kiyayama (Eds.), *The heart's eye: Emotional influences in perception and attention* (pp. 167–196). San Diego, CA: Academic Press.

Dorpat, T. L. (2001). Primary process communication. *Psychoanalytic Inquiry*, *3*, 448–463.

Freud, S. (1953). The interpretation of dreams. In J. Strachey (Ed. & Trans.), *The standard edition of the complete works of Sigmund Freud*. London, UK: Hogarth Press. (Original work published 1900)

Freud, S. (1958). Recommendations to physicians practicing psycho-analysis. In J. Strachey (Ed. & Trans.), *Standard edition* (Vol. 12, pp. 109–120). London, UK: Hogarth Press. (Original work published 1912)

Freud, S. (1966). Project for a scientific psychology. In J. Strachey (Ed. & Trans.), *Standard edition of the complete psychological works of Sigmund Freud* (Vol. 1, pp. 295–397). London, UK: Hogarth Press. (Original work published 1895)

Hecht, D. (2014). Cerebral lateralization of pro- and anti-social tendencies. *Experimental Neurobiology*, *23*, 1–27.

Knickmeyer, R. C., Gouttard, S., Kang, C., Evans, D., Wilber, K., Smith, J. K., . . . Gilmore, J. H. (2008). A structural MRI study of human brain development from birth to 2 years. *Journal of Neuroscience*, *28*, 12176–12182.

Kohut, H. (1971). *The analysis of the self*. New York, NY: International Universities Press.

Kuchinke, L., Jacobs, A. M., Vo, M. L. H., Conrad, M., Grubich, C., & Herrmann, M. (2006). Modulation of prefrontal cortex by emotional words in recognition memory. *NeuroReport*, *17*, 1037–1041.

Lagercrantz, H., & Ringstedt, T. (2001). Organization of the neuronal circuits in the central nervous system during development. *Acta Paediatrica*, *90*, 707–715.

Lyons-Ruth, K. (2000). "I sense that you sense that I sense. . .": Sander's recognition process and the specificity of relational moves in the psychotherapeutic setting. *Infant Mental Health Journal, 21,* 85–98.

Marks-Tarlow, T. (2012). *Clinical intuition in psychotherapy: The neurobiology of embodied response.* New York, NY: Norton.

McGilchrist, I. (2009). *The master and his emissary.* New Haven, CT: Yale University Press.

Meares, R. (2012). *A dissociation model of borderline personality disorder.* New York, NY: W.W. Norton.

Montgomery, A. (2013). *Neurobiology essentials for clinicians: What every therapist needs to know.* New York, NY: Norton.

Rogers, C. (1951). *Client-centered therapy: Its current practice, implications, and theory.* London, UK: Constable.

Ross, E. D., & Monnot, M. (2008). Neurology of affective prosody and its functional anatomic organization in right hemisphere. *Brain and Language, 104,* 51–74.

Schore, A. N. (1994). *Affect regulation and the origin of the self.* Mahwah, NJ: Erlbaum.

Schore, A. N. (2001). The effects of relational trauma on right brain development, affect/regulation, and infant mental health. *Infant Mental Health Journal, 22,* 201–269.

Schore, A. N. (2003). *Affect regulation and the repair of the self.* New York, NY: Norton.

Schore, A. N. (2012). *The science of the art of psychotherapy,* New York, NY: Norton.

Schore, A. N. (2013a). Bowlby's "environment of evolutionary adaptedness": Recent studies on the interpersonal neurobiology of attachment and emotional development. In D. Narvaez, J. Panksepp, A. Schore, & T. R. Gleason (Eds.), *Evolution, early experience and human development. From research to practice to policy* (pp. 31–67). New York, NY: Oxford University Press.

Schore, A. N. (2013b). Regulation theory and the early assessment of attachment and autistic spectrum disorders: A response to Voran's clinical case. *Journal of Infant, Child, and Adolescent Psychotherapy, 12,* 164–189.

Schore, J. R. (2012). Using concepts from interpersonal neurobiology in revisiting psychodynamic theory. *Smith College Studies in Social Work, 82,* 90–111.

Schore, J. R., & Schore, A. N. (2008). Modern attachment theory: The central role of affect regulation in development and treatment. *Clinical Social Work Journal, 36,* 9–20.

Schore, J. R., & Schore, A. N. (2010). Clinical social work and regulation theory: Implications of neurobiological models of attachment. In S. Bennett & J. K. Nelson (Eds.), *Adult attachment in clinical social work* (pp. 57–75). New York, NY: Springer.

Semrud-Clikeman, M., Fine, J. G., & Zhu, D. C. (2011). The role of the right hemisphere for processing of social interactions in normal adults using functional magnetic resonance imaging. *Neuropsychobiology, 64,* 47–51.

Valentine, L., & Gabbard, G. O. (2014). Can the use of humor in psychotherapy be taught? *Academic Psychiatry, 38,* 75–81.

Watt, D. F. (2003). Psychotherapy in an age of neuroscience: bridges to affective neuroscience. In J. Corrigal & H. Wilkinson (Eds.), *Revolutionary connections: Psychotherapy and neuroscience* (pp. 79–115). London, UK: Karnac.

Wittling, W., & Roschmann, R. (1993). Emotion-related hemisphere asymmetry: Subjective emotional responses to laterally presented films. *Cortex, 29*, 431–448.

Selected Neurobiological Arousal Issues as Manifested in a Clinical Case Illustration

ARLENE MONTGOMERY

The University of Texas School of Social Work, Austin, Texas, USA;
Smith College School for Social Work, Northampton, Massachusetts, USA

Attachment patterns and defense mechanisms are profoundly affected by arousal systems within the brain and body to express in-born emotional circuits. Disordered personality functioning and the use and abuse of substances may augment or substitute for a compromised arousal system, leading to meeting criteria for psychiatric diagnoses. These arousal management and regulation issues are illustrated by a case history and session notes, including many of the neurobiological functions described in the introductory article of this journal issue.

INTRODUCTION

A therapy case is presented illustrating many of the concepts described in Miehls and Applegate's (2014/this issue) introductory chapter as well as some additional neurobiological phenomena elaborated on briefly in the next section. The interactions between the clinician and the client are examined line-by-line to exemplify what typically occurs in a therapeutic encounter, emphasizing arousal components.

The intention is not to suggest particular techniques or strategies for addressing the client's concerns but, instead, take a moment to "freeze-frame" the experience to suggest what is likely occurring intrapsychically and interpersonally as a result of the action of selected neurobiologically driven arousal experiences. Arousal experiences that are regulated by the autonomic nervous system (ANS) and the polyvagal system (PS) are implicit in attachment patterns, defense mechanisms, and selected psychiatric diagnoses, including substance use and abuse, are particularly obvious.

More subtle indications of arousal embedded in other structures and functions of the brain and nervous system are mentioned as they appear in the case material; these are treated in detail in the introductory chapter (Miehls & Applegate, 2014/this issue). Some of that material includes the following: the differences as well as integration between the right and left hemispheres of the brain, some structures of the limbic system including the hippocampus and amygdala, and certain phenomena critical to clinical work, such as attachment, resilience, plasticity of the brain, and memory particularly as affected by stress and/or trauma. The client in the illustration was profoundly affected by trauma, leading to borderline functioning, addictive use of alcohol, shame leading to being socially anxious with the attendant anticipation of negativity from others, and heightened fight, flight, freeze, and submit responses—all of which are also described in the introductory chapter. The material is somewhat a composite as well as being heavily disguised for confidentiality reasons.

As the clinician of this 20-year treatment effort, I only became aware of the exciting research findings regarding the neurobiological interactions implicit in clinical work about half-way though our therapeutic involvement, so the commentary about the early therapy regarding the brain function(s) were not in my mind at that time. All speculations must be qualified with the caveat that we do not know for absolute certainty that particular behaviors, and so on, may be explained by the neurobiological underpinnings that we think may be present. However, it seems important to take advantage of the knowledge now available about the functioning of a single brain and that brain in interaction with other brains and to make such speculations.

At this point, it must be said that the client has passed away. Every effort has been made to protect her identity and yet have important and instructive themes emerge for educational purposes. Although the client's subculture may be unfamiliar to the rest of the United States, many details of the history and childhood experiences are quite common in Texas and other southwestern states that border Mexico. Without such background, the reader may be puzzled about many of the shared meanings of the clinical encounter.

OVERVIEW OF STRUCTURES AND FUNCTIONS OF THE BRAIN AND NERVOUS SYSTEM THAT AFFECT AROUSAL REGULATION

Brain-based arousal issues are heavily involved with behavioral and emotional expression. A brief overview follows of the interface among two neurobiological arousal systems (the ANS and the PS) and the recent research on the seven in-born emotional circuits, attachment patterns, the perception of safety–danger (neuroception), defense mechanisms, and certain psychiatric conditions.

Two Neurobiological Arousal Systems: The Autonomic Nervous System and the Polyvagal System

The human nervous system "consists of two major divisions: the brain and spinal cord . . . and the peripheral nervous system consists of all the nervous tissue outside the central nervous system" (Buelow, Hebert, & Buelow, 2000, pp. 151 & 153). The peripheral nervous system is further divided into sensory and motor divisions, and the motor division is divided into the somatic nervous system (five senses) and the autonomic system (arousal), which is further divided into the sympathetic branch (excitatory) and the parasympathetic branch (inhibiting) (Brody, 1992; Buelow et al., 2000). High, low, or balanced arousal experiences are exquisitely controlled by the sympathetic (up-regulated) and parasympathetic (down-regulated) branches that operate in tandem. Of critical importance is that the environment sculpts and trains, so to speak, the ways arousal is expressed; expression of the intensity of affect is not in-born, rather it is experience dependent (Schore, 2003a).

Stephen Porges (2011) described a process, neuroception, in the brain that registers safety–danger in the environment via the vagus nerve (PS). The evaluation of risk via neuroception involves sensitivity of the vagus nerve, which works in concert with the ANS, particularly the parasympathetic branch. At times, in the face of extreme stress or danger, arousal can be almost completely inhibited such that social interaction is unlikely under such conditions. The low arousal may lead to dissociation, death feigning, or even actual death. A more benign response of the parasympathetic–vagus nerve interaction is to engender a calm social approach by the release of the "vagal brake" that spares overuse of the sympathetic branch. Too much activation of the stress response may have a global and negative effect on health.

Emotional Circuitry

Particular early interactions with the environment will shape the brain to express the seven in-born emotional circuits which include the following: seeking, rage, fear, lust, care, panic/grief, and play (Panksepp, 2011) that are found in the same part of the brain of all animals thus far studied and are speculated to also be in the same place in the human brain. According to Panksepp and Watt (2011), depression is intimately related to overactivity of the separation-distress panic system and, if prolonged, can lead to despair, which, in turn, leads to abnormally low activity of the seeking system; this environmentally influenced depression creates psychological pain, which can be shut down by brain opioids.

Attachment and Arousal: Dyadic Regulation of Affect

The attachment patterns learned through interaction with the milieu (particularly the one-to-one dyadic interchanges with primary caregivers) from birth onward are essentially unconscious and nonconscious affect-management strategies; *unconscious* means within the brain of a person and *nonconscious* means two brains synchronously in communion with one another, often nonverbally, but not always (Schore, 2003a, 2003b). The nonconscious transfer of affect may occur between structures of two brains, that is, people may have brain stem-to-brain stem connections, amygdala-to-amygdala connections, right hemisphere-to-right hemisphere connections, or left hemisphere-to-left hemisphere connections. The attachment strategies are managed by the ANS's excitatory and inhibitory branches.

The four childhood and adulthood strategies of attachment and relation to the ANS include the following:

1. Secure attachment is a balance between the excitatory and inhibitory branches, according to context (in adulthood, also termed secure).
2. The three insecure attachment patterns are not affected by context, and two strategies (a. and b. below) have been sculpted by interactions with the environment to be governed by one branch of ANS whereas the other one (c. below) is unpredictable in expression of excitatory or inhibitory arousal.
   a. The ambivalent/resistant attachment of childhood and the preoccupied attachment of adulthood manage affect and behavior primarily by excitatory branch.
   b. The avoidant attachment of childhood and the dismissive of adulthood manage affect and behavior by the inhibitory branch.
   c. The disorganized/disoriented/"Type D" attachment of childhood and the unresolved of adulthood have erratic excitatory or inhibitory activation or both activated simultaneously (Schore, 2003a; Siegel, 1999, p. 74).

Arousal and Defense Mechanisms

Defenses can be separated into three types of arousal strategies. The more adaptive defenses employ the two branches of the ANS as appropriate to the situation. Each defense may use the excitatory or inhibitory branches. These defenses include but are not limited to the following:

affiliation, altruism, self-assertion, self-observation, sublimation, and suppression (American Psychiatric Association [APA], 2000, pp. 811–813) and altruism and humor (Valliant, 1977, pp. 383–386). Defenses that may be managed primarily by the parasympathetic branch include but are not limited to the following: intellectualization, passive-aggression, dissociation (APA, 2000, pp. 811–813) and ascetism, blocking, controlling, denial, displacement, introjection, and repression (Vaillant, 1977, pp. 383–386). Defenses that may be managed primarily by the sympathetic branch include but are not limited to the following: delusions and hallucinations, help-rejecting complaining, derealization, distortion, externalization, projection, reaction formation, repression, splitting, undoing (APA, 2000, pp. 811–813); acting out/regression and devaluation (Kernberg, 1979); identification with the aggressor (Freud, 1936/1966, p. 112); identification (Leowald, 1973); projective identification (Schore, 2003b); psychotic denial, sexualization, hypochrondriasis, externalization, distortion (Valliant, 1977, pp. 383–386); and mania (Winnicott, 1965, p. 132). Further discussion and definitions of the above defense mechanisms can be found in Montgomery (2013).

Arousal Systems and Selected Psychiatric Conditions

Disordered personalities have as a problematic element of the diagnostic criteria the management of levels of arousal and control of behaviors that are not within average expectable range for the culture or subculture. In addition to the disorders of personality, an important aspect of each criterion of the following psychiatric conditions is a clinically worrisome issue with arousal management (i.e., affect management): mood and anxiety disorders, for those disorders that have traumatic stress as the etiology, and substance use and abuse. The person in the following case illustration had a severe trauma history and struggled with social anxiety, depression, substance use and abuse, disordered personality functioning (likely borderline features), and a psychiatric diagnosis of one of the bipolar conditions.

Case Example: Sabina

[Note: For clarity, the commentary on neurobiological considerations is formatted as blocked text/extracts to set it apart from the text relating the client's history.]

Sabina died in her early fifties of causes unknown to me. I only learned of her death when she missed an appointment and I called her cell phone to check up on her. She often missed appointments. Her adult son who lived with her answered her phone and said that she had passed away. I did not attempt to contact her family further and though I looked online, I did not find more information about her death. No cause of death was mentioned in the obituary and memorial page the family had put on the Internet.

I first met Sabina when she was in her late twenties. We worked at a large social service agency though I never actually had interactions with her at that time. I did see her with her elementary school child, Rene, at the agency once. Several years later, she contacted me for individual therapy services. Over the years until her recent death she would erratically come for therapy and disappear sometimes for years.

> I eventually began to believe that her episodic use of therapy was a function of both her mood swings over the course of a year as well as her defense (acting out) against the disturbance of experiencing certain emotions (sympathetic branch of the ANS) and, possibly, inviting unbearably painful traumatic reminders (sympathetic activation) followed by the shut-down (dissociation) of that high arousal (parasympathetic branch and vagus nerve).

Early in our work, I learned bit by bit of her tumultuous childhood and adolescence. Her parents were Mexican American, each having around 10 siblings. Sabina was the youngest of eight children. Although her parents and grandparents had been born in the United States, they had deep ties to northern Mexico, particularly influenced by the Native American culture. Additionally, Sabina became emotionally and, in some years, actually involved with the Native American culture in the United States, especially those figures of the late 20th century. For example, she participated in many symbolic events and marches commemorating accomplishments of Native American peoples and in opposition to the treatment of native people who were resisting the Bureau of Indian Affairs, or protesting the Wounded Knee events or the celebration of Columbus Day. Her first husband was also involved in some of those events. She was also involved with a spiritual leader from Mexico who linked back to some of the Aztec traditions, slightly intermixed with Catholicism.

However, after two children, she divorced her husband. He was little help coparenting as he was addicted to various drugs and lived with his parents. She was the primary support of her two sons until her death. One son, Rene, is diagnosed with schizophrenia and lived with her and the other son, Guillermo, is married and has two children with a woman who is also diagnosed with schizophrenia and drug addictions.

> She had energy for her responsibilities, likely guided by the highly adaptive defense mechanisms of altruism, anticipation, affiliation, humor, self-assertion, sublimation, and suppression, all balanced between two branches of the ANS, meaning that the behaviors reflected by these defenses could be up- or down-regulated, depending on the situation.

During most of her childhood and early elementary school, Sabina's family lived on the same lot with her grandparents and other siblings of her father in a compound in a part of the city where many similar living arrangements were common in a large neighborhood with others of Mexican heritage or recent immigrants from Mexico. In Sabina's generation, Spanish was the first language learned, and it was possible to have an insular existence in the nonintegrated neighborhood and local schools. Although poor, everyone worked and shared. The family experiences were organized around the Catholic Church, food, gardening, multiple caretakers who all seemed to have equal authority over the children, the many cousins, pets, and fiestas. From this relatively stable home life, Sabina was an excellent student.

> Although her early life was filled with many caretakers and activities, it is possible that Sabina had opportunities to build a somewhat secure relationship, such that she was able to manage the appropriate tasks for her developmental level. A secure relationship is reflected in behaviors in which there is flexibility in regulating the intensity of emotional expression (a balanced ANS) by oneself or one has others to whom to turn for temporary affect regulation, thus conferring resilience (thought to have a large arousal management component; Schore, 2003b, p. 11). A secure relationship with concomitant resilience is also marked by an abundance of the highly adaptive defense mechanisms Sabina employed, mentioned above.

This life came to an abrupt halt when her father was sent to prison for drug dealing. Her mother never got along with the father's mother. At a time of dire need, the family had to move out of the compound into the near-by housing project, which was quite dangerous. Over the years, Sabina was the only sibling who went with the mother to visit the father in the prison, many hours away by car.

> The move was a traumatic loss that might challenge the most adaptive of arousal regulation strategies encoded by Sabina's brain throughout her early childhood and elementary years.

Sabina was age 10 years and frightened all the time. An older sibling was "in charge" of the others as the mother worked long hours. The sibling enforced whatever rules that were broken with physical violence. Additionally, Sabina witnessed many gang fights, had sisters who were raped, constantly was around drug and alcohol use, and was physically assaulted multiple times having her lunch money stolen from her. School became her refuge, and she continued to excel. Home was dangerous, and she began to have nightmares after the move. Although married at 18 and a mother soon afterward, she continued to attend the local community college as well as work.

> Neuroception (risk evaluation) was constantly occurring, with few chances for calm, safe approaching. In fact, anything that looked calm could easily mask danger to a little girl who was alone. Not having any help or protection from her immediate milieu, except for teachers at times, her somewhat secure attachment might have been overlaid by either the ambivalent/resistant insecure attachment or elements of the disorganized/disoriented/"Type" D insecure attachment style.

> Both attachment styles are up-regulated, with watchfulness and vigilant behaviors automatically employed to detect the possibility of getting something from the environment as well as possible sources of danger around them (and from within, as well). Although both have dissociative times, the "Type D" has more erratic and unpredictable swings from highly excitable to extremely low arousal; there is a heavy reliance on dissociation to manage the painfully high arousal. The vagal system in conjunction with the parasympathetic branch may have been creating the extreme dissociative experiences required to avoid a state of extreme sympathetic activation awake and sleeping.

Sabina was in her early thirties when she sought therapy. At that point she was unhappily married with two boys, working, and taking a class or two a semester.

SESSION #1

    TX: Hi, Sabina. Do you remember that we worked at ***** years ago?
Sabina: Yes, that is why I am here. I heard that you were divorcing and in a court battle for your two sons and thought that you might not judge me for doing the same thing.

> The highly adaptive defense mechanism, affiliation, is employed in the attempt to establish similarity, to have something in common. Additionally, with her Catholic background, divorce may have elicited judgment from others, possibly a distressing up-regulated experience of shame or guilt.

    TX: I do remember seeing you with your older child, Rene, but I do not remember ever really meeting each other.
Sabina: No, we did not work in the same building.
    TX: I do remember knowing that you and your husband were activists in the Chicano rights movement and that he traveled to Central America as part of that.

Sabina: Yeah, but I did not travel because of the kids . . . actually, that was the way it always was, he left me to do it all with them.

TX: I just wanted to see if we had any conflict with knowing each other or the same people, and like that.

Sabina: No problem. But I did think you were friendly to the Chicanos working there . . . not everybody was, especially to the clerical staff like me. By everybody, I mean the Whites.

Until the comment about Whites, the emotional tone was fairly neutral and matter-of-fact, an expectable intensity of affect called for by the content of the material. However, with the comment about Whites, there was a little spike in the arousal of the therapist, a wariness, that is up-regulated somewhat. As there was no acting on the up-regulation, suppression may have been employed by therapist to achieve somewhat lower affect state.

TX: Oh. Well. [Long pause] I am thinking that your deliberately choosing a White therapist should be talked about right now.

Therapist was thinking hard (left hemisphere, cooler emotions) and in a slightly aroused state (right hemisphere, higher intensity emotions), trying to be cautious and vigilant, all up-regulated states.

Sabina: Well, I knew you had a lot of experience and I am not automatically prejudiced against Whites; it just depends on how they act. Do you have a problem with seeing me?

A little forward and confrontational, but not too much, the behavior expressed an up-regulated state, possibly her trauma-sensitized amygdala was more in an aroused flight mode temporarily.

TX: No, but I do feel a little off balance and worry that somehow I might offend you without knowing it. I wonder if you would let me know if that happens?

Therapist finds a balanced, authentic way to answer her; a little up-regulated, but not out of a comfortable range, using the sublimation defense; therapist being authentic about own worries, perhaps as way to regulate by channeling affect into productive interaction?

Sabina: I am known for being blunt, so probably so. But let's get on with talking about my kids.

Sabina meets therapist with similar intensity of affect, which is matter of fact.

We began an off-and-on-again relationship during which she worried about the effect of the divorce on her boys, particularly the first son, who seemed "weak" as the father said. She stayed around 18 months that time. She continued to work in various social service agencies. Her bilingual, bicultural abilities were heavily utilized for the Spanish-only speaking clients. After a hiatus of several years, she wanted some more help. This time, her father had just died and she was depressed, beyond bereavement. She was hospitalized briefly, and electroshock therapy was recommended. She had no family member able to interface with the mental health professionals. She did not understand that electroshock was recommended and actually scheduled. I took a lot of time to explain the treatment option, and she ultimately refused it. She was given medication for depression and sent home.

> Sabina was in a terribly intense unbearable depressive episode certainly due to grief about her father, likely reviving earlier traumatic losses of him due to legal problems, her mother's refusal to live with her father, and his descent into addiction culminating in his overdosing out in the elements. This depression and other episodes as well were arousing, painful, and unremitting. Was it a mood disorder swing? Was it revival of traumatic memories? Or a combination? Whatever the case, the level of arousal was high, not low, which meant that the sympathetic branch of the ANS was not being attenuated or stopped by Sabina's brain's arousal management networks. She was not, however, in a manic episode. Rather, Sabina was in an intense, up-regulated state of grief.
>
> Sabina's panic system may have been activated by the separation-distress that seemed painfully endless, clearly painfully up-regulated. It generally required great internal and/or external pressure for her to seek help from anyone. Her counter-dependent character style (i.e., giving the appearance of extremely independent and soldier-like functioning even though, like most people, she sometimes needed to rely on others). Although she did have features of borderline personality functioning, her behaviors were likely better accounted for by posttraumatic stress disorder, but no psychiatrists ever gave her that diagnosis. Certainly, for each diagnosis, extremes of arousal of affect are emblematic, as is true of the bipolar condition with which she would eventually be diagnosed.

We did begin to patch together a history of her depressive episodes, most of them around midsummer, especially August, beginning in late high school. These depressive episodes generally did include fatigue, low affect, and sleeping too much. Although we did attempt to link the episodes to events (of which there were many traumatic ones), ultimately it appeared that she might have a mood disorder. At various times she was prescribed medications for the shifting moods, but she had experienced many side effects, such a sudden weight gain and severe acne.

Sabina was an unusual looking woman, with an exotic somewhat Asian look and fit figure. Her boys were also unusually beautiful. She dressed in striking clothes with a Native American/Mexican flavor, garments easy to find in Texas. Her main source of self-esteem, her appearance, was quickly taken from her, which was even more depressing. She was accustomed to being intensely attractive to men.

For several years, she struggled to get psychiatric help with her mood disorder, largely a failure. She had little money for the expensive medical services including frequent blood draws to monitor some of the medications for bipolar symptoms; her insurance covered little or no medical care; she had low-wage jobs which did not allow time off; and the medications tried over time either did not work, had side effects, or could not be afforded long enough to give them a good trial. Discontinuing the medications for mood disorder made the weight loss possible and the skin condition vanished.

There was no help for her with her family responsibilities except occasionally from her mother and one sister. She did manage to work and take classes. She would come and go with therapy in part related to her mood swings. She would tend to come back as the summer approached and dwindle off after a few months. Some of the years when I did not see her were marked with some better luck with antidepressants. She had refused to take the medications for the mood swings.

> She made it clear that she was ambivalent about coming to therapy. She was not noncompliant with her medications because of the side effects. She had to function, had a job where she interacted with the public, and her appearance was important. She did not particularly value her good intellect, however. When her emotional system was regulated enough to think clearly about her medical situation, it is clear that her left-hemisphere (cognition, learning) could function well with a little emotional stability. The highly adaptive defense mechanisms of anticipation, self-observation, and suppression were evident.

During her thirties she had relationships with men who were either from Mexico (some not legal immigrants) or had ties to the activist community. From her late twenties until her death, Sabina also was involved with several groups whose mission was to preserve Mexican native peoples' music, dance, and religious ceremonies. At some point in her late thirties she married a man, a Mexican citizen, who was a decade or more younger than she was. Although still married at the time of her death, they never lived together. He was able to begin his efforts toward becoming an American citizen due to their marriage, but that was not the reason for the legal union. However, they had emotionally violent, angry arguments. They looked like siblings; though she would often declare that she would divorce him, she never could do so. She and I wondered together about this bond to him. He certainly looked like her father's relatives and re-created having an important man in her life, yet not being able to be with him, much like her imprisoned father.

> Her near 20-year marriage re-created elements of her past that were stressful and traumatic in some instances. The frequent angry interactions were a displacement and externalization of early internal and external experiences as she projected onto her second husband the father who dramatically left and returned, with many tearful separations and reunions. At one point I referred them to a Spanish speaking therapist who finally suggested that they should divorce. Projection, projective identification, and externalization (up-regulated) and displacement (seeking a down-regulated experience) made possible chronically reexperiencing her original separation anguish.

As she was finishing her community college degree, I began to suggest that she apply to one of the 4-year universities in the area. She was accepted into a bachelor of social work program, received student loans, and moved into student housing with her younger early teenage son. During this fairly stable time in her life, her son, Guillermo, began a relationship with a girl who would become his wife. She was an abused, neglected, and traumatized girl whose parents did not care that she had begun living with Sabina and her son. Sabina did begin to receive better medical care from the services available to college students. After graduation she began a series of case manager jobs with the non-English speaking, indigent, immigrant (legal and illegal) population who were HIV positive or who had AIDS.

SESSION FOLLOWING GRADUATION FROM UNIVERSITY

    TX: Congratulations on your graduation.
Sabina: I was glad to see you there.
    TX: I was trying not to be too obvious.
Sabina: Oh, for God's sake, they all know who you are. And the ones who don't do not speak English anyway.
    TX: Well . . . OK, I was happy to see your children and grandchild and mother and sisters and husband and whoever else was there.

> So far, that was a low-key, social interaction managed by the PS (calm approach) rather than either the sympathetic or parasympathetic branches of the ANS with the exception of the barbed comment, "Oh, for god's sake . . . " that was typical of her sarcasm and blunt manner at times. A little up-regulated with a slightly aggressive tone.

Sabina: What a day! Not one of my sibs or cousins have done this, so it was complicated. They are not all proud of me. But my kids are. I was hoping that Guillermo would go even though he is married now. You know he was admitted to this university?

TX: Yes, I do remember that he was automatically admitted because he graduated in top 10% of his high school.

Her response went from proud of herself (an up-beat, but not highly aroused affect)to sadness that all were not proud of her (a little lower affect) to pleased over her kids' reaction (a little up-regulated) and back to sadness that Guillermo did not take advantage of admission and financing that would accompany his college opportunity. This is a good example of the undulating rise and fall of the intensity of affect expression within normal limits. With a compromised ANS, the vacillations can be extreme and not necessarily related to the present moment, but reminiscent of past moments being reexperienced. I believe that my brain was in synchrony with the ebb and flow of the intensity of her emotions. That Sabina could have such regulated exchanges from time to time makes me think that her original but nonconscious secure relationship arousal regulation strategy was activated.

Sabina: [Regretfully] Yeah, well, Rene is really smart, too, but he can't get along with people. He always thinks someone is watching him or thinking bad thoughts about him. He hit someone again last week in the Wal-Mart. He thought they were talking about him.

The regret brings about a matter-of-fact presentation (contained arousal), but I could sense the undercurrent of disturbance about his situation; transfer of affect from our lower right brains, as our brains synchronized with one another.

TX: I know he is too old to be on your insurance, but maybe MHMR could help him.

Sabina: Nooo. He won't go. But maybe he could go to my Nurse Practitioner . . . she is a nurse and he might go for that.

We both are in "fix-it" mode, trying to combat the helplessness (right hemisphere) Rene's situation invites with two social workers whose left hemispheres are searching for options, generating ideas, and planning which are all up-regulated behaviors.

TX: It seems that your meds are finally working OK. What are you taking?

Sabina: *****

I am still in fact-gathering mode (left hemisphere) though bringing up a tender topic for her, that is, her emotional stability and its management (right hemisphere).

TX: I wonder how this summer has gone for you, with August often being a hard month for you.

Sabina: [Tears up. Looks away. Looks blank. Says slowly.] You know I think the meds help, but I wish my dad had lived to see me get a degree. People don't really know how he was.

Sabina is not interested in my topic, her medications (my left hemisphere way of distancing from the sadness associated with her graduation) and brings up a tender subject important to her, her dad.

TX: What do you mean?

Sabina: [Looks away again.] He never got out of the 3rd grade before he had to help out with money. It was nothing in the old neighborhood to move drugs around for money. The police never bothered with our neighborhood. It was some rivals who got him sent off. But, even though he OD'd, he is still respected around where we used to live. His name still means something. I just . . . .

TX: [Waiting for her to finish her thought, but she did not.] What did you mean, "People did not really know how he was"?

I am trying to find a narrative thread, a left hemisphere endeavor, but with assistance with the right hemisphere emotional connection I experience with her via the adaptive defense mechanism of affiliation.

Sabina: Well, his English was better than my mother's, actually, she barely speaks English today . . . anyway, she never looked at our grade cards from kinder on, but he did and would sneak me a little Mexican candy for my grades. And he was home a lot, (she makes air quotes) "working from home, you know" [sarcastically] . . . [trails off] what was I saying? Oh, oh, so he loved cards and dominos and would play with whichever of us would sit still and play with him. And he knew all the old songs from back in Mexico. He never got mad or yelled at us. But my mother, well, another story. And Gramma, she scared the shit out of us, always telling us that if we did not do what she wanted, she would die. So we minded her. Always.

Sabina's affect was sad, yet contained (not dissociated, except at the beginning of her remarks when she lost track of her own narrative), obviously painful, as ordinary moments from childhood were imbued with tragic over-tones.

Sabina generally allowed only a little time for difficult topics and affect, so this interaction was atypical in that she stopped my effort to focus on what I was wondering about and redirected the discussion to her father (self-assertion). I always sensed that she wanted to connect more fully with me (right hemisphere-to-right hemisphere synchrony), but had many ways to avoid what it seemed she desperately wanted, authentic connection. She would change the subject, crack a clever joke, leave early, or simply miss appointments after an emotional discussion (acting out). I was often wary and on-guard myself (neuroceoption, detecting safety–danger), even though we had moments of laughter, connection, and shared feminist outrage, especially around issues of racism. I was grateful for those times, as her erratic contact worried me and I had the belief (fantasy?) that some good was coming from our work together.

For a few months she would come off and on and then I did not hear from her for several years. When I did, she had gained considerable weight and did not look healthy. She had begun to drink alcohol every evening, her older son had been in and out of psychiatric hospitals with psychotic episodes, her other son was parenting two toddlers with his schizophrenic wife, and she had some arrests for driving while intoxicated, and was jailed for several months for engaging in a fist fight with a neighbor when they were both drunk.

She did become increasingly socially anxious, suspicious, and negative in social encounters perhaps due to extreme stress and shame (a painful affect involving the sympathetic branch). Being highly activated was often followed by the parasympathetic branch plunging the arousal system to low, often dissociative moments (Schore, 2003a). The social anxiety, approaching phobic at times, may have been triggered by public humiliation likely stimulating memories of her family's shame over her father being imprisoned. These traumatic amygdalar memories did take the form of flashbacks at times. She may have experienced decreasing function of the hippocampus, which is partly involved with limbic action that neutralizes impulsive urges.

A FEW YEARS LATER

She began by relaying the multiple problems she and her family were experiencing.

Sabina: So, in short, well, I am a wreck. I need to keep coming to therapy.
    TX: Sounds like you have a lot of responsibility for one person.

Sabina: True, but some of this is my own fault. Rene can't help it, he is so bad off sometimes. And I have to help Guillermo and the babies. Sometimes she (her daughter-in-law) is way off and won't let me come over, even though I am giving them money and my car. But, whatever, I have to be nice to her or I won't be able to see the kids.

> She barely allows an empathic connection about the hardship on her. Guilt (left hemisphere) and shame (right hemisphere) are easily activated, validated by her psychological and behavioral deterioration. I speculate that the alcohol is a much more reliable source of emotional regulation than another person's attunement and certainly, far out-weighing dissociation for escaping inner pain. Although likely a genetic component for substance use and abuse is at play, to the extent that psychological influences exist, drinking may be an identification (up-regulated) with her father, as well, a way to be close to him, albeit unconsciously.

    TX: I would be glad to see you regularly, you know that, right?

Sabina: I know, but, I got mad at you.

    TX: What?

Sabina: When you said the babies' mother would always need medical care for her schizophrenia, you made me feel hopeless. But, you were right, she only got worse, trying to kill herself and all. It's my dad all over again.

    TX: How so?

Sabina: Hopeless, everyone but me gave up on him.

    TX: Did you feel like we couldn't talk about this?

Sabina: No, I knew we could and that's just the problem. This is the only place where I can even think about some things and it, it, it . . . it's too weird. [Starts crying.]

    TX: Weird?

Sabina: [Really crying hard, which is unusual and in contrast to her flippant and often funny, sarcastic way of expressing herself. Some minutes pass.]

Finally, she says, "I know we have talked about the blank looks, and yes, I know that is dissociative [sarcastically again], but either I do that or I drink. But I want to take better care of my health. Even though you torture me with your questions, I do better somehow."

> Sabina is connecting, though with difficulty, as she "confesses" not only being mad at me but, importantly, the meaning to her of being mad at me. She can be psychologically sophisticated. However, given the unrelenting environmental stress, insight (left hemisphere) does not keep her from drinking and acting out at times (poor control by limbic system and

upper right hemisphere of impulses originating from lower right brain, the amygdala; the fight, flight, freeze actions were triggered by fear, in this case, of her own painfully aroused emotions). Yet, despite the chaos, she still supports a fragile family somewhat adequately. Thankfully, her case-manager skills benefit her children and grandchildren. All along, I had been hoping for a corrective emotional experience for her; at rare instances there were indications of change, validating the plasticity of the brain. Additionally, perhaps being a "good enough" therapist may have at times allowed her to retrieve early more adequate functioning of childhood. I must admit, however, I struggled with my critical thoughts about her drinking and being needed by the family so desperately. It was hard to stay empathically attuned to her at times given such strong counter-transferential reactions (uncomfortably aroused).

For a few years life was a little better. We worked together to get Rene disability income, home visits for social work services and psychiatric services; her extremely difficult job was bearable; and her older son's family life settled somewhat as the children got older and wife was on disability income. Clearly, however the family went, so went Sabina. And then in the same month two important people died. One was a coworker and the other her sister who was "the one in charge" when the family lived in the "projects"; her sister died of cirrhosis of the liver and her close friend of a progressive neurological condition.

Although most of her life she had experienced nightmares, sleeping problems, anxiety, and depression, these symptoms worsened. She had carried out the plans for her sister's memorial service in accordance with some of the spiritual traditions they had observed as children. Afterward, according to tradition, she kept her sister's ashes on an altar in her bedroom. Rene was "freaked out" from time to time over the altar, and she would become really upset when he would move the items, such as the beer or dried flowers. She finally told him in anger that he could live somewhere else if he "so much as touched those things again." He did not, though at times he would become so paranoid in his own room, that he would make a pallet on the floor of her room and sleep there. He was afraid of the sister's spirit.

She had dreams of her sister, who would talk to her, let Sabina know she was okay, and was not in pain. Those were not nightmares to Sabina, as they were comforting. In the past Sabina would have frightening "dreams" or perhaps hallucinations when she would wake up from a disturbed sleep. The dreams were of evil, dangerous spirits or situations and of a religious nature. She was always influenced by the spirituality of some of the Aztec-Mexican-Catholic beliefs, so did not consider the "visions" as a sign of mental illness, but a real phenomenon which many others had also experienced.

The last year of her life she vacillated between trying to take better care of her health (joining a gym, taking vitamins) and then drinking too much, even though she had the recent example of her sister's death from alcohol-related causes. She was struggling with severe sleep apnea, pains in her "side" (her upper right side), nausea, fatigue, sleeping problems of various kinds, and worry about Rene's going off his medications for psychosis. He was hospitalized several more times for psychotic episodes, always following medication noncompliance. She told him that if he did not cooperate with his medication instructions, he would have to move. She had missed a great deal of work around Rene's decompensations, police having to be called for his aggressive behavior, and subsequent hospitalizations.

The last session we had concerned the spreading of the ashes of her sister. Sabina described in great detail an experience the week before involving a loud banging outside her apartment originating from where there was no porch or patio, only a windowless wall two stories high. This was accompanied by loud moaning, sighing, and crying. She was fairly sure that it was her sister, trying to send a message to Sabina. After giving it some thought, Sabina believed that her sister was ready to be "let go" and have her ashes spread to the winds and water.

Sabina: So you can see from where the sounds came from, there was no shared wall with the neighbors or no way for anyone to get up the brick wall to make the noise. I know it was her voice and it is time to plan to take down the altar. She has been with me for long enough [laughing]. Rene will be glad to take apart the altar. He is sick of it.

TX: What about other relatives, like her kids.

I have a matter-of-fact response (contained by upper right hemisphere) to her understanding of the noises in the night. Although not in any way socialized into the Native American traditions, both my West Texas grandparents were rumored to be part "Indian," as some aunts said. That was always disputed due to racist attitudes in my family, but there is a lot of evidence that might be so. Sabina knew that about me many years ago, as she began to let me know about her family background. Whether revealing that was a good idea or not, it did make for a connection that over-rode my "White" appearance and likely helped me distance from those whom she considered racist (perhaps a way for me to manage "White guilt or shame," an unpleasant up-regulated state of arousal?).

Sabina: I will try, but they live far away and I think my sister wants to go soon. It will have to be on the weekend. The ceremony will take a while, [abruptly changing the subject] Besides, I need to get some health appointments. A sleep study has been ordered and that will take time off work. Whatever, and we got some better insurance. I can get the liver enzyme tests the doctor has been pushing me to get, too. Not that you haven't.

TX: Are you worried?

Sabina: [Blank stare, briefly looks away (dissociative moment).] There you go again. I am trying to just do it and think about it later. I have cut back on the wine.

TX: Would your new insurance cover some in-patient detox for you?

Sabina: [Begins to cry.] I don't want to end up like my sister. I thought if I could keep her by me, then she would not be gone. But now she wants to go. Was she trying to tell me something?

TX: I am listening to her and feel emotionally connected to her, though say virtually nothing.

> These interchanges are emblematic of her reflexive defensive maneuvers. She is able to stay on the almost unbearable topic of her sister's ashes by talking about the logistics and time constraints involved in spreading the ashes (left hemisphere planning (lower arousal) and right hemisphere defenses of anticipation, and suppression, adapative defenses), then quickly segues to the association she cannot help but make to herself, who may suffer the same fate (fear managed by self-assertion in going to the doctor). I am doing the same thing in making suggestions and advice-giving (left hemisphere). At the end, she gets back to herself with heart-felt expression of the meaning she ascribes to the night noises. I am present. Both of us are experiencing a low right hemisphere to low right-hemisphere connection.

We wrapped what would be our last session and made a further appointment.

DISCUSSION

Describing Sabina's life experiences, including our interactions, provides a window into the subtle ways we can not only understand the neurobiological underpinnings of apparently ordinary exchanges between two persons, but also have a sense of the impact of stress and trauma within those same interactions. There is a progression from relatively normal functioning in childhood and elementary school indicating that she had, perhaps, a somewhat secure attachment; perhaps even normative for her subculture. She depicted herself, before the time before her father went to prison, as relatively confident that the (multiple) parent figures would be responsive, available, comforting, and protective, particularly under distressful circumstances, permitting exploration of the environment, the description of a secure attachment (Ainsworth et al., as cited in Florsheim, Henry, & Benjamin, 1996, p. 84). The ANS would, therefore, be flexible and able to adapt to most situations, with the up- or down-regulation branches activating behavior as a situation required. The operational right-hemisphere-managed attachment strategy permitted the left hemisphere to therefore function well in school tasks for the early years and indeed set the stage for continued capacity to function academically in her later life.

However, when the family was no longer able to live in the family compound due to strife between Sabina's mother and paternal grandmother, the move to the housing project with the constant stress and actual danger began to influence her employing measures of all sorts to protect herself. I speculate that her attachment category of secure (ANS balanced) began to be overlaid with elements of the anxious-ambivalent attachment style. This ambivalent attachment style may influence the brain of a child to be uncertain whether the parent will be responsive, available, or protective when needed, and who tends to be clingy, greatly distressed by separation, and often fearful of their environments (Ainsworth et al., as cited in Florsheim et al., 1996, p. 84).The chronically more highly aroused states activated the aggressive self-protective behaviors described later. She experienced conflicts as leading to separations between people and reacted as if she were being abandoned.

The defense mechanisms that are more balanced between the excitatory and inhibitory branches of the ANS are employed early in her life (by history) and include affiliation (involvement with kin), self-assertion (doing well in school), and sublimation and suppression (impulses harnessed to complete tasks, such as schoolwork or chores at home). Throughout my contact with her, those same defenses were clearly evident, also including self-observation (self-deprecating humor or acerbic wit directed at herself about her foibles) and altruism (deep love and concern for vulnerable others and efforts to help them, not limited to her family, but including friends, family, and the HIV-positive and AIDs patients on her caseload).

As she was exposed to increasingly stressful and traumatic events, the up-regulated attachment style (excitatory branch of ANS) began to dominate as a survival strategy. Although she could keep up in school, her behavior became increasingly pugilistic, vigilant, watchful, obstreperous, and, at times, violent to insure some safety. She began to utilize splitting primarily (good/bad others), externalization (experiencing outside world as like her fearful internal experience), identification (with her father, who was feared and respected), acting out/regression (examples above), projection (ultra-sensitive to racism), devaluation (impatient with "stupid people" who made her life more miserable than it already was), and, even, perhaps, hallucinations (hearing her sister's voice and noises outside her apartment).

When the painful arousal of the excitatory defenses brought about the unrelenting stress and at times, actual trauma, overwhelming her brain's capacity to tolerate, that arousal began to be managed by the inhibitory (parasympathetic branch of ANS) and the PS (in concert with the parasympathetic nervous system to extremely decrease, dampen, and numb the intensity of emotionality). Defenses such as repression, isolation of affect, dissociation, depersonalization, and derealization (all inhibiting) were more and more heavily utilized. When she discovered that alcohol was a more reliable avenue to numbing, it either augmented or became a substitute for the psychological defenses. She began to have an emotional management strategy in her brain more like the disorganized category of childhood and unresolved of adulthood with the erratic extremes of excitatory behaviors and plummeting to extremes of inhibitory behaviors. As such, she met all criteria for the borderline condition and one of the bipolar conditions, as well.

The diagnostic criteria for both conditions include problematically extreme arousal, either too excitatory or too inhibitory. The current understanding of the etiology of the disordered personalities, in this case, borderline functioning, is in the realm of the milieu. However, many of the mood disorders are thought to have a genetic predisposition, in her case one of the bipolar conditions. Sabina had many close relatives who struggled with drug and alcohol use and abuse problems. It is reasonable to assume that she also had a genetic predisposition to have difficulties with substance use and abuse, even had she not lived in chaos and trauma.

The significance of speculating on the etiology involves the treatment. With the mood disorder, medication was a necessity and helpful. She did try Alcoholics Anonymous but found it culturally too "White" and Christian for her. She did occasionally attend a Spanish speaking meeting, but that was short lived. She never would find a sponsor, an indication of her counter-dependent character style, I think. Perhaps my being able to focus on her drinking was helpful, as, well, but I received no direct indication that this was the case. However, the lability and variability of the behaviors described by the borderline behaviors were amenable to psychotherapy.

Viewing the treatment relationship through the lens of projective identification and transference/counter-transference, I think Sabina mainly projected toward me the emotions of care, panic, anger, and seeking. I identified (counter-transference) with those particular emotional circuits (Panksepp, 2011) and nonconsciously responded like the caretakers of her early life. Even though she was a caretaker in her family and professionally, her reaction-formed behaviors disallowed her open expression of her own need to depend on others. I was invited (via her transferring certain affects to me; Schore, 2003b) to experience, hold, contain, and express some of her intolerable emotions, which included concern, worry, sadness, upset for her health and safety, and anger about various unfair events. As her mind registered that I was resonating with her disowned affects, she could become fairly oblivious to them, and subtly either make fun of me for worrying or be somewhat blank (dissociative) to such emotions, as if I were somehow naïve. These episodes of transference/counter-transference would occur unexpectedly, as the discussion stirred up past or present difficult emotions, thoughts, or memories. Neuroception of internal danger (Porges, 2011) was allowing her to register the painful prospect of her directly experiencing the unbearable affects and, so to speak, handed them off to another mind, mine, in this instance. As she increasingly utilized alcohol as her primary defensive maneuver for regulation of affect arousal, her defenses became more maladaptive in their extremes and the projective identification intensified, becoming defensive projective identification, rather than adaptive projective identification (Montgomery, 2013; Schore, 2003b).

Even though Sabina came to sessions erratically with long stretches of time in between times of therapy, I have always wondered if the fact of my availability, even though she missed so many appointments, was in itself therapeutic (attunement leading to changes via brain plasticity). I knew she was doing the best she could do. She kept the appointment card in the ashtray in her car, so it was always with her, even if she forgot to look at it. I think of Winnicott's "transitional object" (Ogden, 1993, p. 228) as a nontraumatic reminder of an "other" out there somewhere whom you can always see if you want. The card may have been a reminder of the dyadic regulation of affect, our synchronous engagements, which, though less than what she deserved, may have been sustaining over time.

REFERENCES

American Psychiatric Association. (2000). *Diagnostic and statistical manual of mental disorders* (4th ed.). Washington, DC: Author.

Brody, P. (1992). *The central nervous system: Structure and function.* New York, NY: Oxford University Press.

Buelow, G., Hebert, S., & Buelow, S. (2000). *Psychotherapist's resource on psychiatric medications: Issues of treatment and referral.* Belmont, CA: Brooks/Cole Thompson Learning.

Florsheim, P., Henry, W. P., & Benjamin, L. S. (1996). Integrating individual and interpersonal approaches to diagnosis: The structural analysis of social behavior and attachment theory. In F. W. Kaslow (Eds.), *Handbook of relational diagnosis and dysfunctional family patterns* (pp. 81–101). New York, NY: Wiley.

Freud, A. (1966). *The ego and mechanisms of defense. The writings of Anna Freud Volume II*. New York, NY: International Universities Press. (Original work published 1936)

Kernberg, O. F. (1979). Regression in organizational leadership. *Psychiatry, 42,* 24–39.

Loewald, H. W. (1973). On internalization. *International Journal of Psychoanalytic Association, 554,* 9–17.

Miehls, D., & Applegate, J. (2014/this issue). Introduction to neurobiology and clinical work. *Smith College Studies in Social Work, 84*(2–3), 145–156.

Montgomery, A. (2013). *Neurobiology essentials for clinicians: What every therapist needs to know.* New York, NY: Norton.

Ogden, T. (1993). On potential space. In D. Goldman (Ed.), *In one's bones: The clinical genius of Winnicott* (pp. 223–240). Northvale, NJ: Aronson.

Panksepp, J. (2011). Cross-species affective neuroscience decoding of the primal affective experience of humans and related animals. *PloS ONE, 6*(8), 1–15. doi:10.1371/journal.pone.0021236

Panksepp, J., & Watt, J. (2011). Why does depression hurt? Ancestral primary-process separation-distress (PANIC) and diminished reward (SEEKING) processes in the genesis of depressive affect. *Psychiatry, 74,* 5–14.

Porges, S. W. (2011). Music therapy, trauma, the polyvagal theory. In S. W. Porges (Ed.), *The polyvagal theory: Neurophysiological foundation s of emotions, attachment, communication and self-regulation* (pp. 246–254). New York, NY: Norton.

Schore, A. N. (2003a). *Affect dysregulation and disorders of the self*. New York, NY: Norton.

Schore, A. N. (2003b). *Affect regulation and the repair of the self*. New York, NY: Norton.

Siegel, D. J. (1999). *The mindful brain: Reflection and attunement in the cultivation of well-being*. New York, NY: Norton.

Vaillant, G. E. (1977). *Adaptation to life*. Boston, MA: Little, Brown.

Winnicott, D. W. (1965). *The maturational processes and the facilitating environment: Studies in the theory of emotional development*. London, UK: Hogarth Press.

The Interpersonal Neurobiology of Clinical Intuition

TERRY MARKS-TARLOW

Reiss Davis Child Study Center, Los Angeles, California, USA

This article addresses clinical intuition from the standpoint of interpersonal neurobiology, the study of how brains, minds, and bodies are shaped through relationship. First, clinical intuition is placed in a developmental framework consistent with nonlinear science. Then, the operation of intuition is described in terms of implicit processes, which operate automatically in bottom-up fashion, as guided by the right brain, under the radar of conscious awareness. A case example of intuition in action demonstrates the holistic potential of a single image to illuminate the nature of a problem plus point the way toward resolution. This article ends with a cautionary note about the limitations of clinical intuition.

Not long ago, clinical social work journals and mainstream psychotherapy conferences rejected neurobiology. Psychoanalytically minded practitioners clung to a hermeneutic vantage point, claiming that intersubjective levels of meaning making trump all objective attempts to step outside the relationship. Meanwhile, postmodern theorists dismissed neurobiology as mere scientism, or just another language no more privileged than any other form of discourse. Practically minded clinicians expressed concerns about the dangers of biological reductionism—the tendency to reduce psychological phenomena to underlying neurochemistry or brain structures. Taken to extremes, biological reductionism threatens the "talking cure" altogether, if the value of the therapeutic bond is dismissed in favor of genetic explanations or pharmacological treatments.

Happily, there exists a way to inject brain science into the art of psychotherapy, while avoiding pitfalls of reductionism. To do so requires highlighting distinctions between linear and nonlinear approaches to science (Marks-Tarlow, 2008). The danger of reducing psychological, social, or cultural levels to underlying mechanical, electrical, or chemical events exists primarily from a linear perspective. Linear chains allow researchers to collapse complex phenomena into their component pieces, processes, or precursors. By contrast, nonlinear approaches preserve natural complexity, partly by incorporating circular models of causality that permit bidirectional loops of interaction. Minds can alter brains (through top-down mental dynamics) at the very same time that brains can alter minds (through bottom-up physiological processes). As an example, culture shapes emotional expression through accompanying brain changes (e.g., Markus & Kitayama, 1991); meanwhile changes in brain chemistry affect how we feel and, in turn, how we shape culture. Things get even more complex when circular models include multiple brain–mind–body systems. This is indispensable to modeling psychotherapeutic exchanges, where to preserve full complexity means to recognize the centrality of relationship.

Enter the nascent discipline of interpersonal neurobiology (Badenoch, 2008; Cozolino, 2002, 2006; Marks-Tarlow, 2012; Schore, 2003a, 2003b, 2012; Siegel, 1999), an interdisciplinary field that seeks to understand people's minds, brains, and relationships through multiple, convergent perspectives. From a linear point of view, people are separate beings who come together to form relationships, whereas a nonlinear point of view reverses this formulation. The individual is seen to "emerge out" of a relationship with a significant "other." Considering that all babies begin life inside their mother's body, and at birth remain physically and emotionally dependent, a nonlinear formulation dovetails well with actual stages of development.

There is increasing recognition of the importance of a developmental framework to the clinician's eye (e.g., Seligman, 2012). Even when working with adults, clinical practice is best informed by understanding optimal growth patterns plus their potential derailments. Regulation theory as conceived by Allan Schore (2003a, 2003b) is especially important in this regard. Regulation theory marries Bowlby's (1969, 1973) attachment theory—where babies need the security of healthy bonds with critical caretakers—with underlying dynamics in the brain and nervous system. By underscoring the centrality of early attuned or misattuned caretaking to later healthy or unhealthy states of the brain–mind–body system, regulation theory affords a developmental perspective. Regulation theory also is intrinsically nonlinear, by emphasizing critical windows of development plus the disproportionate power of tiny relational traumas to wreak long-term devastation in brains, bodies, and nervous systems. Generally, the earlier an emotional disruption occurs, the more serious, subcortical, far-reaching, and potentially irreversible the outcome. To adopt a developmental framework lends psychotherapists a more nuanced understanding of patient problems and constraints.

ATTUNED RESPONSE AND IMPLICIT PROCESSES

From the perspective of Schore's regulation theory, regardless of orientation, all forms of psychotherapy inevitably deal with problems of emotional dysregulation. Clinical intuition is better suited to treat emotional dysregulation than a more cognitive focus on problem solving, changing thought processes or behavioral prescriptions. This is because clinical intuition draws upon the same natural faculties that evolved many millennia ago to maximize attuned responses to babies. In all mammals, a mother's attuned care is indispensable to self-care. This means that interactive regulation (the use of attuned relationship to down-regulate high arousal or negative emotion or up-regulate low arousal and positive emotion) precedes the capacity for self-regulation. Whether dealing with children or adults during psychotherapy, precisely because interactive regulation is instinctual, no preset formula or manualized approach can dictate the form each moment will take. Attuned response changes so rapidly, down to the microsecond, based on ever-shifting contours of emotion and arousal, as picked up unconsciously by body-to-body cues.

Within talk therapy, attunement relates less to the content of speech, or what we say, and more to the processes of speech, or how we say it—tone and rhythm of voice (prosody), posture, body movements, facial expression, and eye gaze. These paralinguistic vocal, visual, facial, and postural cues are all part of the implicit relational knowing (Lyons-Ruth, 1998; Seligman, 2012), the primary form of learning and memory a baby uses for the first 2 years of life. Implicit knowledge involves emotional, relational, and body-based experiences that draw upon different underlying brain areas than later developing, explicit, cognitive and verbal faculties. Implicit processes shape Bowlby's internal working models, by forming social expectations and coloring the emotional tone of ongoing experience. It is possible that the implicit level accounts for the quality and landscape of repetitive dreams.

Whether working with children or adults, to pick up on these tiny, multimodal, implicit cues, context is everything. During early development and in psychotherapy, the full context is always too complex for any complete verbal description or prescription. This is one reason why parental and clinical intuition take on such significance and how-to books pale by comparison. Only through intuitive channels can we register the full spectrum of interpersonal data by drawing upon immediate sensory, emotional, and imaginal cues. Because clinical intuition responds to nuance implicitly and subcortically, this is a fully embodied mode of perceiving, relating, and responding. By contrast to explicit levels of processing (e.g., thinking, analyzing, deciding), implicit responses are fast acting and effortless; they operate automatically, in context, beneath the level of conscious awareness (Claxton, 1997). The importance of implicit relational learning to psychotherapy has been underscored by clinical theorists like Daniel Stern (1985, 2004), members of the Boston Change Process Study Group (2008), and infant researcher Beatrice Beebe (2010; Beebe, Lachmann, Markese, & Bahrick, 2012). Beebe (2010) documented how tiny contingent moments of discordance or synchrony between caretakers and infants affect future attachment status.

During psychotherapy, when clinicians become immersed in flow states (Csikszentmihalyi, 1990, 1996) with patients, they get caught up in the throes of implicit processes as intuitively guided. Here, there may be emotional challenge, yet often little sense of effort. When therapists and patients ride the waves of interrelatedness, it becomes easy to find smooth rhythms of exchange. Time flies by. Psychotherapy can take on an all-enveloping quality of wholeness. This sometimes feels like a dance where exquisitely coordinated movements are choreographed by no one and both people at once. Or, it may feel like a song of syncopated call and response. When psychotherapists are lucky enough to spend long periods intuitively immersed, despite intense often negative emotional involvement, they can nonetheless leave work feeling energized and refreshed. Amid deep intuitive engagement, the relationship itself becomes vitalized, pulling each person along, ideally nudging both into spontaneous, unexpected places.

Due to the primacy of this mode during psychotherapy, I assert that clinical intuition is what fills the gap between theory and practice (Marks-Tarlow, 2012, 2014). Where theory is static, intuition is alive. Where theory exists outside of real time, intuition involves immersion within the lived moment. Where theory attends to similarities between groups of people, clinical intuition attends to the particulars of this person, in this room, during this moment, given this developmental history. Because of the implicit, exquisite attention to detail and distinctions, I believe clinical intuition is a necessary, though not sufficient, ingredient for deep change during psychotherapy.

Given such a central role proposed, it seems rather peculiar that clinical intuition has received so little attention in clinical theory and studies. When researching my book *Clinical Intuition in Psychotherapy*, I found only one other devoted to the topic (Charles, 2005). Its author was as surprised and dismayed as I at the dearth of empirical material. I speculate that this hole in the literature exists due to the easy association of intuition with that which is mystical, magical, paranormal, airy-fairy, and in short, nonscientific. Fortunately, these misconceptions largely dissipate when intuition is examined through lenses of interpersonal neurobiology as materially grounded in implicit faculties.

RADICAL UNIQUENESS

Whereas explicit learning can be had from books or classrooms, implicit learning cannot; it is too highly sensitive to the particulars of context. Instead, implicit learning requires direct experience. This is the point of practicums and internships during clinical training. Effective psychotherapy implicates implicit relational learning by requiring close attention to the particulars. As mentioned, we must notice what is unique about this person, involved in this conversation, during this moment. But it is not just psychotherapy patients who are unique; so is each practitioner. This lends an individualized "chemistry" to each therapeutic dyad. Indeed, the chemistry itself, that is, the quality of the relationship between any given patient and therapist dyad appears to be more important to the outcome of the therapy than either the orientation or training of the therapist (Geller & Greenberg, 2002; Messer, 2002).

Given that each practitioner's genetics, history, and developmental experience are highly individualized, it is no surprise that each clinician sports his or her own highly individualized intuitive repertoire. Whether emerging in the form of flashes, hunches, or gut feelings, radical uniqueness holds true for ordinary levels of attuned response, as well as for more extraordinary forms of knowing (Mayer, 2007). An example of extraordinary knowing was relayed to me by a psychoanalyst at a conference several years ago (Marks-Tarlow, 2012). The female therapist had picked up her male patient in the waiting room. The man preceded the therapist down a long hall toward the office. He turned the corner and went out of sight. As he sat down, the patient let out a long sigh that sparked the therapist's sudden concern, "Uh oh! I hope he doesn't need CPR." After the therapist rounded the corner to join him, the patient relayed his horrendous tale from that week. He had been playing basketball with his best friend, who suddenly fell to the floor unconscious. The friend needed CPR but wound up dying anyway.

The psychotherapist was astounded. How did she pick up ahead of time on such a central thread in the patient's narrative? Although it may not be possible to know exactly how this happened, most psychotherapists have remarkable war stories like this one; yet many keep such stories private, if not secret, for fear of judgment or disbelief. The more seminal the moment, the higher the emotional intensity, and the greater our capacity to tune into invisible strings that continually interconnect the minds, brains, and bodies of people we love and care for. It is quite possible that dangerous, fearful circumstances heighten receptivity, perhaps communicated through body-to-body channels, amygdala to amygdala. For one psychotherapist, an intuitive moment might arrive as a flash of insight—an image or visual capacity to "see" an interpersonal pattern in a way that conveys new understanding or meaning. The clinical case described later involves a visual metaphor of this variety. For another practitioner, clinical intuition may take the form of a hunch, that is, a cognitive sense of knowing that arrives fully fleshed out, as if out of nowhere. As in the example above, a sense of concern or certainty might surround information that is invisible to the naked eye or seemingly beyond the scope of our reach.

At times, our intuitive repertoire appears not only unique, but down-right idiosyncratic. One clinical psychologist I know is also a musician. He reports hearing music as an ongoing, almost continuous backdrop during psychotherapy. Ominous music might signal a sense of emotional danger in the room, whereas joyful tones might signal an intimate moment or recognition of progress achieved.

CLINICAL INTUITION IS EMBODIED

In all forms of intuition, the body aspect is key. Because intuition is subcortically driven and originates in early developing, somatically based sensing and feeling, all kinds of intuition involve embodied perception and knowledge. Because intuition processes social and emotional cues below the threshold of awareness, its implicit operations tap into Freud's concept of the unconscious. The burgeoning field of neuropsychoanalysis (e.g., Kaplan-Solms & Solms, 2000) translates classical psychoanalytic concepts into brain structures and circuitry, as grounded in empirical research and speculation. To articulate an underlying neurophysiology is to fulfill Freud's (1895/1953) dream as expressed in "Project for a Scientific Psychology," but for which the requisite technology did not yet exist during Freud's time.

Schore (2003b, 2010, 2011) offered the fascinating possibility that Freud's unconscious can be localized within the right-brain's early developing, implicit self. In a model that is inherently more relational than Freud's, Schore's deepest subcortical layer of processing social and emotional cues begins with the amygdala, which is functional at birth. Able to read primitive states of danger and safety while tracking negative and positive emotions, this bottom level corresponds to Freud's deep unconscious as well as to Jung's archetypes. The second level, which comes online around age 3 or 4 months, contains midlevel cortical structures of the anterior cingulate and insula that mediate attachment bonds plus process pain and social conflict. This middle level corresponds to Freud's preconscious level of processing. The third tier of the hierarchy enters in around age 12 months, when the orbital frontal cortex and other prefrontal areas loop into the limbic circuitry. This highest layer of implicit self carries conscious awareness. It also mediates humor and personality, imagery and metaphor, dreams and symbolism, while incorporating multimodal information to integrate inside and outside environments.

Because intuition is fully attuned to the body's autonomic nervous system (which regulates arousal) and to limbic structures like the insula (which reads internal body states), it makes sense that clinical intuition can also arrive in the form of gut feelings. Sometimes called somatic countertransference (Lewis, 1986) or projective identification (Waska, 1999), psychotherapists can experience what amounts to minisymptoms in response to dysregulated states in patients. Somatic signals clue us into the deep unconscious of others. A knot in the stomach might signal dysregulated anger, an ache in the chest, dysregulated grief. Somatic symptoms such as these are particularly prevalent in cases of dissociated, unconscious emotion not yet accessible to patients (Marks-Tarlow, 2014; Schore, 2012). When dissociated emotions are experienced by sensitive therapists, our bodies function like resonant tuning forks (Stone, 2006).

The seemingly mysterious phenomenon of somatic countertransference is partly demystified by recent research into the neurobiology of empathy (e.g., Decety, 2011; Decety & Ickes, 2009). From the perspective of the brain, empathy has two aspects—one emotional, the other cognitive, each with different underlying neural correlates. The emotional aspect of empathy involves a contagion effect, that is, sharing an attenuated version of the feeling states of another. The cognitive dimension of empathy involves mentalizing (Fonagy, Gergely, Jurist, & Target, 2004), that is, cognitively understanding the mind of another, while registering differences between self and other. Decety (2011) emphasized the importance of balance. If emotional resonance runs too high, the resulting personal distress actually trumps the capacity for true empathy. Perhaps psychotherapist burnout and compassion fatigue represent the sort of imbalance where clinicians' bodies are too highly resonant for our own health.

An important reason to pay attention to gut feelings during psychotherapy is because the guts have a brain of their own, being part of the enteric nervous system (in charge of digesting food)—which is the third division of the autonomic nervous system that operates relatively autonomously alongside sympathetic and parasympathetic branches. The enteric nervous system is evolutionarily older than the central nervous system (brain and spinal cord). With respect to survival, this makes sense, for it is more important to eat than to register emotion, pain, or any other sensation. The enteric nervous system contains more than 100 million nerves that transmit messages through the spinal cord via all the major neurotransmitters: dopamine, serotonin, acetyl choline, nitric oxide, and norepinephrine.

Recent research (Welgan & Meshkinpour, 2000) reveals exquisite social sensitivities of the gut. When emotionally tinged words were presented to participants, increased intestinal contractions and changes in rectal tone were measured in response to angry, sad, or anxious words, especially for people with irritable bowel syndrome. It appears that the mind is embodied in the brain, though the brain is embedded in the body; and the embodied nature of clinical intuition is precisely how clinicians tune into nuance, variability, and the full complexity of relationship, as expressed moment to moment.

INTUITION IS A TWO-WAY STREET

Whatever form it may take, clinical intuition often runs in both directions during psychotherapy. The notion of all-knowing psychotherapists who deliver insight to patients dates back to classical psychoanalysis. At its inception, psychoanalysis was deeply influenced by the medical model in which it arose. The psychoanalyst (predominantly male) was imbued with power and authority to provide insight to his patients (often female). Insight took the form of interpretations designed to bring unconscious conflicts and motivations to conscious awareness. Interpretations regarding forbidden wishes and repressed fears frequently did prove therapeutic. Yet in hindsight, we see how historically insulated and culture-bound such transference–countertransference dynamics were, as derived from the Victorian era of suppressed sexuality and prefeminist thought.

Contemporary schools of psychoanalysis have altered the power structure of the therapist–patient dyad. In present day, more highly relational practice, the model is less hierarchical and nonauthoritative. Therapists and patients serve as copartners. Each is expected to bring authentic presence and full faculties to the enterprise of emotional healing. No matter what the intuitive prowess of the psychotherapist, patients retain final authority over the sovereignty of their subjectivity. Horizontal models of power enable clinical intuition to extend bidirectionally—not only from therapist to patient, but also from patient to therapist. Yet the issue is even subtler, especially when one takes into account the priming time and emotional preparation that so often precedes intuitively guided insights. From the truly intersubjective perspective of interpenetrating subjectivities, it may be wisest to consider all acts of intuition, no matter in whom they originate, as acts of cocreativity. Perhaps all intuitions emerge from the relational unconscious that is shared between therapists and patients (Gerson, 2004).

RIGHT- VERSUS LEFT-BRAIN MODES

Although implicit, intuitive learning and memory are guided by the early developing right brain, conscious deliberation is orchestrated by the later developing left brain. When looking at hemispheric differences, a popular misconception places particular activities like solving a math problem or playing the violin squarely inside one hemisphere or the other. The resulting controversy prompts some neuroscientists to refute the concept of hemispheric specialization altogether. For example, Kosslyn and Miller (2013) favored a horizontal division into "top brain" and "bottom brain." Surely, as these researches suggest, cortical versus subcortical distinctions in brain function are significant. Nonetheless, all reptilian and mammalian brains are physically divided into left and right halves for important reasons, although a more nuanced view of brain lateralization is needed.

Psychiatrist Iain McGilchrist has devoted himself to the study and significance of hemispheric specialization. In his masterful, empirically grounded book on the topic, McGilchrist (2009) asserted that both sides of the human brain can approach just about any activity. Yet each hemisphere offers a different quality of subjectivity that brings into being a whole different world. The right brain specializes in the global picture, taking into account an overview of the world. By contrast, the left brain hones in on the details, often in service of exerting its will. This part/whole difference in how each hemisphere attends to the world is reflected perceptually in how each side regulates the visual field. The left hemisphere attends to the right side of space only. By contrast, the right hemisphere specializes not only in the left side of space, but also in combining visual information from both sides of space.

The right hemisphere's perspective is holistic, whereas that of the left hemisphere is piecemeal. Clinical intuition is a function of the right hemisphere precisely because its holistic operation preserves the entire, embodied context. Clinical intuition allows clinicians to take in the overview to hone in on what is most salient. Indeed, as McGilchrist (2009) emphasized, the right brain regulates what type of attention we are using, plus when and how we switch modes. The type most relevant to clinical intuition is open attention or broadband focus. This mode is reminiscent of Freud's (1912/1958) "evenly hovering attention" as well as Bion's (1967) suggestion that the most effective way to enter a session involves putting aside all memory and desire. Because broadband attention takes in the whole of things, it provides the widest lens for sensing and subsequently zooming closer in on what is most important at any given time. When we zoom in on a detail during psychotherapy, sometimes we remain close to a right-brain focus, such as when the object of our attention includes the body. For example, we may notice that a patient's facial expression reveals something that his words do not. But just as easily, we may shuttle over to a left-brain focus on a tiny detail or on explicit content, as when we get absorbed in a patient's narrative about a recent incident.

When the left brain is in the forefront of consciousness, its verbal and logical processes tend to operate in a vacuum, by removing its object of focus from context. This is easy to see with language. When I write the word *desk*, I strip out the entire sensory context of any particular desk. The more abstract the arena of reflection, the more important that left-brain analysis and deliberation be fully grounded by the right-brain's concrete and holistic sensibilities. Otherwise, it becomes all too easy for awareness to slip into delusion and falsity, including utter fabrication. Michael Gazzaniga was an early neuroscientist to study split-brain patients, whose corpus callosum (the huge brain tracts connecting right and left hemispheres) was severed to prevent the spread of grand mal seizures. Gazzaniga (2005) nicknamed the left-brain as "the interpreter" due to its story telling capacities plus relentless quest for explanations and making sense of whatever it encounters.

Translated into clinical terms, the left brain's need for a complete and coherent story easily becomes the stuff of higher order defenses, like intellectualization, rationalization, and denial. This is why effective therapy requires that left-brain, detailed focus and narratives be grounded in the right-brain intuition plus fully embodied context. As alluded to by McGilchrist's (2009) eloquent title (*The Master and His Emissary*), the right brain (including clinical intuition) is the master, whereas the left brain (including clinical deliberation) is its emissary. Proper whole-brain functioning requires close communication between the two sides.

McGilchrist (2009) identified a natural hierarchy of attention that moves right-left-right. First, the primacy of the right brain capitalizes on open, global attention. Then, as something strikes our interest, clinicians may shuttle to the left for a more detailed zoom, only to return to the right to free associate, find a metaphor, let an image emerge, or return to an open view. As clinicians, we use this order of attention naturally and intuitively, as I demonstrate shortly with a case example.

IN PURSUIT OF NOVELTY

When examining the role of right-brain intuition versus left-brain deliberation during psychotherapy, it helps to understand the conditions under which clinical intuition functions better than clinical deliberation. These include uncertain or ambiguous circumstances; when there is incomplete information; situations of emergency or urgency; when time is of the essence; or in situations of intense arousal and high emotionality. By contrast, deliberate reasoning is more useful when full information is available, under emotionally neutral circumstances, and when no urgency or time pressure exists.

This understanding emerged partly from research in critical care nursing (e.g., King & Appleton, 1997). Clearly, the emergency room is a place of great urgency and intense pressure. Life and death matters are common, requiring immediate response, with little time for research or questions. To complicate matters, emergency room patients may be unconscious or unable to respond verbally for other reasons. In the context of critical care nursing, remarkable stories of clinical intuition abound.

Psychotherapy usually presents less drama than the emergency room. Yet, in attenuated form, conditions in our offices can be quite similar. This especially holds true if we work with highly traumatized individuals, at the edges of regulatory boundaries. All factors considered, clinical intuition is the primary mode of response in psychotherapy for multiple reasons. Because clinical work deals with high levels of complexity, it is important to consider the full context. It is better for ideas to emerge from observations and direct experience, rather than to walk into the room with a preset theory or set of ideas, in search of supporting evidence. Despite operating with ambiguous information, conditions of uncertainty, and emotional urgency, we must detect what is most salient in hopes of stimulating and exploring novel territory. And with respect to novelty, the right brain is again foundational.

Because division of labor across the two sides of the brain is quite ancient, an evolutionary perspective is useful. Brain lateralization extends back more than 500 million years to early vertebrate development, long before the appearance of warm-blooded animals (MacNeilage, Rogers, & Vallortigara, 2009). In reptiles and birds, the left side of the brain became specialized for tasks that are routine, such as eating a meal or building a nest. By contrast, the right side of the brain became specialized for tasks that involve novelty, such as detecting danger or seeking shelter. We easily detect this difference in predator/prey relationships. Predators stalk their prey using the right visual field (as mediated by the left hemisphere), which allows them to zoom in on potential food sources. By contrasts, prey perceive predators most easily through the left visual field (as mediated by the right hemisphere). The ease of detecting danger on the left undoubtedly has led to widespread prejudice against left-handed people. For example, words like "sinister," which translates in Latin to mean left-handed, associates the left side with things that are evil or threatening, like the devil.

With respect to clinical concerns, this distinction between hemispheres based on novel versus routine concerns broadens our context for understanding why intuition is so important during psychotherapy. To effect deep change, therapists and patients must be open to what is new, which is inherently the domain of the right brain. Although the left brain can help people analyze problems, spell out choices, or make conscious predictions about what might come next, only the right side carries the creative capacity for something entirely novel, spontaneous, or unpredictable to emerge.

CLINICAL EXAMPLE

I choose this clinical example in order to describe a right-left-right-left clinical sequence. I begin with an open stance (right); from there, I zoom in on a significant detail (left); out of the ensuing exploration came a useful image (right), that provided a core metaphor to be fleshed out again and again in future sessions.

In a recent session, a patient I'll call Greta[1] doubted her capacities to be creative at work the way she perceived her colleagues to be. As my patient got more and more caught up in comparisons to her coworkers, she started slumping further and further down on my couch. Greta appeared to be in the throes of the same kind of "sinking" feeling she was describing at work.

My attention intuitively shifted from what Greta was saying to what was happening in her body. Drawn to Greta's rather collapsed posture, I seized the opportunity to work holistically and somatically by asking where and how Greta experienced that sinking feeling in her body, in real time.

Greta responded, "I feel as if I'm standing in quicksand. The more I struggle to get out, the deeper I sink in." This image of standing in quicksand was brief and simple, yet over the ensuing weeks, Greta and I came to appreciate how brilliant this image was as an embodied metaphor that allowed us to unpack more and more from within it.

Here is some background. My patient worked in a hypercompetitive, hypermale, highly alpha, professional environment. In response to these conditions, Greta's initial instinct was to compete like the others. Although this strategy is easy to understand, unfortunately this mode of relating to others did not suit Greta at all. Instead of thriving on the competition, as many of her colleagues appeared to do, Greta became ever more fearful of being less than others and left only in a one-down position. Greta responded to ongoing work pressures and deadlines with a kind of internal running. Because there was no resolution to be had, the faster Greta moved on the inside, the more she scrambled on the outside. She became defensively aggressive, and in turn more impatient and impulsive with others. Greta started barking out orders and spitting out criticisms to colleagues. After each episode of loss of self-control, Greta would grow horrified and regretful at her own outburst. She would then dissolve into a fit of fear that no one liked her or wanted to work with her. This culminated in Greta's self-proclaimed "paranoia," an obsessive worry about being publicly shamed and fired.

Translated into neurobiological terms, Greta's amygdala was chronically signaling emotional danger, to which the sympathetic branch of her autonomic nervous system responded with a perpetual state of hyperarousal. Feeling like prey among predators, Greta became hypervigilant. Her attention was turned outwards, often riveted on the facial expressions and vocal prosody of her colleagues, especially the partners in her firm. Greta began having trouble sleeping. She suffered from headaches, stomach aches, and started catching colds more often. These stress symptoms are common when the body is flooded by cortisol, the major stress hormone. High sympathetic arousal diverts circulation away from inner organs and functions, including digestion and immune response. Rather than attend to the inner viscera, blood is sent instead to the outer limbs to ready the organism for fight/flight responses. But in this modern era, there is often no one to fight and nowhere to flee. When stress floods the body but cannot be alleviated, this leads to allostatic load (McEwen, 2002), making it impossible to clear out problems, rest up, or restore balance.

Physiologically and emotionally, Greta was caught in a negative loop from which she could not exit. The more fearful and "paranoid" she became, the more out of control Greta acted. The harder Greta tried to get out of her plight, the deeper she sank in. Greta was trapped in a vicious cycle that indeed bore an uncanny resemblance to quicksand!

Whether originating in patients or psychotherapists, there is often great beauty and paradox to be found within intuitive flashes. Although it seems perverse to find aesthetic pleasure surrounding "ugly" truths, the recognition of deep pattern is vital to therapists and patients alike. Because intuition recognizes the whole in the part, intuition is particularly adept at uncovering deep pattern. Precisely because imagistic products of the right brain are holistic, they point toward an overview, often by linking inner conditions with outer circumstances. When we attend carefully enough to spontaneously produced images such as the quicksand image, we can seek broader wisdom, and sometimes solutions emerge naturalistically.

By meditating on Greta's dilemma of sinking in quicksand, the natural response of stillness and reflection was obvious. This is exactly what Greta lacked in her sense of urgency and impulsive responses. Instead of her hypervigilant, hyperactive external focus on the deeds of other, which further triggered her reactivity, Greta would benefit from pulling her attention back into her own body and her own psyche. She needed to prioritize calming down above all else. Only by stilling Greta's impulse to run could she ground herself sufficiently to find her own inner authority and bring the whole of who she is into work. To truly shine Greta needed to pay attention to her own sources of integrity and to her priority of relating well to others, even if this meant countering the predominant culture of her firm. By gathering her wits in stillness, Greta could maximize her chances to utilize all of her resources, inner and outer, to step out of the quicksand of fear, frustration, and impulsivity.

FLASHES IN THE DARK

Part of the utility of intuitive flashes like Greta's is an opportunity to revisit them again and again in psychotherapy. Images like the quicksand serve as through lines for tying together broad themes and key moments from the past. A session or two after her quicksand image emerged, Greta spontaneously recalled a memory. As a rebellious teenager, Greta's parents sent her to psychotherapy, hoping for a quick fix to the problem of Greta's relentless anger. During an early session, the therapist asked Greta to draw a picture of a man and a woman. When Greta completed the drawing, the therapist noted an absence of feet in both figures. Looking back, Greta mused, "Perhaps those figures *did* have feet after all, but they were hidden under the quicksand." At this point of self-reflection, it became clear to Greta and myself that sinking feelings of being stuck and immobilized had a long history.

In this session and in many more to follow, psychotherapy took on a different feel. Our conversations sunk deeper, further under the surface. A year and a half into the work, Greta now focused less on recalling and rehashing events of the week and more on unearthing her dark, shadowy side that had been living for decades under the mud. Greta slowed down her frantic efforts to purge this side of herself. She even allowed me to stand alongside her in the muck. Instead of fighting this unpleasant side while sinking ever deeper into it, Greta began confronting the inner perfectionist who was too intolerant to face her own blemishes. As Greta's interest in her internal world increased, her outer drama decreased. Greta's fear lessened significantly that anyone would discover, skewer, or fire her for her defects.

As Greta's clinical imagination opened up, it allowed her to face and synthesize internal truths. All of this occurred in tiny shifts. Meanwhile, I was acutely aware of an irony at the heart of Greta's potent image. At the very same instant that she had protested her lack of creativity, Greta's unconscious had been wonderfully clever. Greta's symbolic, "high right" had delivered the perfect image in response. Not only did it capture the problem, but it also offered the solution in a single flash. Although this sequence of events felt amazing to me, they did not to Greta. Instead, the original image and its capacity to cohere previous feelings, knowledge, and experiences felt mundane, like the mud itself. When I inquired if anything felt more magical to Greta, she noted some previous occasions when I had delivered interpretations offering insights she had never before considered. I suppose at those times, my intuitions helped Greta to feel lifted out of the mud. By contrast, Greta's own vision delivered both of us into the mud. But so be it. Such was the difference in our perspectives.

THERAPIST BEWARE

After touting the benefits of clinical intuition and providing a clinical example, a word of caution is now in order. Within psychotherapy, it is always important to hold intuitive sensibilities lightly and with humility. Just as left-brain, conscious thought can bleed into delusional thought and lies without the grounding of right-brain intuition, so too can clinical intuition infuse wrong information and misguided impulses into psychotherapy, if its operations proceed unchecked, without supporting evidence provided by careful deliberation.

The line between helpful intuition and harmful countertransference is thin and ever shifting. Intuitions should always be scrutinized for projections, impulsive actions, or toxic instincts. Never assume an intuition is correct without seeking corroboration, either by checking in with patients or by seeking other sources of observation or reflection. The dangers of the intuitive mode are brought home by Daniel Kahneman, the only psychologist who has ever won a Nobel Prize (for economics, as there are no prizes for psychologists). Kahneman (2002) detailed risks of overconfidence surrounding intuition's felt-sense of certainty. In Kahneman's experiments, in response to math questions, people easily go astray by answering impulsively and prematurely, without taking the time to cross-check validity.

During psychotherapy, it would be wise to slow things down and think things through if any of the following experiences occur: great urgency to respond; frequent feelings of defensiveness; unrelenting repetition in patient/therapist dynamics; long trajectories of deterioration, either in the patient's condition or the therapeutic bond; chronic feelings of fatigue or being drained. Should any of these conditions hold, especially over a long period of time, it is vital to step out of intuitive mode and use conscious deliberation instead. Relentlessly seek feedback, within yourself and from your patient; and if doubts persist, be sure to seek supervision or consultation.

Here is some advice for the prudent clinician. Always watch to see how your intuitions fold into the clinical dialogue. Ask patients whether they feel a resonance with what you are saying. Especially when speculating about unconscious feelings or motives, patients cannot always attain certainty about unconscious truths. Often they have to look at the issue sideways, as if gazing with peripheral vision or through opaque lenses. With respect to clinical intuitions concerning the deep unconscious, keep in mind that by definition patients cannot have full access. The best that can be expected is a fuzzy feeling of resonance, a "sort-of-knowing" (Petrucelli, 2010). Most importantly—if a patient insists something is off or holds no resonance at all, then let it go—at least for now.

Remember that deliberation and intuition are dual aspects of psychotherapy that work hand in hand. Both are important, and we continually shuttle back and forth between these two modes. Where clinical intuition facilitates the art of psychotherapy, conscious deliberation facilitates a more scientific, empirical approach. We use intuition to take leaps into the unknown and deliberation to check their impact and relevance. To shuttle back and forth between modes requires looking and asking for feedback to check the accuracy or utility of all intuitive leaps. The more we use our skills of observation and inquiry in service of gathering feedback and checking accuracy rather than assuming we are correct, the more sensitively honed we will be as therapeutic instruments.

CONCLUSION

This article illuminates the utility and power of clinical intuition as a primary mode during psychotherapy. The topic deserves much more attention in clinical research and writing than it has gotten to date. Clinical intuition is an embodied, holistic faculty of perception and response during psychotherapy. Intuition is a right-brain mode that both attends to the big picture, as well as sticks to the tiny details of emotion and its relational fluctuations. Clinical intuition operates by tapping into implicit learning and memory, while drawing upon the full embodied context, as it shifts from microsecond to microsecond.

An intuitive mode of perception and response operates automatically and effortlessly under the surface of awareness, lending ease, achieving flow, making connections, and finding interpersonal pattern. In contrast to left-brain, clinical deliberation, right-brain clinical intuition guides attention to what is most salient, thereby expanding our potential for entering novel territory. Whether an image or other intuitive production arises initially in the therapist or patient is of little importance. Given its priming time and context-dependent nature, it may be most useful to view all intuitive products as intersubjective products of the relational unconscious. No matter how it arises or in whom, intuition should be cherished as necessary, though not sufficient, to deep change within psychotherapy.

NOTE

1. Patient permission obtained; all identifying data disguised.

REFERENCES

Badenoch, B. (2008). *Being a brain-wise therapist: A practical guide to interpersonal neurobiology*. New York, NY: W.W. Norton.

Beebe, B. (2010). The origins of 12-month attachment: A microanalysis of 4-month mother-infant attachment. *Attachment & Human Development, 12*(1/2), 3–141.

Beebe, B., Lachmann, F., Markese, S., & Bahrick, L. (2012). On the origins of disorganized attachment and internal working models: Paper I. A dyadic systems approach. *Psychoanalytic Dialogues, 22*, 253–272.

Bion, W. R. (1967). *Second thoughts*. London, UK: William Heinemann.

Boston Change Process Study Group. (2008). Forms of relational meaning: Issues in the relations between the implicit and reflective-verbal domains. *Psychoanalytic Dialogues, 18*, 125–148.

Bowlby, J. (1969). *Attachment (volume 1)*. New York, NY: Basic Books.

Bowlby, J. (1973). *Separation: Anxiety & anger (Vol. 2: Attachment and loss)* (International Psycho-Analytical Library No. 95). London, UK: Hogarth Press.

Charles, R. (2005). *Intuition, counseling and psychotherapy*. New York, NY: Wiley.

Claxton, G. (1997). *Hare brain, tortoise mind: How intelligence increases when you think less*. New York, NY: Ecco Press.

Cozolino, L. (2002). *The neuroscience of psychotherapy: Building & re-building the human brain*. New York, NY: W.W. Norton.

Cozolino, L. (2006). *The neuroscience of human relationships: Attachment and the developing social brain*. New York, NY: W.W. Norton.

Csikszentmihalyi, M. (1990). *Flow: The psychology of optimal experience*. New York, NY: Harper and Row.

Csikszentmihalyi, M. (1996). *Creativity: Flow and the psychology of discovery and invention*. New York, NY: HarperCollins.

Decety, J. (2011). The neuroevolution of empathy. *Annals of the New York Academy of Sciences, 1231*, 35–45.

Decety, J., & Ickes, W. (2009). *The social neuroscience of empathy*. Cambridge, MA: MIT Press.

Fonagy, P., Gergely, G., Jurist, E., & Target, M. (2004). *Affect regulation, mentalization, and the development of the self*. London, UK: Karnac Books.

Freud, S. (1953). Project for a scientific psychology. In J. Strachey (Ed. & Trans.), *The standard edition of the complete psychological works of Sigmund Freud* (Vol. 1, pp. 283–397). London, UK: Hogarth Press. (Original work published 1895)

Freud, S. (1958). Recommendation to physicians practicing psychoanalysis. In J. Strachey (Ed. & Trans.), *The standard edition of the complete psychological works of Sigmund Freud* (Vol. 7, pp. 109–120). London, UK: Hogarth Press. (Original work published 1912)

Gazzaniga, M. (2005). Forty-five years of split-brain research and still going strong. *Nature Reviews Neuroscience, 6*, 653–659.

Geller, S., & Greenberg, L. (2002). Therapeutic presence: Therapists experience of presence in the psychotherapy encounter in psychotherapy. *Person Centered & Experiential Psychotherapies, 1*, 71–86.

Gerson, S. (2004). The relational unconscious: A core element of intersubjectivity, thirdness, and clinical process, *Psychoanalytic Quarterly, 73*(1), 63–98.

Kahneman, D. (2002, December 8). *Maps of bounded rationality: A perspective on intuitive judgment and choice* (Nobel Prize Lecture, Aula Magna, Stockholm University). Retrieved from http://www.nobelprize.org/nobel_prizes/economic-sciences/laureates/2002/kahnemann-lecture.pdf

Kaplan-Solms, K., & Solms, M. (2000). *Clinical studies in neuro-psychoanalysis*. London, UK: Karnac Books.

King, L., & Appleton, J. (1997). Intuition: A critical review of the research and rhetoric. *Journal of Advanced Nursing, 26*, 194–202.

Kosslyn, S., & Miller, G. (2013). *Top brain, bottom brain: Surprising insights into how you think*. New York, NY: Simon & Schuster.

Lewis, P. (1986). *The somatic countertransference*. Chicago, IL: American Dance Therapy Association Conference.

Lyons-Ruth, K. (1998). Implicit relational knowing: Its role in development and psychoanalytic treatment. *Infant Mental Health Journal, 19*(3), 282–289.

MacNeilage, P., Rogers, L., & Vallortigara, G. (2009). Origins of the left and right brain. *Scientific American, 301*(1), 60–67.

Marks-Tarlow, T. (2008). *Psyche's veil: Psychotherapy, fractals and complexity*. London, UK: Routledge.

Marks-Tarlow, T. (2012). *Clinical intuition in psychotherapy: The neurobiology of embodied response*. New York, NY: W.W. Norton.

Marks-Tarlow, T. (2014). *Awakening clinical intuition: An experiential workbook.* New York, NY: W.W. Norton.

Markus, H., & Kitayama, S. (1991). Culture and the self: Implications for cognition, emotion, and motivation. *Psychological Review, 98*(2), 242–253.

Mayer, E. (2007). *Extraordinary knowing: Science, skepticism, and the inexplicable powers of the human mind.* New York, NY: Bantam.

McEwen, B. (2002). Sex, stress and the hippocampus: allostasis, allostatic load and the aging process. *Neurobiology of Aging, 23*(5), 921–939.

McGilchrist, I. (2009). *The master and his emissary: The divided brain and the making of the western world.* New Haven, CT: Yale University Press.

Messer, S. (2002). Let's face facts: Common factors are more potent than specific therapy ingredients. *American Psychologist, 9*(1), 21–25.

Petrucelli, J. (Ed). (2010). *Knowing, not-knowing and sort-of-knowing: Psychoanalysis and the experience of uncertainty.* London, UK: Routledge.

Schore, A. (2003a). *Affect dysregulation & disorders of the self.* New York, NY: W.W. Norton.

Schore, A. (2003b). *Affect regulation & the repair of the self.* New York, NY: W.W. Norton.

Schore, A. (2010). The right-brain implicit self: A central mechanism of the psychotherapy change process. In J. Petrucelli (Ed.), *Knowing, not-knowing and sort of knowing: Psychoanalysis and the experience of uncertainty* (pp. 177–202). London, UK: Karnac.

Schore, A. (2011). The right brain implicit self lies at the core of psychoanalytic psychotherapy. *Psychoanalytic Dialogues, 21,* 75–100.

Schore, A. (2012). *The science of the art of psychotherapy.* New York, NY: W.W. Norton.

Seligman, S. (2012). The baby out of the bathwater: Microseconds, psychic structure, and psychotherapy. *Psychoanalytic Dialogues, 22,* 499–509.

Siegel, D. (1999). *The developing mind.* New York, NY: Guilford Press.

Stern, D. (1985). *The interpersonal world of the infant.* New York, NY: Basic Books.

Stern, D. (2004). *The present moment in psychotherapy and everyday life.* New York, NY: W.W. Norton.

Stone, M. (2006). The analyst's body as tuning fork: Embodied resonance in countertransference, *Journal of Analytical Psychology, 51*(1), 109–124.

Waska, R. (1999). Projective identification, countertransference, and the struggle for understanding over acting out. *Journal of Psychotherapy Practice and Research, 8*(2), 155–161.

Welgan, P., & Meshkinpour, H. (2000). Role of anger in antral motor activity in irritable bowel syndrome. *Digestive Diseases and Sciences, 45*(2), 248–251.

Working Implicitly in Couples Therapy: Improving Right Hemisphere Affect-Regulating Capabilities

FRANCINE LAPIDES

Santa Cruz Psychoanalytic Psychotherapy Society, Santa Cruz, California, USA

Attachment theory, viewed through the lens of neurobiology, explains how infants learn, through unconscious, rapid, nonverbal interactions with caretaking adults, to successfully manage their own emotional energy. These neurological affect-regulating mechanisms formed in early childhood shape later-forming attachment relationships, including those of adult romantic dyads which depend, for intimacy and stability, on the same right-brain, nonverbal, modulating capacities. Psychoanalytic researchers have identified healing, implicit, unconscious psychobiological mechanisms, other than verbal insight, explanation, and interpretation, that can be learned remedially in couples therapy. This article examines an implicit, emotion-focused approach to couples work that brings unconscious affect center stage.

Psychotherapy is physiology . . . a somatic state of Relatedness. Mammals become attuned to one another's evocative signals and alter the structure of one another's nervous systems . . . . Speech is a fancy neocortical skill, but therapy belongs to the older realm of the emotional mind, the limbic brain. (T. Lewis, Amin, & Lannon, 2002, pp. 168–169)

ATTACHMENT THEORY THROUGH A NEUROBIOLOGICAL LENS: EXPERIENCE-DEPENDENT MATURATION OF THE BRAIN

The infant's capacity to regulate affect emerges within a delicate, nonverbal, interactive dance, choreographed unconsciously, between her parents and herself (Beebe & Lachmann, 1998) as parents contingently match and attune with their infant's changing affect states. When parents fail to do this with enough consistency, the infant's capacity to regulate affect is compromised.

These early relational experiences have dramatic consequences for later development because affect-regulating circuits of the fetal/neonatal brain are developing rapidly between the third trimester of pregnancy and the second year of life, a period of time when the total volume of the brain more than doubles (Knickmeyer et al., 2008). Much of this growth, especially of the white matter (the myelinated tracks connecting and communicating between structural centers in the brain), is driven by experience (Schore, 2009b). Neurological circuits of emotional regulation including the insula, the anterior cingulate (AC), and the orbital frontal cortex (OFC), create cortical and subcortical pathways down into the amygdala; these circuits, especially in the right hemisphere (RH), calm the child by turning down the neuromodulating autonomic nervous system (ANS) and the neurosteroidal hormones of the hypothalamus–pituitary–adrenal axis (HPA) stress response (Schore, 1994, 1997, 2001a).

When the earliest attachment relationships are insecure (not sufficiently contingent or attuned) less-than-optimal axonal connections are developed between these higher regulation and the lower arousal centers in the brain. As a result, more periods and higher frequencies of dysregulation ensue (Schore, 1994, 1996, 2003a). When chronically hyperactivated and hypersensitized in critical periods of infancy, an individual's stress response, especially in reaction to relational injuries, launches more readily, escalates to higher levels of intensity, and persists (Schore, 2003a) setting the stage for rapid bouts of dysregulated conflict and distressed adult partner relationships. These eruptions are marked by anger, blame, and defensiveness and may jeopardize or destroy relational intimacy and trust. Years later, therapists see these residual distortions in the couples who seek our help (Johnson, 2004).

A single human skull houses two virtually separate brains and though many mental activities utilize both hemispheres, their dominant capacities are quite unique. Among the difference between the hemispheres is that the RH is dominant for empathy, attunement, and affect regulation and stores an internal working model of the earliest attachment relationships and the strategies of affect regulation that were learned in them (A. N. Schore, personal communication, November 19, 2005). More of the human cortex is devoted to these RH modalities of face and voice and touch than to the verbal language specialty of the left hemisphere (LH) (Damasio, 1999). This language of the RH, affective and body based, transmitted by the primary process communications of face, gesture, posture, touch and prosody (the vocal qualities of volume, rhythm, pitch, timber, tone, and speed), is nature's first and primary vocabulary. Parents use these RH nonverbal modalities to communicate with their children around bodily needs and affective states. When the parental response is timely and attuned, the child thrives and the relationship develops as secure.

In the absence of this attuned resonance, the child is left in extended states of dysregulated affect (Beebe, 2000), and the attachment system evolves as insecure, or worse—when the parent is frightening, abusive, or neglectful—as disorganized (Lyons-Ruth, Bronfman, & Parsons, 1999). In the latter case, the infant left in extended states of disrupted affect eventually learns to defend himself through bursts of dysregulated energy followed often by a dissociative shutting down (Tronick & Weinberg, 1997). Thus without adequate attunement, the early developing regulating structures of the infant's brain fail to mature appropriately (Schore, 1994, 2001b) leaving the child personally and socially impaired, unable to regulate his own, or other's arousal states.

These deep subcortical RH templates of affective experience continue to exert influence over behavioral and emotional aspects of our lives, though they remain largely outside our conscious awareness, encoded in implicit (unconscious) procedural (body) memory (Schore, 2003b). They shape the choices that we make (Damasio, 1999) including our selection of potential mates, and the means by which we manage conflicts in these intimate relationships.

Romantic love has been, for some time, conceptualized as an attachment relationship (Hazan & Shaver, 1987; Johnson, 1996, 2004; Johnson & Denton, 2002; Shaver & Hazan, 1993), and theories designed to treat adult relationships have drawn heavily from these attachment paradigms (Erel & Burman, 1995; Johnson, 2004). Although the earliest attachment relationships initially wire the brain for affect regulation (Schore, 1994; Trevarthen, 2001), new attachment relationships can reorganize neural circuits, enhancing this capacity. This wiring of one brain through resonant interaction with another brain is the psychoneurobiological basis for the healing potential of important adult relationships, including romantic partnerships, the deeply attuned dyad in psychotherapy (Safran & Muran, 2000) and the triad of a couple and their psychotherapist. Thus, effective couples therapy uses the same processes that occur between parents and infants in secure attachments (attunement, empathy, healthy boundary setting, and resonance) to reactivate and rewire RH procedural templates from childhood (Atkinson, 1999, 2002; Cozolino, 2002; De Bellis et al., 2002; Schore, 2003b). Because most affect-regulating capacities reside in the RH, and because the subcortical RH can change only when it is activated and engaged in real time (Schore, 2003b), this article elaborates on the important corollary that emotionally charged conflicts must be experienced (or reexperienced), during the couples therapy hour and not just discussed (Goldman & Greenberg, 1992; Johnson, 2004; Makinen & Johnson, 2006; Tatkin, 2005b).

THE NEUROPHYSIOLOGY OF AFFECT REGULATION IN COUPLES THERAPY

The brain is constructed to save and support our lives. In an emergency where split-second assessments and reactions can make the difference between life and death, the subcortical areas of our brain prepare us for instant, life-preserving reactions of fight, flight, or freeze. These regions within the RH are fast enough to appraise potential threat and able to mobilize massive neuromodulatory responses through the sympathetic nervous system (SNS) and via the release of stress chemicals (catecholamines and glucocorticoids).

When couples merely disagree, the brain has time to route its findings cortically where they can be assessed more carefully, permitting attentive listening and the capacity to empathetically hold the partner's point of view (Fonagy, Gergely, Jurist, & Target, 2002). At such times, communication occurs more or less calmly frontal lobe to frontal lobe. But relational conflict, especially in the primary attachment of a romantic pair, can feel deeply threatening and can trigger an emergency response that shuts down the frontal lobes leaving only a subcortical appraisal system with no input from higher cortical centers to evaluate or regulate that energy. The amygdala has, in essence, hijacked the brain into a self-protective flight, flight, or freeze response (LeDoux, 2002) that threatens the couple's intimacy. Here partners likely fall back upon their more primitive internal working models of relationship learned in childhood (Bowlby, 1988).

Gottman (1999) used the term *diffused physiological arousal* (DPA) to illustrate such a surge of hyperactivation sufficient to shut down cortical appraisal and problem-solving strategies, rational thought, and impulse control. Repeated failures to curb such escalations can result in the emergence of destructive rage and expressions of disgust, contempt, and blame (Gottman & Gottman, 2008; Ogden & Minton, 2000). In the absence of successful efforts at repair, these eruptions eventually damage the couple's empathic bond (Tatkin, 2005a).

This capacity for repair requires that at least one person in the couple regain his or her own intention and capacity to regulate. With neither able to self-regulate, interactive strategies for calming down can fail, especially if they are too dissimilar. Some individuals, for example, may want desperately to stay engaged, to express their hurt or fears in hopes of finding an understanding and a sympathetic ear. Their ability to self-regulate, that is, to hold arousal and regulate their feelings independent of their partner, may be minimal. Others become emotionally overwhelmed and need time to withdraw and settle down before they can once again think and talk coherently. Given these disparate coping styles, one member looks precipitously for interactive repair to a partner who has focused internally to self- or auto-regulate; the former may feel abandoned and the latter invaded or intruded upon, escalating rather than reducing their mutual dysregulated energy. When both are quick to hyperactivate, conflict erupts frequently; when both move reflexively toward hypoactivation, the relationship will likely have a deadened quality as conflicts are collusively avoided and conversations kept superficial and polite (Tatkin, 2007). And where the neuroaffective styles are mixed, we might see a fearful or angry pursuit of a partner who is perceived as abandoning, and/or an avoidant retreat away from a partner who threatens or actually manages to overwhelm. Where tendencies toward hyperactivation are present in both members of the romantic pair, they likely manifest in mutual irritability, quick tempers, and disagreements marked by aggression and defensiveness. If energy surges too high too rapidly it can trigger states of dissociated rage where violence can, and sometimes does, ensue. But for many people, when these exchanges of mutual escalating rage reach a critical level, the brain protects itself by launching a neuronal circuit breaker. Neural connections are disrupted between the prefrontal cortical and subcortical limbic structures, particularly in the RH (Schore, 2009a) trapping the intense energy beneath a deadened or numbed dissociative state (Porges, 2001). These reactions develop as survival strategies mediated unconsciously in lower centers of the brain. If repeated frequently, such dissociative patterns can become chronic traits (Perry, Pollard, Blakely, Baker, & Vigilante, 1995).

APPLICATIONS: USING THE NEUROLOGICAL LITERATURE ON RIGHT HEMISPHERE–BASED AFFECT AROUSAL, AFFECT REGULATION, AND REGULATION THEORY TO WORK WITH DYSREGULATION IN COUPLES THERAPY

Couples enter therapy with betrayals and affairs, bouts of eruptive emotionality, or deadening distance that has defensively grown up over repeated ruptures without repair. Therapists are frequently presented with enormous discrepancies in the stories that are told, and newer therapists may feel pulled to take sides or referee. With these couples, therapists often see the limitations of a purely cognitive approach. Tools of negotiation, compromise and improved communication skills presuppose separate nervous systems that can operate independently and that can, in high arousal states, follow helpful guidelines that encourage listening well and communicating nondefensively. This is neurologically beyond many couples who present for therapy.

Neuroscience, in a variation on systems theory, offers a paradigm shift from the idea of separate individuals in conflict, to what Allan Schore (personal communication, September 17, 2005) calls a "single fused neural circuitry":

Rather than viewing the couple as two separate people, the contemporary neuroscience picture is of a single, emotionally-fused system whose coupled chemistry tunes the brains and minds of each. Just as a caretaker's precise responses tune the brain and mind of a newborn baby, so too do the dynamics of the couple ... set the stage either for well-regulated or dysregulated emotion within individuals.

In moments of high emotionality, cortical centers in the RH and LH disconnect, and couples lock into their subcortical RHs, reverting to primitive styles of defensiveness. What we "know" and what we "intend to do," like lists of good communication skills, are processed through words in the neocortex of the LH and become inaccessible during heightened arousal states.

Partners in most couples who seek therapy grew up insecurely attached and sensitized to threat. A scowl, a cutting tone of voice, or a rolling of the eyes can evoke anger, blame, and defensiveness at lightning speed in that "bottom-up hijacking" of the brain by the amygdala (LeDoux, 2002). This pours powerful stress chemicals into the bodies of each, leaving them trapped in subcortical structures in the RH. Although this occurs in secure and insecure systems alike, the latter cannot repair and interactively regulate these breeches, and so they become heightened and long-lasting states of shared emotional reactivity.

Couples therapy must activate those deep subcortical recesses of our unconscious mind where affect resides, trauma has been stored, and preverbal, implicit attachment templates have been laid down. Such RH activation within distressed relationships implies the need for therapeutic approaches that are affective and deeply relational, with an emphasis on RH resonance, rather than cognitively constructed LH interventions and analysis (Schore, 2003b). Therapists who want to modify those early neural patterns must work in RH modalities, utilizing the same affective primary-process attunement, mediated by facial expressions, eye contact, verbal-prosody, body posture, gestures, and general vitality that are being rapidly and unconsciously exchanged. We slow the interactive pace and refocus couples from the verbal content to the process that is occurring beneath the verbal dialogue. Here we track the meaning conveyed in prosodic tones of voice that easily carry fear, anger, sarcasm, or contempt. We watch for eye contact or its absence and for the subtle or rapid flashes of facial expressions that communicate affect so powerfully. We interrupt patterns of mutually escalating anger and defensiveness and may ask clients to focus on us briefly so that we can help them to calm down. And if escalation feels runaway we may ask the calmer of the two to briefly leave the room so that we can work with the partner who most needs our help to regulate, until it is safe for the partner to return. We take them into the meanings behind their words and into a closer relationship with the arousal in their bodies, and with their own feeling states. It's important that we access and increase their capacity for accurately picking up facial, vocal, and bodily cues from their partner, stopping to check out assumptions they have made, and reading their own interoceptive cues that are available once they can tune in (Tatkin, 2013). We use well-timed interventions to create a sense of safety in the room, helping them to access and speak from more vulnerable states, to give reassurances with their face and tone as well as with their words, to take in offers of regret, and to recognize and name nonverbal expressions of their partner's pain. And, so importantly, to be able to hold contact with their partners' eyes during moments of vulnerability so that coregulation between the couple can more easily occur.

Evidence is mounting for the efficacy of such implicit and affect-based approaches in couples therapy (Byrne, Carr, & Clark, 2004; Denton, Burleson, Clark, Rodriguez, & Hobbs, 2000; Greenman & Johnson, 2012; Johnson, 2005, 2013; Johnson & Talitman, 1997). Collectively they point to the need to enhance the ability for affect regulation in our patients with approaches that activate and reorganize higher and lower centers on the right side of the brain.

IMPLEMENTING RH IMPLICIT AND AFFECT-BASED APPROACHES IN COUPLES THERAPY

Because distressed relationships are characterized by repeated ruptures that are not repaired, it is essential that, once dysregulated, couples be able to successfully repair and reconnect. Partners must learn to track externally- and internally arising energies, by recognizing environmental triggers and their own internal, visceral-response-arousal signs. As somatic approaches demonstrate (Levine, 1997, 2010; Ogden & Minton, 2000; Ogden, Minton, & Pain, 2006) the body knows how to do this automatically, provided the escalating or falling energy can be contained.

In the initial stages of therapy, the couple's therapist functions as the external regulator, providing containment by helping them to recognize arousal in their bodies, and wait to talk or act until they're calm enough to think. We assist them to get their entire brain turned on, arousal and regulating centers functioning simultaneously. This strengthens affect-regulating centers in the prefrontal cortices with their modulating pathways to lower, emotional centers in the brain. These are the very functions, and subsequently structures, that, as infants, they did not internalize and grow. In the vignette below, the husband, in a moment of agonizing pain, manages to slip momentarily into an OFC-mediated observer state and separate his past trauma from the present dysregulating exchange. In that instant, his whole brain is activated and functioning in an integrated way and his affect shifts immediately, though temporarily, toward calm.

SELF AND COREGULATION STRATEGIES: TEACHING INTERPERSONAL REGULATION SKILLS

Dysregulated couples require considerable coaching at first, with less intervention on our part as they acquire the more sophisticated self and coregulatory capacities they would have ideally developed in childhood. Our initial goal is to actively assist, then to teach them how to regulate themselves and, finally, to help them coregulate with one another at moments of distress. Through practice, higher neural regions on the right become better at turning down more primitive centers of arousal, improving the individual's capacity for regulation, discernment, and impulse control (Beer & Lombardo, 2007).

Coregulation bids for soothing and repair made by one intimate partner to another are generally more powerful than attempts by either to self-regulate, and often more effective than those made by the therapist to soothe. They do, however, require that at least one member of the couple at a time be able to set their own emotions temporarily aside, to listen to what their partner is saying affectively, and to hear the pain beneath their partner's defensiveness. They must learn to track their partner's nonverbal material, and understand the triggers that serve to dysregulate their partners and themselves.

It helps to position them face-to-face, inviting them to speak with their posture, their eyes (Demos, Kelly, Ryan, Davis, & Whalen, 2008; Harrison, Singer, Rotshtein, Dolan, & Critchley, 2006; Harrison, Wilson, & Critchley, 2007; Tatkin, 2013), their empathic tears, and their entire face; to use softened expressions, smiles, and calming voices (all RH modalities), as well as their words, to soothe. They must learn to listen deeply, to pace themselves, to wait patiently when their partner turns away, to allow each other time to recover, and then reengage, deepening their empathic bonds and creating a sense of safety in the relationship. Touch is also mediated in the RH; encouraging a couple to hold hands as they struggle through a conflict can calm their nervous systems and make it harder for them to fight.

To be successful, the partner initiating recontact and repair must be able to hold their sense of calm for two, three, or even four repeated bids allowing their partner's nervous system time to soothe so that defensiveness can drop and connection can be resumed. Watch in the second session of the vignette that follows as the wife's, Eleanor, soothing reaching out fails to register and her partner continues to escalate. In this case, she manages to hold on and tries again, the second time more successfully. Therapists working closely with couples' relational distress are immersed in, and occasionally on the receiving end, of powerful energies that may activate reciprocal feelings in response. This can happen when energy erupts precipitously, locking clients into a destructively escalating crescendo of desperation and hostility; when they turn away from one another in a steely silent rage; or when their energy collapses into despair or hopelessness. Fear, reactive anger, shame, or a sense of helplessness can briefly flare in the therapist who might feel overwhelmed by the intensity of the interactions, or even dissociate into distraction or confusion under a momentary sense of threat. The therapist's capacity to track not only the nonverbal social emotional cueing in the couple, but also her own RH-based visceral experiencing, and to reregulate, is paramount to providing the couples with the "container" that Bion (1962) talked about. This work requires a tolerance for excessive and collapsed energy, an ability to attune to subtler affects, and a sound capacity to model and to teach more about "how to be" with one another and with one's own affect and energy than about what "to do" (Safran, 2003), especially about what "to do" to change their partner's affect or behavior rather than their own.

COUPLES VIGNETTE: PRESENTING PATTERNS

Eleanor and Leonard[1] have recently moved to the West Coast for his new executive position, a move that took her away from her family, work, and friends. Eleanor blames Leonard for her loss though she agreed to move and alternates between reactive grief and rage at him. They fight frequently, and he is almost always the one to reapproach and offer to repair. Their 6-year-old son, Eric, is stuttering and has begun to act out aggressively. They know the tensions in their relationship are affecting him, but early relational trauma has left them with highly reactive nervous systems and insufficient affective resiliency.

These are extracts of therapy sessions 2 months part. The couple has been encouraged to have in the therapist's office, rather than to describe, the discord they experience at home, and the first of two sessions begins along a well-rehearsed path as the conflict comes alive in an embodied way.

Session 2

Speaking of her isolation since the move, Eleanor's voice grows shrill. As she repeats this apparently well-rehearsed complaint, her voice rises, her face distorts in anger and her eyes fill with tears. I try to ask a question, but she brushes me aside and continues to escalate. Leonard sits passively, staring straight ahead. He appears to be partly in genuine hypoarousal, and partly to be holding still as a conscious strategy. Watching him for some sign of recognition and finding none, she becomes angrier and yells, "You have your work; you don't know what it's like for me!" He grimaces and turns away. She bites her lip, narrows her eyes, and her rage dissolves in tears. Her bid for interactive regulation fails when she finds no compassion on his face for her and triggers in her a feeling of abandonment. Leonard is "down-regulating" and is apparently unaware of being provocative and a source of dysregulation for her. He later says he believed that by being silent, he was preventing her from becoming angrier and more upset, that is, that he could avoid escalating her.

"I think she needs to know you've heard," I say, encouraging him to turn his body back toward her again. Although she will not look at him, he sees her bent forward in pain and in a softened voice he says, "I'm sorry, I know you miss your parents and your friends and that the move has been hard for you." She is regulated enough to look briefly up then down again. Even in this instant of connection, there is a drop in tension, and she appears more sad than angry now, which seems to further soften him. "No, look at me," he invites. "I do know you've felt lost and are having trouble making friends." They talk together for a minute or two as he continues in a soothing voice, but she has to be frequently cued by me to hold his gaze, and looks down repeatedly. When he says, "I just wish you weren't so sad," she hears an edge of exasperation in his voice, and her tone sharpens instantly with a sarcastic reply, mocking him, "Yes, just smile, Eleanor, and leave me alone!"

The first hyperarousal I have seen in him occurs here when he erupts,

> I'm tired of being blamed. I was miserable in Des Moines. You knew that I was sinking in that job. You're not trying to help yourself or Eric to adjust. You think I should be grateful if you manage 2 days in a row without completely melting down.

These few minutes of dialogue illustrate the level of dysregulation that they, and their child, are subjected to repeatedly.

NEUROLOGICAL COMMENTARY ON SESSION 2

Unable to resolve her loss, Eleanor triggers into hyperaroused states and turns on Leonard in repeated episodes of blame and rage. Typically, he copes by shutting down into unavailable hypoarousal until, under her relentless badgering, he explodes into his own hyperaroused reactive rage that leaves her feeling even more abandoned and shut out (J. Lewis, 2000). In this session, encouraged by the therapist, he begins to coregulate with her, but they have become so hypersensitized that the slightest edge of impatience in his voice sets her off again, and this triggers him. Over the years of marriage, they have become that "emotionally fused system" A. N. Schore (personal communication, September 17, 2005) described, and the thresholds for HPA hyperactivation have dropped in each of them. (Note: The couple has previously agreed that whenever dysregulated arousal occurs, they will allow me to redirect their focus from content to process, that is, from the verbal argument to their physiological arousal and that we will not return to the subject matter at hand until they have calmed enough to listen and to think, i.e. to have their entire brains available to them. his agreement must be enforced repeatedly in early sessions when arousal spikes are frequent and instantaneous.)

Session 6

They enter the room to take their customary places across from one another and instantly the air is ripe with tension. Sensing what feels mildly dangerous in the steely silence, I ask, "When did this one begin?" "Last night," Eleanor snarls. As she begins recounting the details of their fight, I'm listening less to content and more to the metaconversation of her body and her voice. As her face contorts, her voice escalates, the words racing out in pressured speech; bursts of phrases like machine gun fire. She is breathing in gasps, sucking in air, and then holding her breath.

"Eleanor," I say, "I want you to look at me. Can you do that?" Here I have raised my voice so that it is slow, but strong and firm, and repeat myself several times until I break through her escalating crescendo and she looks at me. "Good," I say, "now can you breathe with me? I want to help you slow down a bit, so we can work this out." She can maintain eye contact with me to about the count of 3 when her eyes dart away, her energy shoots back up, and she tries to return to a description of the fight. "Not yet," I say, "This is the time to calm, not to talk. Try to keep my eyes. That's good. I'm right here with you." It takes several more rounds until she will fully engage. And I can begin to walk her through a body scan to anchor her propioceptively.

Neurological commentary on Session 6

In the silence as they enter the room, I can feel my own visceral response, an implicit body knowing, and a subcortical sensing of danger before higher conscious centers have had time to process the incoming stimuli. This somatic-countertransference reaction of fear in me sets off a well-rehearsed sequence of self-regulating shifts as I slow my breathing and let my shoulders drop. Imaging research demonstrates that the right orbitofrontal cortex activates as a mother decodes her infant's emotional cues to respond sensitively to them (Nitschke et al., 2004). My own regulating centers have come on to assess the situation and to calm myself enough to think.

I use my own RH modalities of face and prosody to help her regulate. Getting her to look at me is critical; regulating face-to-face interactions of parents and infants begins bidirectionally around 8 weeks of life as the face-processing centers of the RH come online, and this remains a major regulatory pathway throughout life (Schore, 1994). Another regulating modality is auditory prosody. I have raised my voice to meet her frantic energy until she hears and looks at me, then I stair-step down the activation when I see her able to follow me. I know here to keep my sentences simple as LH processing is impaired at elevated levels of arousal, and to rely on more RH nonverbal means to connect with her. Somatically scanning her own body brings her into her own RH where process information coming up somatically gets "read" first in the higher cortical centers on the right (Schore & Schore, 2008). Her breathing slows and becomes more regular as her parasympathetic nervous system (PNS) turns on.

Session 9

Eleanor begins by complaining that Leonard has been overly critical that week. "I couldn't even do a simple thing like pass out Halloween candy," she says. "I was putting handfuls into the children's bags and in a murderous tone he told me I'm too controlling, to let the children take their own. I thrust the bowl at him and stormed away." I glance at him; he looks ready to explode.

"Where are you right now, Leonard?" I ask. He has practiced self-regulating skills for weeks and manages to step into an observing state of mind. His OFC is turned on, and he can describe the rage, even as it's happening.

"I'm that raging child, trying and not being heard by mom or dad. I feel the same frustration and helplessness. I had only one solution then; they were never going to hear, so I separated out myself." He's tearing up now and his body droops. "When I can distance for a minute like that, and get the association to my parents growing up." But then he dysregulates again, losing the observer stance and slipping back inside the pain. "I could have done it differently with them, if only I could have made it different." The pitch of his voice goes up, his throats tightens, he looks away and down (the classic position of shame), and hunches forward in his chair clutching his stomach as though in agony. His auditory prosody, gestures, and posture—all those nonverbal, RH signals—are flashing pain. I glance at her, prepared to help her regulate her arousal state, but this time she's already there. She leans into him and whisper, "It's all right, sweetheart." But he's swept away and misses the coregulation bid.

He begins to sob,

> I can't take this anymore. I'm not a person, my needs don't get addressed. I'm about to go into a board meeting with my boss, when she calls. She has no awareness of where I am and that I may be nervous or absorbed and not want to deal with this right then.

He's now crying openly.

"You look sad and small," I say. His higher observing centers aren't on just now, so I bring mine in instead. "Notice what's happening," I suggest, "your voice, your body and where and how you feel this pain. And try to look at Eleanor, try to hold her gaze." I sense it's safe to do this because she appears, as I glance at her, to have managed to hear the accusation without losing her focus on his pain. She leans in again, coming close to his face until he looks up and then she smiles reassuringly, and mirrors his sad expression (Fonagy et al., 2002; Winnicott, 1971/1982).

"She has more capacity to respond than my parents did," he concedes. He's able for a moment to discriminate between the current relationship and those of his childhood. "I'm reacting to old neglect," he says.

For the first time in more than 2 months of therapy, they have a tender moment here in front of me. She gathers him in, and he cries and then he apologizes and thanks her for something I cannot quite hear. "You just thanked her Leonard?" I inquire. "Yes," he says, "for letting me be the one who falls apart."

NEUROLOGICAL COMMENTARY ON SESSION 9

From fragments of autobiographical memories stored in Leonard's RH, there awakens an image of him at age 8 or 10 experiencing an implicit whole-body sense of powerlessness in his family of origin. After these months of practice, his higher cortical, regulatory centers stay engaged, and he maintains an awareness of himself at age 40, watching the torrent of emotional despair, and responds to himself with empathetic tenderness. He then brings to bear his well-articulated LH to construct a coherent narrative and gives language to the right-brain flood he is experiencing.

His ability to feel and hold his pain triggers an empathetic softening in Eleanor. She reaches out to him and holds her openness until the repair attempt is heard and used by him to further regulate, and they are able to connect and calm. This capacity to stay connected to herself and to him must be learned and reinforced. So often the first tender offer of repair by one member of the couple fails to reach its mark and the offering partner, feeling dropped or shamed, may escalates and/or retaliate.

Visual contact is a central element for the establishment of a primary attachment. The facial mirroring that Eleanor does for Leonard is reminiscent of the attuned interactions of a mother who not only imitates an emotional display, but also produces an exaggerated "marked" version of his expression (Fonagy et al., 2002), creating an intersubjective resonance, a kind of "biological mirror" (Papousek & Papousek, 1979) or an "amplifying mirror" (Schore, 1994). These high-intensity mirroring exchanges create a "merger" experience between two systems attuned to each other (Sander, 1991). This calming is echoed neurologically and psychophysiologically as A. N. Schore (personal communication, June 9, 2007) reminds us, "The experience of feeling cared about in a relationship reduces the secretion of stress hormones and in shifting the neuroendocrine system toward homeostasis allows for the return of safety and intimacy."

SUMMARY

Couples therapists must learn to work in the immediacy of affective states of repeated ascending and descending spirals of energy. Entering into these shared arousal states, we choreograph consciously and unconsciously, regulating first one member, and then the other, toward a dance of primary-process attunement and into moments of affect synchrony. For it is only in the closeness of intimate encounters, in the deep subcortical recesses of our RHs, when the most primitive of old relational wounds have been touched, and oldest attachment template have come to life, that they can be soothed and healed. It is these repeated experiences that allow couples to regain trust and deepen their empathic bond.

ACKNOWLEDGMENTS

The author wishes to thank Allan Schore and Margaret Rossoff for their helpful comments.

NOTE

1. The case material presented here is a composite of several couples and disguised so as not to violate the confidentiality of any client.

REFERENCES

Atkinson, B. (1999, July/August). Brainstorms: Rewiring the neural circuitry of family conflict. *Family Therapy Networker*, 23–33.

Atkinson, B. (2002, September/October). Brain to brain: New ways to help couples avoid relapse. *Psychotherapy Networker*. Retrieved from thecouplesclinic.com/pdf/brain_to_brain.pdf

Beebe, B. (2000). Coconstructing mother-infant distress: The micro-synchrony of maternal impingement and infant avoidance in the face-to-face encounter. *Psychoanalytic Inquiry, 20*, 412–440.

Beebe, B., & Lachmann, F. (1998). Co-constructing inner and relational processes: Self- and mutual regulation in infant research and adult treatment. *Psychoanalytic Psychology, 15*(4), 480–516.

Beer, J. S., & Lombardo, M. V. (2007). Insights into emotion regulation from neuropsychology. In J. J. Gross (Ed.), *Handbook of emotion regulation* (pp. 69–86). New York, NY: Guilford Press.

Bion, W. R. (1962). *Learning from experience*. London, UK: Heinemann.

Bowlby, J. (1988). *A secure base: Clinical applications of attachment theory*. London, UK: Routledge.

Byrne, M., Carr, A., & Clark, M. (2004). The efficacy of behavioral couples therapy and emotionally focused therapy for couple distress. *Contemporary Family Therapy*, *26*(4), 361–387.

Cozolino, L. (2002). *The neuroscience of psychotherapy: Building and rebuilding the human brain*. New York, NY: W. W. Norton.

Damasio, A. (1999). *The feeling of what happens: Body and emotion in the making consciousness*. New York, NY: Harcourt Brace.

De Bellis, M. D., Keshavan, M. S., Shifflett, H., Iyengar, S., Beers, S. R., Hall, J., & Moritz, G. (2002). Brain structures in pediatric maltreatment-related post-traumatic stress disorders: A sociodemographically matched study. *Biological Psychiatry*, *52*(11), 1066–1078.

Demos, K., Kelly, W., Ryan, S., Davis, F., & Whalen, P. (2008). Human amygdala sensitivity to the pupil size of others. *Cerebral Cortex*, *18*, 2729–2734.

Denton, W. H., Burleson, B. R., Clark, T. E., Rodriguez, C. P., & Hobbs, B. (2000). A randomized trial of emotion-focused therapy for couples in a training clinic. *Journal of Marital and Family Therapy*, *26*, 65–78.

Erel, O., & Burman, B. (1995). Interrelatedness of marital relations and parent-child relations: A meta-analytic review. *Psychological Bulletin*, *118*, 108–132.

Fonagy, P., Gergely, G., Jurist, E. L., & Target, M. (2002). *Affect regulation, mentalization, and the development of the self*. New York, NY: Other Press.

Goldman, A., & Greenberg, L. (1992). Comparison of integrated systemic and emotionally. *Journal of Consulting and Clinical Psychology*, *60*, 962–969.

Gottman, J. M. (1999). *The seven principles for making marriage work*. New York, NY: Crown Publishing Group.

Gottman, J. M., & Gottman, J. S. (2008). Gottman method couple therapy. In A. S. Gurman (Ed.), *Clinical handbook of couple therapy* (pp. 138–166). New York, NY: Guilford Press.

Greenman, P. S., & Johnson, S. M. (2012). United we stand: Emotionally focused therapy (EFT) for couples in the treatment of posttraumatic stress disorder. *Journal of Clinical Psychology: In Session*, *68*(5), 561–569.

Harrison, N., Singer, T., Rotshtein, P., Dolan, R., & Critchley, H. (2006). Pupillary contagion: Central mechanisms engaged in sadness processing. *Scan*, *1*, 5–17.

Harrison, N., Wilson, C., & Critchley, H. (2007). Processing of observed pupil size modulates perception of sadness and predicts empathy. *Emotion*, *7*, 724–729.

Hazan, C., & Shaver, P. R. (1987). Romantic love conceptualized as an attachment process. *Journal of Personality and Social Psychology*, *52*, 511–524.

Johnson, S. (1996). *The practice of emotionally focused marital therapy: Creating*. New York, NY: Brunner-Routledge.

Johnson, S. (2004). Attachment theory a guide for healing couple relationships. In W. S. Rholes & A. Simpson (Eds.), *Adult attachment* (pp. 367–387). New York, NY: Guilford Press.

Johnson, S. (2005). The evolution of couples therapy: A new era. *The Psychologist: British Psychological Association*, *18*, 538–539.

Johnson, S. (2013). *Love sense: The revolutionary new science of romantic relationships*. New York, NY: Little, Brown and Co.

Johnson, S., & Denton, W. (2002). Emotionally focused couple therapy: Creating secure. In A. Gurman & N. Jacobson (Eds.), *Clinical handbook of couple therapy* (3rd ed., pp. 221–250). New York, NY: Guilford Press.

Johnson, S., & Talitman, E. (1997). Predictors of success in emotionally focused marital therapy. *Journal of Marital and Family Therapy*, *23*, 135–152.

Knickmeyer, R. C., Gouttard, S., Kang, C., Evans, D., Wilber, K., Smith, J. K., . . . Gilmore, J. H. (2008). A structural MRI study of human brain development from birth to 2 years. *Journal of Neuroscience*, *28*(47), 12176–12182.

LeDoux, J. (2002). *Synaptic self: How our brains become who we are*. New York, NY: Viking.

Levine, P. (1997). *Waking the tiger: Healing trauma*. Berkeley, CA: North Atlantic Books.

Levine, P. (2010). *In an unspoken voice: How the body releases trauma and restores goodness*. Berkeley, CA: North Atlantic Books.

Lewis, J. (2000). Repairing the bond in important relationships: A dynamic for personality maturation. *American Journal of Psychiatry*, *157*, 1375–1378.

Lewis, T., Amin, F., & Lannon, R. (2002). *A general theory of love*. New York, NY: Random House.

Lyons-Ruth, K., Bronfman, E., & Parsons, E. (1999). Atypical attachment in infancy and early childhood among children at developmental risk. IV. Maternal frightened, frightening, or atypical behavior and disorganized infant attachment patterns. *Monographs of the Society for Research in Child Development*, *64*(3), 67–96.

Makinen, J., & Johnson, S. (2006). Resolving attachment injuries in couples using EFT: Steps towards forgiveness and reconciliation. *Journal of Consulting and Clinical Psychology*, *74*, 1055–1064.

Nitschke, J. B., Nelson, E. E., Rusch, B. D., Fox, A. S., Oakes, T. R., & Davidson, R. J. (2004). Orbitofrontal cortex tracks positive mood in mothers viewing pictures of their newborn infants. *NeuroImage*, *21*(2), 583–592.

Ogden, P., & Minton, K. (2000). Sensorimotor psychotherapy: One method for processing traumatic memory. *Traumatology*, *6*(3), Article 3. Retrieved from https://www.sensorimotorpsychotherapy.org/articles.html

Ogden, P., Minton, K., & Pain, C. (2006). *Trauma and the body: A sensorimotor approach to psychotherapy*. New York, NY: W. W. Norton.

Papousek, H., & Papousek, M. (1979). Early ontogeny of human social interaction: Its biological roots and social dimensions. In M. von Cranach, K. Foppa, W. Lepenies, & D. Ploog (Eds.), *Human ethology: Claims and limits of a new discipline* (pp. 456–478). New York, NY: Cambridge University Press.

Perry, B. D., Pollard, R. A., Blakely, T. L., Baker, W. L., & Vigilante, D. (1995). Childhood trauma, the neurobiology of adaptation, and "use dependent" development in the brain: How "states" become "traits." *Infant Mental Health Journal*, *16*, 271–291.

Porges, S. W. (2001). The polyvagal theory: Phylogenetic substrates of a social. *International Journal of Psychophysiology, 42,* 123–146.

Safran, J. D. (Ed.). (2003). *Psychoanalysis and Buddhism: An unfolding dialogue.* Boston, MA: Wisdom Publications.

Safran, J. D., & Muran, J. C. (2000). *Negotiating the therapeutic alliance: A relational treatment guide.* New York, NY: Guilford Press.

Sander, L. (1991, June). *Recognition process: Specificity and organization in early human development.* Paper presented at the University of Massachusetts Conference on the Psychic Life of the Infant, Amherst, MA.

Schore, A. N. (1994). *Affect regulation and the origin of the self; the neurobiology of emotional development.* Mahwah, NJ: Erlbaum Associates.

Schore, A. N. (1996). The experience-dependent maturation of a regulatory system in the orbital prefrontal cortex and the origin of developmental psychopathology. *Development and Psychopathology, 8,* 59–87.

Schore, A. N. (1997). Early organization of the nonlinear right brain and development of a predisposition to psychiatric disorders. *Development and Psychopathology, 9,* 595–631.

Schore, A. N. (2001a). The effects of a secure attachment relationship on right brain development, affect regulation, and infant mental health. *Infant Mental Health Journal, 22,* 7–66.

Schore, A. N. (2001b). The effects of relational trauma on right brain development, affect regulation, and infant mental health. *Infant Mental Health Journal, 22,* 201–269.

Schore, A. N. (2003a). *Affect dysregulation and disorders of the self.* New York, NY: W.W. Norton.

Schore, A. N. (2003b). *Affect dysregulation and the repair of the self.* New York, NY: W.W. Norton.

Schore, A. N. (2009a). Relational trauma and the developing right brain: The neurobiology of broken attachment bonds. In T. Baradon (Ed.), *Relational trauma in infancy* (pp. 19–46). East Sussex, UK: Routledge.

Schore, A. N. (2009b). Attachment trauma and the developing right brain: Origins. In P. Dell & J. O'Neil (Eds.), *Dissociation and dissociative disorders* (pp. 107–141). New York, NY: Taylor & Francis Group.

Schore, J. R., & Schore, A. N. (2008). Modern attachment theory: The central role of affect regulation in development and treatment. *Clinical Social Work Journal, 36,* 9–20.

Shaver, P. R., & Hazan, C. (1993). Adult romantic attachment: Theory and evidence. In D. Perlman & W. Jones (Eds.), *Advances in personal relationships* (pp. 29–70). London, UK: Kingsley.

Tatkin, S. (2005a, January–February). Marital therapy and the psychobiology of turning toward and turning away. *The Therapist, 15,* 75–78.

Tatkin, S. (2005b). Psychobiological conflict management of marital couples. *Psychologist-Psychoanalyst, 25*(1), 20–22.

Tatkin, S. (2007, December). *The pseudo-secure couple (aka false-self couple).* Paper presented at the Milton H. Erickson Foundation Couples Conference, Anaheim, CA.

Tatkin, S. (2013) Applying a psychobiological approach to the identification and treatment of social-emotional deficits in couple therapy. *Psychotherapy in Australia, 17*(4), 1–21.

Trevarthen, C. (2001). The neurobiology of early communication: Intersubjective regulations in human brain development. In A. F. Kalverboer & A. Gramsbergen (Eds.), *Handbook on brain and behavior in human development* (pp. 841–882). Dordrecht, The Netherlands: Kluwer.

Tronick, E. Z., & Weinberg, M. K. (1997). Depressed mothers and infants: Failure to form dyadic states of consciousness. In L. Murray & P. I. Cooper (Eds.), *Postpartum depression in child development* (pp. 54–81). New York, NY: Guilford Press.

Winnicott, D. W. (1982). *Playing and reality*. New York, NY: Tavistock. (Original work published 1971)

Interface Between Psychotropic Medications, Neurobiology, and Mental Illnesses

ROSEMARY L. FARMER

School of Social Work, Virginia Commonwealth University, Richmond, Virginia, USA

The interface between psychotropic medication, neurobiology, and mental illnesses should be more adequately recognized by clinical and other social workers. This article argues for this claim by examining its consistency with current policies of the National Institute of Mental Health and by discussing understandings about the relationship between neurobiology and mental illness and medication.

INTRODUCTION

Is the interface between psychotropic medications, neurobiology, and mental illnesses adequately recognized and understood by social workers? This article argues that it is not. The intertwining of these three constructs should be better understood. There is such a close connection between the three—between psychotropic medications, neurobiology, and mental illnesses—that it can be argued that the neurobiological becomes the psychosocial. The interface between psychotropic medications, neurobiology, and mental illnesses is crucial to our practice as clinical social workers.

The more one reads and learns about the neurosciences and mental illness, the more is the realization that the biopsychosocial-spiritual (BPSS) framework is the core from which all understanding and interventions emanate. This framework, which is central to social work theorizing and practice, will serve as the organizing feature for our discussion of medication, neurobiology, and mental illness. But at the same time, we need to be wary of overestimating or underestimating the strength of the biological component. In an age of neuroscience, where focus on the brain is pervasive, it is easy to do the former. Although the neurobiological aspects of illness at first glance appear to be specifically ensconced in the biological domain, we see how this is only partially accurate. For example, when we talk about epigenetics (how the genome responds to the environment) we see that genes are blueprints for the making of proteins (Lipton, 2005). And then there are the nongenetic factors that cause our genes to express themselves differently. There are genes, and then proteins, and then genes are turned on or off based on environmental things like stress, diet, behavior, toxins, and so on that activate chemical switches that regulate gene expression. Therefore, we are not totally controlled by our genes, and the psychosocial aspects of our existence are also important. Likewise neural plasticity is a biosocial concept that says that the brain alters in response to what it experiences. By learning new information, we can reshape our brain via changes at the nerve cell level. Thinking, learning, and acting change the brain's functioning and its structure (Andreasen, 2001; Restak, 2003). Even neurogenesis (how new neurons are created) is now understood to continue to occur in the adult brain. We used to think that the brain matured in adolescence and then stopped growing. But we now know that brain changes are lifelong, and even the aging brain can rejuvenate and improve itself (Taupin, 2005).

This article is divided into three sections. The first section is about consistency with policies of the National Institute of Mental Health (NIMH). It indicates that there is agreement about the need for greater understanding of the etiology of mental illnesses and the NIMH's reemphasis on the need for more neurobiologically based research to reach this goal. The second is about medication and neurobiology, and it includes discussion of some of the basic tenets of psychopharmacology and of diversity in medication effects based on race and ethnicity. The third section is on mental illness and neurobiology. It returns to showing how the BPSS perspective used by social workers requires that neurobiological knowledge provides the missing link for what is necessary to assist persons with their mental illnesses and provide effective clinical interventions. It demonstrates how the neurobiological becomes the psychosocial because neurobiological understandings cannot be used in isolation, and environment is now an important part of our knowledge about the brain (viz. neuroplasticity and epigenetics).

CONSISTENCY WITH NATIONAL INSTITUTE OF MENTAL HEALTH

These claims about the interface between psychotropic medications, neurobiology, and mental illnesses are consistent with the NIMH's reemphasis on the need for more neurobiologically based research to eventually find the etiology of mental illnesses. During the past year clinical social workers have been trying to familiarize themselves with the newly arrived *Diagnostic and Statistical Manual of Mental Disorders, 5th edition* (*DSM-5*; American Psychiatric Association, 2013), and some of us are actually teaching the new diagnostic nomenclature to masters' of social work (MSW) students. As we struggle with the changes, and try to understand how the new diagnostic categories and lack of axes will affect our practice, we are reminded of the fact that not only social workers are wondering about this new diagnostic system.

Just prior to the publication of the *DSM-5* in May 2013, Dr. Thomas Insel, director of the NIMH, reported that the new manual of mental disorders lacked scientific validity and therefore should not be used in designing research studies, which is currently the case (Belluck & Carey, 2013). Instead, Insel saw the need to focus on biology, genetics, and neuroscience, which will better incorporate the complexity of disorders (Belluck & Carey, 2013). Although Insel appreciates the need of clinicians to categorize mental disorders, there is a lack of specificity in our understanding of disorders, and some symptoms are found across different categories of illness. We are left with a labeling of persons who have a certain disorder, but with no clear idea about the causes of the disorder. To remedy the way we think about mental illnesses, and address some core critiques of the *DSM*, in 2009 NIMH began a new project, the Research Domain Criteria (RDoC), which would incorporate data on pathophysiology, especially related to genomics and neuroscience. The RDoC is intended to ensure that diagnoses are reliable and valid (Insel et al., 2010). To achieve this goal, and with regard to research funding, *DSM* categories will be disregarded and focus will be placed on investigating the biological underpinnings of disorders (Bullock & Carey, 2013). Instead of relying on clinical observation and patient report of symptoms, the new approach will define basic dimensions of functioning such as negative valence systems (fear, anxiety, loss), positive valence systems (reward learning, reward valuation), cognitive systems (attention, perception, working memory, cognitive control), systems for social processes (attachment formation, social communication, perception of self and others), and arousal/modulatory systems (arousal, circadian rhythm, sleep and wakefulness). Each of these domains will be studied by using several units of analysis, that is, genes, molecules, cells, neural circuits, physiology, behaviors, and self-reports (NIMH, 2013).

Although Insel's comments concerning the *DSM-5* will be looked upon with disfavor by some, it can be argued that leaders of the NIMH are making a bold and portentous statement about the huge importance of neurobiology for understanding and treating mental illnesses. As the largest group of clinical providers of care, social workers are on the front lines of working with individuals who have mental illnesses, and their families. As such, we need to be knowledgeable about the neurobiological understandings of human behavior and what can lead to the development of illness. And, not only do we need knowledge for practice, but social workers' unique approach and lens can and should be incorporated into neuroscience research. Although this is beginning to occur in research universities around the country, we all need to be cognizant of how to participate with neuroscientists in the development of hypotheses and implementation of studies. Social workers have a great deal to offer if we are willing to expand our thinking and ways of knowing and engage with multidisciplinary teams that are exploring genetic, behavioral, physiological, neural circuit, and cellular aspects of mental illness. On what is this belief based? Social workers are educated to always look at the person-in-environment, and as the definition of the term *environment* is expanding, we are the ones who have the tools to appreciate and incorporate the variety of environments that exist. As social workers, we use the *DSM*, but we also develop fuller BPSS assessments. As we add more of the bio to our BPSS assessments, we are getting closer to a full understanding of our clients, their strengths and vulnerabilities.

MEDICATION AND NEUROBIOLOGY

Beginning in the 1950s, when thorazine was serendipitously discovered to have antipsychotic effects, social workers and other mental health professionals became hopeful that psychotropic medications might provide effective treatment for various mental illnesses. Monoamine oxidase inhibitors (MAOIs) and cyclic antidepressants were also commonly prescribed to treat depression. But the conventional or first-generation antipsychotics had some unpleasant and serious side effects such as extra pyramidal symptoms (EPS) and tardive dyskinesia (TD). Some of the antidepressants also had problematic side effects (e.g., the MAOIs) and though the cyclic antidepressants were the most commonly prescribed antidepressants from the late 1950s through the 1980s, they had many negative side effects and did not adequately treat depression in every person who had it. During the 1970s and 1980s pharmaceutical companies engaged in much research and development, in an attempt to find new antipsychotics and antidepressants that were more effective, for more patients, and with fewer negative side effects. In 1987 the selective serotonin reuptake inhibitors (SSRIs) were introduced into the U.S. market, and they were heralded as being much more consumer friendly in that they would have fewer side effects and less overdose potential. In 1988, when the "atypical" or second-generation antipsychotics were approved for use in the United States, there was tremendous excitement and huge anticipation that these newer medications would lead to fewer negative side effects, and especially that they would not lead to TD, which is seen as an irreversible and serious condition. It was also anticipated that the new antipsychotics would be effective in the treatment of negative symptoms such as social withdrawal, anhedonia, and flat or blunted affect. Although the earlier studies of the second-generation antipsychotics like risperidone and clozapine seemed to point to less EPS and TD (Hunter, Kennedy, Song, Gadon, & Irving, 2003), more long-term studies show similar effectiveness to the first-generation medications but equivocal results related to side effects (Komossa et al., 2009; Komossa et al., 2011). Some of the newer antipsychotics showed fewer negative symptoms and less EPS, but many led to increased weight gain, sedation, orthostatic hypotension, and decreased sexual drive. SSRIs and the more recent selective norepinephrine reuptake inhibitors (SNRIs) have become the most commonly prescribed antidepressants, and they are also used to treat anxiety and eating disorders. They produce fewer adverse side effects though constipation, dry mouth, anxiety, and restlessness, and so on remain problematic for some users. Additionally, the SSRIs have been found to be 60% to 70% effective, which leaves almost one third of patients who do not benefit from these medications.

It seems like our earlier anticipation and excitement about finding psychotropic medications that would effectively treat all the major mental illnesses is now waning. Pharmaceutical companies that for years engaged in research to find the drug that was most selective in its effects (i.e., adequately treated symptoms but did not influence other brain areas that resulted in negative side effects) have more recently discontinued these efforts. According to one physician, Big Pharma has apparently decided that it is just too risky and too costly to develop new psychotropics, and instead they are focusing their research efforts on finding new drugs to treat cancer, heart disease, and diabetes (Friedman, 2013). Friedman (2013) noted that during the past 30 years there have been no really new psychotropics developed; rather, newer drugs may be safer and have fewer side effects, but they work in the brain in the same way as the original 1950s medications did. We still do not know the basic etiology of most mental illnesses, and the psychotropics we use today are no more effective than, for example, thorazine. As neuroscience knowledge and technologies grow, it is now more common for scientists to focus on brain research that is trying to understand neural networks and to identify and modify key brain circuits (Bell, 2013). This is in line with the new federal initiative mentioned earlier (i.e., the Research Domain Criteria Project; NIMH, 2013) that is encouraging brain research that investigates how brain networks contribute to problems that are shared by several different diagnoses.

Clinical social workers frequently work with clients who are taking one or more psychotropic medications, but one can still hear some social workers say that they "do not have anything to do with that" and they often do not know which medication the client has been prescribed. In my view, these attitudes border on professional malpractice and need to be addressed. As social workers, we need to be very clear as to our role vis-á-vis our clients and their prescribed medications. We are not medical professionals and do not prescribe medications or tell clients which medication they should be using. But we legitimately assume the roles of physician assistant, consultant, counselor, monitor, advocate, educator, and researcher (Bentley & Walsh, 2014). In the fourth edition of their popular book on social workers and psychotropic medication, Bentley and Walsh (2014) provided detailed descriptions of the various roles and the situations in which they are performed. These authors also discussed social work roles in the context of the social work discipline, which focuses on the perspectives of person-in-environment, social justice, strengths, and empowerment. Collaboration with other health care providers, clients, and their families is also crucial for effective social work practice with regard to medications. In a national study that surveyed social workers about the roles and activities they performed related to psychiatric medication, it was found that the social workers' beliefs about being competent and performing an appropriate role were positively associated with frequency of the activities performed (Bentley, Walsh, & Farmer, 2005). Therefore, it would seem that we must continue to educate social workers about medications, how and why they work in the brain, and what are the psychosocial aspects of medication use, to ensure that social workers are and feel competent in this area of their practice. To assume a knowledgeable role in work with clients who use psychotropics, social workers need to know basic information about the structure and functioning of the brain, what is neurotransmission, how do medications work, what are pharmacokinetics and what is pharmacodynamics, and what are the various classes of medications.

Basic information about medications that affect a person's thinking, emotions, and behavior could easily be incorporated into social work classes or presented to social workers in the community. An outline of such a module could consist of the following nine items:

1. Psychotropics work in the brain and central nervous system (brain and spinal cord) to effect the level of the neurotransmitter (NT).
2. Brain diagram to show structures (e.g., prefrontal cortex, amygdala, hippocampus, hypothalamus, brain stem) and functions of the brain; there are numerous diagrams available on the Internet, which show the structures.
3. Neuron—a cell and functional unit of the brain; specializes in information processing; diagrams of the neuron can be shown, which describe axons, dendrites, synapses, and so on.
4. Neurotransmission—all human behaviors, including thoughts and emotions, are the result of neural activity; axon sends chemical and electrical messages to receiving neurons; synapse is communication point between neurons and where the action is.
5. How medications work: (a) NT released by presynaptic neuron and directly binds to receptor site, either stimulating receptor (an agonist)

or blocking effect of naturally occurring NT (an antagonist); (b) medication works by causing release of more NT and thereby increases effect of the system; (c) medication works by blocking reuptake of NT back into presynaptic neuron, and effect is to increase neurotransmission; (d) medications may increase or decrease number of receptor sites or change sensitivity of receptors.

6. Major neurotransmitters implicated in psychotropic drug activity: acetylcholine, norepinephrine, dopamine, serotonin, gamma aminobutyric acid, glutamate.

7. Pharmacokinetics—how the body responds to the presence of a medication; it includes absorption (process by which the drug moves from site of administration into the bloodstream), distribution (process by which drug travels to desired site of action), metabolism (process by which the body breaks down the chemical structure of a drug into derivatives that can be eliminated from body), and excretion (process by which drug is eliminated from body, primarily done by kidneys).

8. Pharmacodynamics—the effects of a drug on the body (desirable and undesirable effects); it includes *therapeutic index* (ratio of lowest average concentration needed to produce desired effect and lowest average concentration that produces toxic effects), dose response (measure of therapeutic effect as a function of increasing dose), lag time (time a medication takes to affect targeted behavior), tolerance (body's reduced responsiveness to a drug because the sensitivity of receptors changes over time), and adverse or side effects (any effects of a drug that are unintentional and unrelated to its desired therapeutic effect).

9. Types of psychotropics: antipsychotics (first- and second-generation), antidepressants (MAOIs, tricyclic antidepressants [TCAs], SSRIs, SNRIs), antianxiety medications (benzodiazepines, beta blockers, buspirone), mood stabilizers (lithium, carbamazepine, depakote, tegretol), psychostimulants (ritalin, adderall), cognitive enhancers (cognex, aricept, metrifonate).

The above outline provides the major categories of neurobiological knowledge that help to prepare social workers for working with clients who are taking psychotropics, that they will be prepared to educate clients and their families, to assist with monitoring of medications, and to communicate effectively with team members. This knowledge can be taught in a 2- to 3-hour session, using Internet diagrams and handouts and allowing for discussion between social workers and instructor.

Returning to our BPSS framework, it is crucial that we appreciate that the taking of medications has not only physiological effects but also psychosocial effects. The attitude of the professional (be it the nurse, doctor, or social worker) with regard to medications can have a direct influence on whether and how a client takes prescribed medication. For example, if the practitioner has a negative attitude about medications, this can unconsciously be transmitted to the client, unless the practitioner is aware of her attitude and can manage it. The attitude of the client toward medications, including that of family members, also has an impact. If the client feels stigmatized by having a mental illness, and needing to take a psychotropic medication, negative feelings may occur, and the client will stop taking the prescribed medication. Attitude and stigma are also related to the meaning of taking medication for any specific person, and meaning often derives from one's culture. Meaning can be understood as part of the spiritual component of the BPSS framework. In recent years, social workers have made a major contribution to the literature on meaning of medications. Bentley (2010) conducted a qualitative research study with 21 adults with serious mental illness and found seven themes around medication being a pervasive positive force, a tolerated fact of life, an internal and individual experience, a prominent part of the story and evolution of one's mental illness, a basis of gratitude and source of victory over past struggles, a necessary protection of a personal sense of humanness, and a symbol of differentness and dependency. Floersch et al. (2009) studied children and adolescents and found that themes of expectation and hope were especially prominent among the youth.

Diversity in Medication Effects

It has been known for many years that medications have different effects based on a person's age, gender, race and ethnicity; these differences are based on pharmacokinetic and pharmacodynamic processes. Since the 1970s there has been more interest in finding out how race and ethnicity may affect medication effects, with especially greater interest expressed during the 1990s, though the participation of minorities in clinical drug trials remains small. Pharmacokinetics and pharmacodynamics, as described above, are controlled by genetic factors, but in recent years we have come to understand that environment is also involved in the expression of our genes. In this context, environment includes lifestyle, behavioral patterns, and social interactions, which reflect one's culture (Chen, Chen, & Lin, 2008). Therefore, any one person's response to a medication will be determined by gene–environment interactions, which for social workers is especially relevant because they are very knowledgeable about working with environments. Pharmacokinetics includes the processes of absorption, distribution, metabolism, and excretion, which together determine the optimal dosage and dosage regimen for a particular medication. Metabolism is especially important because it usually determines interindividual and cross-ethnic variation in drug response (Lin, Smith, & Ortiz, 2001). Enzymes, which are proteins that facilitate chemical changes, are important for the metabolism of medications, and the most important for metabolism of psychotropic medications are the cytochrome P-450 enzymes.

There are at least 57 different CYP-450 enzymes, but only several of these are involved in the metabolism of psychotropics. Genes control these enzymes, and the genetic differences are called genetic polymorphisms or mutations, which alter the way the enzyme functions. Mutations lead to much variability in the way the enzymes function, and this becomes evident in different populations; the mutations are ethnically specific. The mutations help us to classify persons into four groups, which are called "inherited metabolizer status." The four groups are poor metabolizers (PM), intermediate metabolizers (IM), extensive metabolizers (EM), and ultrarapid metabolizers (UM). Because the rate of metabolism determines how long a medication remains in the body before being excreted, it is important for how effective a medication may be. For example, a poor or intermediate metabolizer will have difficulty metabolizing medications such as nortriptyline and haldol and may be more likely to experience side effects as a result of elevated plasma levels of the drug. An extensive or ultrarapid metabolizer may require more than the usual dosage to benefit from the medication (Daly et al., 1996). Although there is currently mixed evidence for whether the CYP-450 genetic polymorphisms influence metabolizer status, some genotyping of the CYP-450 enzymes is being conducted, especially in situations where finding an effective medication for a patient has been challenging (Caley, 2011).

Pharmacogenomics, which is the study of how a person's genetic inheritance affects response to medications, has led to some beginning understanding of how different ethnic and racial groups respond to psychotropics. For example, African Americans have been found to need lower doses of most medications, and to be at greater risk for experiencing side effects, when compared with Whites (Malik, Lake, Lawson, & Joshi, 2010). Whites are considered to be the standard population with which others are compared, because most drug research has been conducted using White participants. More specifically, African Americans are poor metabolizers of antidepressant and antianxiety drugs (Burroughs, Maxey, & Levy, 2002) and therefore require lower doses, but they have faster response when given an appropriate dose. Because African Americans have a low baseline white blood cell count, they cannot be prescribed clozapine, the atypical antipsychotic that can lead to the serious side effect of agranulocytosis. Lithium appears to be excreted more slowly by African Americans, and therefore they experience more side effects with typical doses (Bentley & Walsh, 2014). Although it is important to be aware of the research results for persons of different races and ethnicities, we need to bear in mind that due to the mixed lineage of so many people a study may not be representative of all in that racial or ethnic group (Pena, 2011).

Asians have been found to require lower doses of antipsychotics and antidepressants because they tend to be poor metabolizers of many medications. Among East Asians (i.e., Chinese, Japanese, Korean) up to 70% are intermediate metabolizers, meaning that they have a slower rate of metabolism and may experience side effects at higher doses (Lin et al., 2001; Smith, 2006). Lin et al. (2001) found that up to 25% of East Asians are poor metabolizers of one of the CYP-450 enzymes involved with the metabolism of valium and several of the SSRIs. As a result, these persons would be especially sensitive to such medications. With regard to lithium, the research is mixed. Some studies have found that smaller doses are needed for Asians, and other studies find that lithium is metabolized at a similar rate to White (Wing, Chan, Chan, Lee, & Shek, 1997).

Persons of Hispanic ancestry, which would include persons from Spain, Mexico, Cuba, Puerto Rico, Central America, and South America, also have genetically determined responses to medications, though there is even less research conducted with these groups.

There is some evidence that Hispanics require lower doses of antidepressants and antipsychotic medications like risperidone and experience more adverse effects (Lawson, 2000). Studies of Mexican Americans have shown faster rates of some enzyme activity due to fewer gene mutations, as compared with African Americans, Whites, and Asians (Luo, Poland, Lin, & Wan, 2006). The result is normal metabolism and response to medications and fewer Mexican Americans who could be classified as poor metabolizers (Mendoza et al., 2001).

As mentioned previously, gene–environment interactions also influence one's response to a psychotropic medication. One example is cigarette smoking, as tobacco causes one of the CYP-450 enzymes to function in a way that the blood concentrations of most antipsychotics and antidepressants are reduced by about 50% (Smith, 2006). This is a little-known fact, among the general public and mental health professionals, and it can have a large impact, because many persons who experience depression or psychotic symptoms also smoke cigarettes. The foods we eat also can influence the enzymes that affect psychotropics. For example, a high-protein diet increases the speed of metabolism of certain medications, whereas a high-carbohydrate diet slows the rate of metabolism. In studies of immigrant populations, it has been found that groups of people who move from their home country to another and change their diet as a result (usually to a higher-protein diet) are found to metabolize drugs differently, based on their new diet (Lin et al., 2001). This is a good example of the importance of environmental factors for whether a prescribed medication will work appropriately for a specific individual. As the environmental expert, it is the role of the social worker to be cognizant of these types of factors, be able to educate the client/user of medication, and perhaps even to alert the prescriber of the medication. Herbal products and vitamins can also influence the metabolism of psychotropics, and some recent data report that between 8% and 57% of psychiatric clients (mainly those with depression and anxiety) use these products

(Sarris, Panossian, Schweitzer, Stough, & Scholey, 2011). Because these products are frequently purchased in "health food stores" they are assumed to be healthy. But this is difficult to determine, because most such products are not regulated by the U.S. Food and Drug Administration, and research on these products, their active ingredients, and their efficacy, is minimal. In the few studies that have been done, results point to some herbal medicines, like St. John's Wort, inducing the expression of the drug-metabolizing enzymes of the CYP-450 system. Other herbal products were found to inhibit enzyme expression (Piscitelli, Burstein, Chaitt, Alfaro, & Falloon, 2000). In the example of St. John's Wort, which induced enzyme activity, this would lead to reduced concentrations of the psychotropic, especially in women.

MENTAL ILLNESS AND NEUROBIOLOGY

We now return to the third subquestion: How does the neurobiological become the psychosocial? A focus on the relationship between neurobiology and mental illness, again using a BPSS lens, will help to respond to this question. It is argued that recent research about the structure and function of the brain provides the missing link to our knowledge and enhances the biological domain of our understanding (Farmer, 2009). It is essential for informing our clinical practice with those persons who experience mental illness. Why? Because neurobiological insights corroborate our psychosocial perspective and help authenticate our therapeutic interventions.

The neuroscience research of the past 30 years demonstrates that a major origin of psychopathology is trauma to the early developing nervous system, which results in affective or emotional dysregulation, that is,. loss of the ability to regulate intensity and duration of affects, especially negative affects (Bradley, 2000). The Adverse Childhood Experiences (ACE) Study, a large epidemiological public health study, which examined the medical, social, and economic consequences of adverse childhood experiences, linked certain childhood experiences with a large number of public health problems, including depression, substance abuse, sexually transmitted diseases, cancer, heart disease, chronic lung disease, and diabetes. The ACE study is an ongoing collaboration between the Centers for Disease Control and Prevention (CDC) and Kaiser Permanente and includes more than 17,000 participants. The adverse childhood experiences (ACEs) that are measured are those which occur in a household prior to age 18. They include the following: recurrent physical or emotional abuse; contact sexual abuse; the presence of an alcohol or drug abuser in the household; an incarcerated household member, someone who is chronically depressed, mentally ill, institutionalized, or suicidal; a mother who is treated violently; one or no parents; and emotional or physical neglect. As the number of ACEs a person experiences increases, the greater is the likelihood of the person becoming an IV drug user, attempting suicide, having coronary artery disease or liver disease, being a smoker, and abusing alcohol. The ACEs experienced during childhood are seen as reflecting exposure of the brain to cumulative stress that leads to impairment in multiple brain structures and functions (Anda et al., 2006). The brain impairment is said to change parts of the brain that mediate mood, anxiety, healthy bonding with others, memory, and where our bodies store fat. It could be argued that these brain areas are related to the development, in later life, of various mental illnesses. More specifically, ACE studies have found that the risk of an adult developing alcoholism and depression increases as the number of adverse childhood experiences increases (Dube, Anda, Felitti, Edwards, & Croft, 2002). Among adult children of alcoholics, depression appears to be largely due to having been raised in a home with alcohol-abusing parents and other ACEs (Anda et al., 2002; Chapman et al., 2004). Also of interest is the finding that prescription medication rates increased among study participants during yearly follow-up as the ACE score increased. This is understood to demonstrate a strong link between childhood experiences and adult mental illness (Anda et al., 2007). Although we need to keep in mind that the research conducted using the ACE scores demonstrates correlations between variables, and not causation, the findings from more than 50 studies do provide very compelling data about how brain development can be linked to mental illnesses. In a recent article written by the two original ACE Study researchers (Robert Anda & Vincent Felitti) the authors described how effective social work practice which prevents ACEs and focuses on resiliency can contribute to overall health improvements (Larkin, Felitti, & Anda, 2014).

The interface between neurobiology and mental illness has also been informed by our understanding of attachment theory, which has been greatly augmented by neuroscience research. We now know about the social nature of the human brain (Eisenberg, 1995), meaning that social relationships (via attachment) are necessary for the development of the brain. The attachment process allows the immature brain of the infant to use the mature brain of the parent to develop emotions (and social relationships) that are regulated. The social experience between caregiver and child shapes the way the brain develops. Fonagy and Target (2005) noted that attachment relationships of infancy serve an evolutionary purpose by ensuring that brain structures that mediate social cognition are adequately organized to make possible relationships with others. The close connection between two brains, which occurs during the attachment process, helps infants or young children to manage their own affective abilities (A. N. Schore, 2003). This is the sense in which attachment theory has shifted into affect and affect regulation. J. R. Schore and Schore (2008) refered to this dyadic regulation of affect as "regulation theory." And yet many of the clients of social workers do not have a secure attachment history, which impairs their affective and relationship abilities. Here again is a main reason why neurobiology serves as the missing link to more effective clinical practice. Longitudinal studies that followed children from infancy to late adolescence have found that disorganized attachment behaviors in infancy are precursors of later dissociative symptomatology and appear to be related to poor parent–infant affective communication (Main, 1996). Borderline disorders are also said to be related to disorganized attachment histories (Gergely, Fonagy, & Target, 2000). Conduct disorder, substance use disorders, narcissistic and antisocial personality disorders are associated with dismissing attachments. Mood disorders and obsessive–compulsive characteristics have been found to be associated with preoccupied attachments Additionally, a study of adolescents who were hospitalized at age 14 for mental illness were reviewed at age 25, and all displayed insecure attachment organization as adults (Dozier, Stovall, & Albus, 1999; Fonagy et al., 1996).

Knowing about brain structure and function provides relevant information for clinical practitioners, especially as this relates to stress and the relationship of stress to mental illness. We know that stress that is predictable and moderate can facilitate resiliency and enhance memory. However, when stress is severe and prolonged, it can damage the hippocampus (involved with memory storage, reality testing, and inhibition of the amygdala) and disrupt the immune system. Glucocorticoid hormones that are released as part of the body's stress response can disrupt immune and inflammatory responses, and cellular growth and reproduction (Cozolino, 2002). Trauma, especially early relational trauma, can be understood as an extreme kind of stress—an emotional/physical wound that is painful, distressful, or shocking, and a wound that can alter the cells, structure, and functioning of the brain. Brain areas disrupted by trauma are those involved in the child's responses to stress and fear (i.e., brain stem, hippocampus, amygdala, frontal cortex). To manage the severe stress, a child will engage in one of two response systems. The hyperarousal response leads to freeze/flight or fight, and the dissociative response leads to detachment, compliance, or being numb to abuse. These responses become imprinted in the right brain and change the brain's structure, which results in inadequate stress coping mechanisms. This damage to the right hemisphere, which is the seat of intuition, creativity, affect regulation, and emotion, results in a children (and later adults) who have great difficulty regulating their emotions. The ACE studies have demonstrated how childhood trauma can adversely affect the developing brain and lead to disrupted neurodevelopment. These early experiences have long-term effects on biological systems that govern one's response to stress, and they can create the necessary conditions for childhood and adult depression, anxiety, and post-traumatic stress symptoms.

Recent discoveries about a specialized kind of neurons called mirror neurons also help us to appreciate the interface between neurobiology and mental illnesses. Discovered in the 1990s in Italy, mirror neurons are a special type of visuo-motor neuron that make it possible for us to learn complex motor skills merely by watching others perform these same skills. Research on the mirror neuron system (MNS) is still in its early stages, but what is currently known is that the MNS links visual and motor experiences and makes possible implicit learning via imitation of what is seen, heard and felt (Grafton, Arbib, Fadiga, & Rizzolatti, 1996; Rizzolatti & Craighero, 2004). Mirror neurons are believed to be involved in the development of empathy and understanding the intentions of others. They are also believed to form the neural substrate for a theory of mind (ToM), which is defined as having an idea about what the other knows, wants, and is likely to do. By example, persons with autism may lack ToM and persons with schizophrenia may also lack a well-developed ToM. As a result, those with schizophrenia may misunderstand the intentions, goals, and beliefs of others, which can lead to inappropriate behavior toward others. Mirror neurons connect the observed and the observer, which creates the neural foundation for social interaction (Cozolino, 2006). They link us to each other, and it can be argued that our MNS is how attunement between client and clinician gets laid down in neural structure. Practice wisdom tells us that the relationship between client and clinician is considered to be the core feature of the helping process. Research corroborates this wisdom as studies on effective therapy have consistently concluded that the therapeutic alliance is the strongest positive factor (Bayliss, 2006; Butler & Strupp, 1986; Horvath & Symonds, 1991). It seems quite possible that our new knowledge about mirror neurons, and how they enhance our understanding of imitative learning, action, and intention understanding, provides some compelling reasons for why and how the therapeutic relationship is effective.

As we work with persons who have a mental illness, we need to keep in mind the possible help that psychotropic medications might provide to alleviate symptoms, but as social workers, our main task is to use our knowledge of brain plasticity and the clinical social work process. Cozolino (2002) noted that the integration of neural networks is essential for mental health because psychopathology results from problems with integration and coordination of these networks. The psychotherapeutic process is seen as the means through which neural network integration and coordination can be restored, since this process brings together emotion and cognition (right and left brain). This is the sense in which clinicians function as "neuro-architects." In other words, via the therapeutic relationship we can reshape our client's brain (we assist with the rewiring of our client's nervous system) (Siegel, 2006). Until the etiology of mental illnesses is discovered, the best we can do is to help clients manage their illness. Thinking about clients who struggle with depression, anxiety, borderline personality disorder, schizophrenia, and others it seems clear that what is frequently needed is assistance with self-regulation. As we return to our understanding of attachment theory postneuroscience, we see that the clinical relationship (which has always been at the core of what social workers do) makes possible a right brain-to-right brain experience.

Just as the right hemisphere of the brain develops first in the infant and is the location where the earliest bonds with another are formed, so in later life, the therapeutic relationship can enhance or replace the original attachment relationship, using the right brain and its continual development in adulthood. As we look at some of the newer therapeutic techniques being used by social workers, we can see more right brain workings, that is, mind–body therapies, guided imagery, relaxation response, meditation, journaling, stress reduction, and mindfulness. These techniques are examples of how the neurobiological, how we understand the workings of the brain, has become the psychosocial.

CONCLUSION

This article argues that the interface between psychotropic medications, neurobiology, and mental illnesses should be adequately recognized and understood by social workers. It has done so by discussing the consistency of such a claim with the policies of the NIMH, and with developments in psychopharmacology and neurobiology, and with understandings about mental illness and neurobiology. It is deepened by the inclusion of the BPSS perspective used by social workers.

The article shows that the interface between psychotropic medications, neurobiology, and mental illnesses is so close that the neurobiological becomes the psychosocial. It pointed to the crucial relevance of this interface to the practice of clinical social work.

REFERENCES

American Psychiatric Association (APA). (2013). *Diagnostic and statistical manual of mental disorders* (5th ed.). Arlington, VA: Author.

Anda, R. F., Brown, D. W., Felitti, V. J., Bremner, J. D., Dube, S. R., & Giles, W. H. (2007). Adverse childhood experiences and prescribed psychotropic medications in adults. *American Journal of Preventive Medicine, 32*(5), 389–394.

Anda, R. F., Felitti, V. J., Walker, J., Whitfield, C. L., Bremner, J. D., Perry, B. D., . . . Giles, W. H. (2006). The enduring effects of abuse and related adverse experiences in childhood: A convergence of evidence from neurobiology and epidemiology. *European Archives of Psychiatry and Clinical Neurosciences, 56*(3), 174–186.

Anda, R. F., Whitfield, C. L., Felitti, V. J., Chapman, D., Edwards, V. J., Dube, S. R., & Williamson, D. F. (2002). Adverse childhood experiences, alcoholic parents, and later risk of alcoholism and depression. *Psychiatric Services, 53*(8), 1001–1009.

Andreasen, N. C. (2001). *Brave new brain: Conquering mental illness in the era of the genome.* New York, NY: Oxford University Press.

Bayliss, P. J. (2006). The neurobiology of affective interventions: A cross theoretical mode. *Clinical Social Work Journal, 34*(1), 61–81.

Bell, V. (2013, October). Changing brains: Why neuroscience is ending the Prozac era. *Brain in the News*, 1–2.

Belluck, P., & Carey, B. (2013, May 6). Psychiatry's guide is out of touch with science, experts say. *The New York Times*. Retrieved from http://www.nytimes.com/2013/05/07/health/psychiatrys-new-guide-falls-short-experts-say.html?_r=0

Bentley, K. J. (2010). The meaning of psychiatric medication in a residential program for adults with serious mental illness. *Qualitative Social Work, 9*(4), 479–499.

Bentley, K. J., & Walsh, J. (2014). *The social worker and psychotropic medication*. Belmont, CA: Brooks/Cole.

Bentley, K. J., Walsh, J., & Farmer, R. L. (2005). Roles and activities of social workers with psychiatric medication: Results of a national survey. *Social Work, 50*, 295–303.

Bradley, S. J. (2000). *Affect regulation and the development of psychopathology*. New York, NY: Guilford.

Burroughs, V. J., Maxey, R. W., & Levy, R. A. (2002). Racial and ethnic differences in response to medicines: Towards individualized pharmaceutical treatment. *Journal of the National Medical Association, 94*(10, Suppl.), 1–26.

Butler, S., & Strupp, H. (1986). Specific and nonspecific factors in psychotherapy: A problematic paradigm for psychotherapy research. *Psychotherapy, 23*(1), 30–40.

Caley, C. F. (2011). Interpreting and applying CYP450 genomic test results to psychotropic medications. *Journal of Pharmacy Practice, 24*(5), 439–446.

Chapman, D. P., Whitfield, C. L., Felitti, V. J., Dube, S. R., Edwards, V. J., & Anda, R. F. (2004). Adverse childhood experiences and the risk of depressive disorders in adulthood. *Journal of Affective Disorders, 82*(2), 217–225.

Chen, C. H., Chen, C. U., & Lin, K. M. (2008). Ethnopsychopharmacology. *International Review of Psychiatry, 20*(5), 452–459.

Cozolino, L. J. (2002). *The neuroscience of psychotherapy: Building and rebuilding the human brain*. New York, NY: W.W. Norton.

Cozolino, L. J. (2006). *The neuroscience of human relationships: Attachment and the developing social brain*. New York, NY: W.W. Norton.

Daly, A. K., Brockmoller, J., Broly, F., Eichelbaum, M., Evans, W. E., Gonzalez, F. J., . . . Zanger, U. M. (1996). Nomenclature for human CYP2D6 alleles. *Pharmacogenetics, 6*, 193–201.

Dozier, M., Stovall, K. C., & Albus, K. (1999). Attachment and psychopathology in adulthood. In J. Cassidy & P. Shaver (Eds.), *The handbook of attachment theory* (pp. 648–673). New York, NY: Guilford Press.

Dube, S. R., Anda, R. F., Felitti, V. J., Edwards, V. J., & Croft, J. B. (2002). Adverse childhood experiences and personal alcohol abuse as an adult. *Addictive Behavior, 27*(5), 713–725.

Eisenberg, L. (1995). The social construction of the human brain. *American Journal of Psychiatry, 152*(11), 1563–1575.

Farmer, R. L. (2009). *Neuroscience and social work practice: The missing link*. Thousand Oaks, CA: Sage.

Floersch, J., Townsend, L., Longhofer, J., Munson, M., Winbush, V., Kranke, D., . . . Findling, R. L. (2009). Adolescent experience of psychotropic treatment. *Transcultural Psychiatry, 46*(1), 157–179.

Fonagy, P., Leigh, T., Steele, M., Steele, H., Kennedy, R., Mattoon, G., . . . Gerber, A. (1996). The relation of attachment status, psychiatric classification and response to psychotherapy. *Journal of Consulting, and Clinical Psychology, 64*(1), 22–31.

Fonagy, P., & Target, M. (2005). Bridging the transmission gap: An end to an important mystery of attachment research? *Attachment and Human Development, 7*(3), 333–343.

Friedman, R. A. (2013). Opinion: A dry pipeline for psychiatric drugs. *Brain in the News, 20*(7), 6–7.

Gergely, G., Fonagy, P., & Target, M. (2000). Attachment and borderline personality disorder: A theory and some evidence. *Psychiatric Clinics of North America, 23*(1), 103–123.

Grafton, S. T., Arbib, M. A., Fadiga, L., & Rizzolatti, G. (1996). Localization of grasp representation in humans by PET: 2. Observation compared with imagination. *Experimental Brain Research, 112*, 103–111.

Horvath, A., & Symonds, D. (1991). Relation between working alliance and outcome in psychotherapy: A meta-analysis. *Journal of Counseling Psychology, 38*(2), 139–149.

Hunter, R., Kennedy, E., Song, F., Gadon, L., & Irving, C. (2003). Risperidone versus typical antipsychotic medication for schizophrenia. *Cochrane Database of Systematic Reviews,* (2), CD000440. doi:10.1002/14651858.CD000440

Insel, T., Cuthbert, B., Garvey, M., Heinssen, R., Pine, D. S., Quinn, K., . . . Wang, P. (2010). Research domain criteria (RDoC): Toward a new classification framework for research on mental disorders. *American Journal of Psychiatry, 167*, 748–751.

Komossa, K., Rummel-Kluge, C., Hunger, H., Schwarz, H., Bhoopathi, P. S., Kissling, W., & Leucht, S. (2009, October 7). Ziprasidone versus other atypical antipsychotics for schizophrenia. *Cochrane Database of Systematic Reviews,* (4), CD006627. doi:10.1002/14651858.CO006627.pub2

Komossa, K., Rummel-Kluge, C., Schwarz, S., Schmid, F., Hunger, H., Kissling, W., & Leucht, S. (2011, January 19). Risperidone versus other atypical antipsychotics for schizophrenia. *Cochrane Database of Systematic Reviews,* (1), CD006626. doi:10.1002/14651858.CD006626.pub.2

Larkin, H., Felitti, V. J., & Anda, R. F. (2014). Social work and adverse childhood experiences research: Implications for practice and health policy. *Social Work Public Health, 29*(1), 1–16.

Lawson, W. B. (2000). Issues in pharmacotherapy for African Americans. In P. Ruiz (Ed.), *Ethnicity and psychopharmacology* (pp. 37–47). Washington, DC: American Psychiatric Press.

Lin, K. M., Smith, M. W., & Ortiz, V. (2001). Culture and psychopharmacology. *Psychiatric Clinics of North America, 24*(3), 523–538.

Lipton, B. (2005). *The biology of belief.* Santa Rosa, CA: Elite Books.

Luo, H. R., Poland, R. E., Lin, K. M., & Wan, Y. J. (2006). Genetic polymorphism of Cytochrome P450 2C19 in Mexican Americans: A cross-ethnic comparative study. *Clinical Pharmacology Therapeutics, 80*(1), 33–40.

Main, M. (1996). Introduction to the special section on attachment and psychopathology: Overview of the field of attachment. *Journal of Consulting and Clinical Psychology*, *64*(2), 237–243.

Malik, M., Lake, J., Lawson, W. B., & Joshi, S. V. (2010). Culturally adapted pharmacotherapy and the integrative formulation. *Child and Adolescent Psychiatric Clinics of North America*, *19*(4), 791–814.

Mendoza, R., Wan, Y. J., Poland, R. E., Smith, M., Zheng, Y., & Berman, N. (2001). CYP2D6 polymorphism in a Mexican American population. *Clinical Pharmacology and Therapeutics*, *70*(6), 552–560.

National Institute of Mental Health. (2013). *Research domain criteria (RDoC)*. Retrieved from http://www.nimh.nih.gov/research-priorities/rdoc/index.shtml

Pena, S. D. J. (2011). The fallacy of racial pharmacogenomics. *Brazilian Journal of Medical and Biological Research*, *44*(4), 268–275.

Piscitelli, S. C., Burstein, A. H., Chaitt, D., Alfaro, R. M., & Falloon, J. (2000). Indinavir concentrations and St. John's wort. *Lancet*, *355*, 547–548.

Restak, R. (2003). *The new brain*. Emmaus, PA: Rodale.

Rizzolatti, G., & Craighero, L. (2004). The mirror neuron system. *Annual Review of Neuroscience*, *27*, 169–192.

Sarris, J., Panossian, A., Schweitzer, I., Stough, C., & Scholey, A. (2011). Herbal medicine for depression, anxiety and insomnia: A review of psychopharmacology and clinical evidence. *European Neuropsychopharmacology*, *21*(12), 841–860.

Schore, A. N. (2003). *Affect dysregulation and disorders of the self*. New York, NY: W.W. Norton.

Schore, J. R., & Schore, A. N. (2008). Modern attachment theory. *Clinical Social Work Journal*, *36*(1), 9–20.

Siegel, D. J. (2006). An interpersonal neurobiology approach to psychotherapy. *Psychiatric Annals*, *36*(4), 248–256.

Smith, M. W. (2006). Ethnopsychopharmacology. In R. F. Lim (Ed.), *Clinical manual of cultural psychiatry* (pp. 207–235). Washington, DC: American Psychiatric Publishing.

Taupin, P. (2005). Adult neurogenesis in the mammalian central nervous system: Functionality and potential clinical interest. *Medical Science Monitor*, *11*(7), RA247–RA252.

Wing, Y. K., Chan, E., Chan, K., Lee, S., & Shek, C. C. (1997). Lithium pharmacokinetics in Chinese manic-depressive patients. *Journal of Clinical Psychopharmacology*, *17*(3), 179–184.

The Neurobiology of Substance Use Disorders: Information for Assessment and Clinical Treatment

SUSANNE BENNETT

National Catholic School of Social Service, The Catholic University of America, Washington, DC, USA

PATRICIA PETRASH

Institute of Contemporary Psychotherapy and Psychoanalysis, Washington, DC, USA

Neuroscientific research on substance use disorders (SUD) suggests addiction is a complex, multifactorial process, resulting in changes in brain circuits and the brain reward system. This article presents definitions and stages of addiction, highlights of known research on SUD's etiology, and an overview of empirically supported integrated approaches to treatment of persons with SUD. Applying current neuroscientific and outcome research to clinical treatment of a patient with alcohol use disorder, a case discussion illustrates the etiology of addiction and the importance of matching appropriate interventions to the patient's stage of addiction and evolving recovery needs. Special emphasis is placed on attending to the physiological cognitive symptoms evident in early recovery. Five recommendations are proposed for clinical treatment of SUD.

Neurobiological research on the study of addictions suggests that substance use disorders (SUD) emerge from a complex interplay of cognitive, behavioral, environmental, genetic, and physiological factors, which lead to underlying changes in brain circuits and the brain reward system (Koob,

2010; Pihl & Stewart, 2013). Since the founding of the National Institute on Alcohol Abuse and Alcoholism (NIAAA) more than 40 years ago, there has been increased emphasis on the effects of drugs and substances on brain functioning and on how neuroscience can inform clinical treatment (Koob, 2010). This wealth of research has led to information suggesting why some individuals develop an addiction, whereas others do not. Nevertheless, there is ongoing discussion about what neurobiology can and cannot tell us about addictions (Kalant, 2009), debate about whether addiction is a brain disease (Levy, 2013), and questions about how neurobiological research can inform best practices and explain treatment outcomes of persons with substance abuse disorders (Koob, 2010; Pihl & Stewart, 2013).

Nonmedical clinicians working with substance users often shy away from understanding the neurobiology of SUD and focus instead on treating common co-occurring behavioral disorders, such as trauma, depression, or anxiety. Some attempt to treat the psychosocial issues that accompany patients with SUD, without understanding the physiological complexities of addiction. Yet neuroscientists have conducted a massive amount of research over the last two decades on the etiology and course of SUD, particularly alcoholism, and this research is increasingly informing treatment. In this article, we present the highlights of current studies on the etiology of SUD, research on SUD treatment, and a case illustration of clinical intervention informed by this research for the treatment of alcohol use disorder (AUD). Definitions of substance use disorders and addiction begin this overview.

ADDICTION AND SUBSTANCE USE DISORDERS DEFINED

In the words of Pihl and Stewart (2013), "The definition of substance use disorders can be sweeping" (p. 242); that assessment is evident in the recent publication of *The Diagnostic and Statistical Manual of Mental Disorders* (5th ed. [*DSM-5*]; American Psychiatric Association [APA], 2013). The *DSM-5* has changed the nomenclature of SUD, dropping previous distinctions between *dependence* and *abuse* and merging these two definitions into a single disorder. Substance use disorders are based on patterns of pathological behaviors and four groupings of criteria (impaired control, social impairment, risky use, and pharmacological criteria). These criteria are related to the use of nine specific substance classes and are coded along a range of severity from mild (two to three symptoms), to moderate (four to five symptoms), to severe (six or more symptoms). In AUD, for example, anyone who meets two out of 11 criteria during a 12-month period is thought to have an AUD. Although there is considerable overlap between the *DSM-5* and earlier editions of the manual, the revised diagnostic terminology reflects recent research by adding *craving* and omitting *legal problems* as criteria. The *DSM-5* (APA,

2013) also removes the word *addiction* as part of the terminology "because of its uncertain definition and its potentially negative connotation" (p. 485).

Despite the elimination of the word addiction from the *DSM-5*, the term is common among clinicians and neuroscientists alike. Generally, *addiction* is defined as a physical dependence that develops through a repeated pattern of large doses of drugs that are self-administered, result in reinforcing psychoactive effects, and lead to difficulty in ceasing use despite the user's strong motivation (Kalant, 2009). Koob (2010), the current director of NIAAA, further defined alcoholism and addiction to other drugs as "a chronic, relapsing disorder" (p. 144) that includes three stages of an addictive process. The first stage is a binge-intoxication stage, in which increasing levels of alcohol and/or other drugs are needed for the brain to feel a positive reward. The second stage is the withdrawal-negative-affect stage, in which the user experiences negative consequences when the substance is discontinued. And, the third stage is the preoccupation-anticipated stage, when the substance user feels an exaggerated craving and motivation to continue substance use. Koob (2010) proposed that these three stages are each "associated with specific changes in the structure and function of various brain-signaling molecule (i.e., neurotransmitter) systems and in the circuits connecting various brain regions to relay information related to a specific function" (p. 144). It is because of these changes in the brain that a chronic substance user "eventually loses behavioral control over drug seeking and drug taking" (Koob, 2010, p. 144). NIAAA's emphasis on research into the underlying neuroscientific mechanisms of addictions has led to the development of new medications for the treatment of alcoholism and to the development of new models for understanding addiction as a brain disease.

Levy (2013) proposed that scientists aim to "elucidate the neuropsychological causes and correlates of addiction" to offer a "compassionate" view of addiction as "a disease that must be treated, not something for which addicts can be blamed" (p. 4). Although addiction clearly has an effect on specific neural pathways that lead to brain adaptation, he argued that it is "misleading" to state that addiction is a brain disease, because "addiction is a disorder of a person, embedded in a social context" (Levy, 2013, p. 4). This is not to say that the sufferer of the disorder is to blame, but that the social environment mediates the development of the disorder and the outcome of effective treatment. Levy (2013) stated, "If we are to understand addiction and respond appropriately to it, we must not focus on just the addicted individual herself, much less her brain. Our focus must be on her, in her social setting" (p. 6). Levy's view is congruent with the growing body of clinical evidence that there is a complex and strong relationship between AUD, stress, and anxiety, demonstrating the important link between social context and neurobiological factors (see Silberman et al., 2009, for overview).

Although we fully accept the importance of social context and believe that psychosocial factors serve as underpinnings or triggers of addictions, we wish to highlight the basic and applied literature on the neurobiology of SUD and the research on integrated treatment. Areas of neurobiological study have focused on the development of addictions (e.g., the role of genetics, the role of dopamine and the reward system, and the role of neurotransmitter signaling causing tolerance and cravings) and on how this body of research informs multidimensional approaches to treatment. The following findings emerge from these areas of study.

HIGHLIGHTS OF NEUROBIOLOGICAL RESEARCH

Research on Etiology of Addiction

GENETIC STUDIES

For centuries, it has been common knowledge that "alcoholism runs in families" (Kalant, 2009, p. 784), leading clinicians and persons with SUD to believe that addiction is genetically based. Indeed, family, twin, and adoption studies show that SUD has high hereditability and that genes play a role in one's risk for developing addictions (Pihl & Stewart, 2013). Studies estimate that 40% to 60% of an individual's vulnerability to addiction is due to genetic factors (National Institute of Drug Abuse [NIDA], 2010). However, Pihl and Stewart (2013) argued it is impossible to generalize these genetic findings, because biological markers vary from family to family and there have been hundreds, if not thousands, of genes identified as contributory to addictions, perhaps indirectly. Some of these genes, such as ones related to impulsivity, are evident in a number of other behavioral disorders and are not specific to addiction. Kalant (2009) also underscored that "a gene does not encode a trait," and genes "are not necessarily continuously active, i.e., they may be switched on ('expressed') or off under different circumstances" (p. 785).

Clearly, genetic factors are not the sole biological influence on substance use. Once a person begins using alcohol and/or other drugs, these substances affect nearly all brain neurotransmitters in complex ways not fully understood (G. Shean, personal communication, January 28, 2014). The following information describes some of the known neurochemical effects of substance use, yet this overview is inevitably oversimplified and subject to elaboration and revision as more knowledge becomes available.

DOPAMINE AND ITS EFFECT ON REWARDS

Dopamine is one of the neurotransmitters present in the numerous areas of the brain that regulate feelings of pleasure and reward, as well as emotion, cognition, motivation, and movement. Scientists now recognize that people take potentially addictive drugs because alcohol and other drugs (AOD) act on cells in the brain's limbic system, an action that leads to the release of dopamine and the subsequent experience of pleasure. This process is involved in the binge-intoxication stage of the cycle of addiction, mentioned earlier (Koob, 2010). Dopamine release motivates a first-time drug user to return to the experience, because the release results in euphoria, increased energy, and generally positive feelings (Kalant, 2009; NIDA, 2010). Although dopamine-containing cells in the brain are activated differentially based on the drug of abuse (e.g., opioid drugs, ethanol, cocaine, or amphetamines), the end result of dopamine activity in the prefrontal cortex of the brain is the same. In the brain's pleasure circuits, the natural rewards of eating and sex actually are dwarfed by the large amount of dopamine produced by drugs of abuse (NIDA, 2010). When dopamine floods the brain circuits, particularly through drugs that are ingested or smoked, the effects also last longer than natural rewards, providing further motivation for repeated use.

CELLULAR SIGNALING AND ITS EFFECT ON TOLERANCE AND CRAVINGS

Alcohol and other drugs are known to have major effects on the normal communication and functioning of the billions of neurons (e.g., individual nerve cells) in the brain (NIDA, 2010). When AODs affect neural functioning, cells attempt to restore equilibrium by adapting in an opposite manner (Kalant, 2009). For example, dopamine surges caused by AODs eventually result in abnormally lower levels of dopamine in the brain, causing the abuser to feel listless. As a result, the individual takes increasing amounts of the drug to boost the dopamine level (NIDA, 2010). These adaptive changes tend to gradually increase tolerance and physical dependence to overcome the effects of the drug's withdrawal.

During this stage of addiction, the body's hypothalamic-pituitary-adrenal (HPA) response (e.g., the stress-response system) is activated (Koob, 2010). When the normal response of the HPA is disrupted because of alcohol and other drugs, dopamine activity decreases and the hypothalamus or pituitary in the brain's limbic system is activated, releasing a molecule called corticotropin-releasing factor (CRF). Eventually, cycles of drinking and withdrawal lead to a weaker HPA response and a more sensitive CRF stress system (Koob, 2010), creating the withdrawal-negative affect stage of addiction. Acute withdrawal reactions occur when the drug is removed suddenly through a receptor blocker. In other words, the brain's adaptive changes create signaling cascades, defined as neurotransmitter molecular events. Over time, the development of tolerance can compromise the brain's long-term health and cognitive functioning, through significant changes in neurons and brain circuits (NIDA, 2010).

Signal transmissions that use the neurotransmitter glutamate also cause brain circuits in several parts of the brain to be affected (Koob, 2010), including the prefrontal cortex, which is the most evolved structure of the brain, affecting behaviors and regulating executive functioning; the amygdala, which affects emotional processing; the insula, which affects disgust; and the hippocampus, which affects memory formation and recall. When AOD use decreases the amount of glutamate needed by the brain, the result is impaired cognitive functioning, problems with learning and memory, and, eventually, uncontrollable cravings (NIDA, 2010). Sound judgment and self-control are eroded, moving the user into the preoccupation-anticipation stage of addiction. At this point, users discover it is extremely challenging to stop using AODs, despite motivation or good intentions. Furthermore, long-term use of alcohol and other drugs has been found to lead to adaptations in a person's conditioned habits. For example, environmental cues that are reminders of past experiences can trigger cravings, even without the drug being present. Scientists have found that "This learned 'reflex' is extremely robust and can emerge even after many years of abstinence" (NIDA, 2010, p. 20). In other words, the changes to the brain caused by alcohol and other drugs remain, long after an individual stops using the substance.

MULTIFACTORIAL INTERACTIONS

Although acknowledging the importance of specific empirical findings emerging from neuroscience, researchers urge caution to avoid a reductionist viewpoint, because of the complexity of neurobiological processes and the multiplicity of factors that trigger neural mechanisms. Many researchers are currently taking a modular approach to understanding the brain, recognizing that the function of a brain region is not due to a specific brain abnormality but to interactions of various brain patterns in a complex network (Shean, 2010). For example, the neurobiological deficits scientists believe are related to AOD are probably distributed throughout many, if not all, areas of the brain, rather than in one localized region. Furthermore, understanding the mechanisms of how one neuron is linked to another and how that mechanism is altered through drug use helps to explain how changes occur in neural functioning, but not why the changes occur (Kalant, 2009). The reward system is actually "a convenient label rather than literal fact, and it provides no insight into the reasons why some drug users become addicted while the great majority of users . . . never pass from use to compulsive use" (Kalant, 2009, p. 784). Numerous other neurotransmitters beside glutamate also interact with dopamine in a complex manner, leading to different cognitive experiences and positive and negative reinforcing effects over time. Finally, it is critical to note that genetic vulnerabilities interact with environmental factors, such as stress, to lead to addiction. In other words, Kalant (2009) said, addiction is "a behavioral disorder generated within an extremely complex interactive system of drug, individual use, environment and changing circumstances. This is no longer the terrain of pharmacology or neurobiology or psychology or sociology, but an amalgam of all of them" (p. 786). Pihl and Stewart (2013) agreed that neurobiological research confirms that SUD is a "multifactorial, multilevel, interactional process" (p. 256) and has "a potentially large number of distinct etiological pathways" (p. 251). They stated, "Complexity is the rule. Which drug, used how and how much, with whom, under what conditions, and most significantly, by whom, all impact the course of the disorder" (Pihl & Stewart, 2013, p. 244).

Clearly, this complex interaction of factors is compounded in co-occurring conditions, such as SUD and major depression (Niciu et al., 2009), SUD and anxiety disorders (Silberman et al., 2009), and SUD and trauma (Brady, Back, & Coffey, 2004). According to Brady et al. (2004), epidemiological studies reveal a particularly high prevalence of SUD among individuals with PTSD; 36% to 50% of individuals seeking treatment for SUD have a lifetime prevalence of PTSD, and 25% to 42% have post-traumatic stress disorder (PTSD) at the time of treatment. Longitudinal studies on the PTSD–SUD link suggest that people use substances to escape painful symptoms by self-medicating. With growing evidence that strong neurobiological commonalities exist between the two disorders, the question is whether chronic substance abuse causes changes in the physiological pathways that then make an individual susceptible to PTSD, or if traumatic experiences, especially in early childhood, make an individual more vulnerable to SUD (Brady et al., 2004). Understanding the interaction of these dynamic processes has implications for treatment.

Research on Treatment of Addictions

PSYCHOPHARMACOLOGY

Just as there are multiple, interactive pathways leading to addiction, there are numerous interventions that address these different pathways. Research on psychopharmacology and brain circuitry suggests a number of medications that are effective for treatment of SUD. Disulfiram, commonly known as antabuse, is a well-known medication that provides aversive treatment for persons with chronic alcoholism (Pihl & Stewart, 2013). It blocks the body's processing of alcohol by causing an unpleasant reaction when alcohol is consumed. The patient experiences nausea, elevated heart rate and respiration, and vomiting—similar to the effects of a severe hangover. A second major biological treatment is antagonist treatment, medications that cancel cravings and the pleasurable effects of the abused substance by blocking the release of dopamine. One such medication is Naltrexone, which is supported by NIAAA clinical trials (Koob, 2010) and is reportedly most effective when used in conjunction with psychotherapeutic treatment approaches. The third form of biological treatment is agonist substitution, which offers a similar drug as a substitute for the more harmful abused drug. Methodone is an example of an agonist substitution used in the treatment of opiate dependence, whereas nicotine gum or patches are examples used in the treatment of cigarette smoking (Pihl & Stewart, 2013). Other medications may be used to manage withdrawal symptoms during detoxification. Acamprosate is an Food and Drug Administration (FDA)-approved medication for treating alcohol dependence to reduce symptoms that accompany withdrawal, such as irritability, depression, restlessness, and anxiety (NIDA, 2009). Although researchers are actively engaged in developing effective biological treatments for SUD, Koob (2010) pointed out that "none of the existing medications are effective in all patients, and additional agents need to be identified and developed that allow for effective treatment of additional patient subgroups" (p. 149).

SOCIAL CONTEXT INTERVENTIONS

Structured "12-Step" self-help groups such as Alcoholic Anonymous (AA) or Narcotics Anonymous (NA) have long been considered "the most popular model for the treatment of substance abuse" (Pihl & Stewart, 2013, p. 261). These 12-Step programs provide participants with needed structure and behavioral techniques that address re-learning and ways to avoid triggers. In addition, 12-Step self-help groups attend to social context, one of the central factors interacting with other variables in the development of addiction (Levy, 2013). The groups reinforce the importance of friends, family members, and feeling a part of a social community of people who share the struggle of recovering from SUD. Research suggests that group treatment (professionally-led and 12-Step groups) forms the most prevalent treatment approach for SUD (Weiss, Jaffee, de Menil, & Cogley, 2004). An analysis of 24 treatment outcome studies on the effectiveness of group treatment for SUD showed no differences in effectiveness between group and individual treatment or between types of group therapy. However, there was some indication from these studies that the effectiveness of "treatment as usual" was enhanced by the addition of specialized group therapy.

INDIVIDUAL PSYCHOTHERAPY

Motivational Interviewing (MI) and Cognitive-Behavioral Treatment (CBT) are two of several forms of individual psychotherapy that have been shown to be effective for particular stages of substance use or for persons with SUD and co-occurring disorders. MI is a collaborative, person-centered model of practice that is an empirically validated intervention considered effective for SUD treatment (Substance Abuse and Mental Health Services Administration [SAMHSA], 2013a). MI is especially beneficial in the early stages of treatment for persons who have co-occurring disorders and may not accept they have SUD, such as someone who is self-medicating with alcohol due to anxiety or bereavement. Nonconfrontational, MI methods enable the clinician to build a therapeutic relationship while assessing and exploring the patient's understanding and/or acceptance of the disorder. MI may be used alone, but research suggests it is most effective for treating SUD when it is a prelude to other forms of treatment or used in conjunction with them (Pihl & Stewart, 2013).

Once a patient accepts that he or she has a SUD and is motivated to change, CBT is often used to address the distorted thinking that accompanies substance abuse and behaviors that lead to addiction. Based on learning theory, CBT is designed to enhance coping skills, increase self-efficacy, and alter thought processes about the risks and rewards of substance use. CBT is beneficial in helping patients deal with stress, a major factor that interacts with neurobiological variables and triggers cravings. According to Pihl and Stewart (2013), "CBT is among the most effective commonly employed treatments for alcohol use disorders" and "there is mounting evidence for the efficacy of CBT in the treatment of nicotine dependence" (p. 260).

INTEGRATED TREATMENT AND TREATMENT MATCHING

The interaction of neurobiological factors with psychosocial factors supports interventions that combine psychopharmacology, social context interventions, and various forms of individual psychotherapy. Integrated treatment is especially critical for individuals who have co-occurring mental and substance abuse disorders. One treatment model called integrated treatment for co-occurring disorders is an empirically supported intervention supported by SAMHSA (2013b) for the treatment of co-occurring mental and substance use disorders. This model incorporates multiple approaches, including MI, CBT, and 12-Step groups, and is considered a "stage-wise treatment." Based on the belief that individuals go through different stages in the recovery process (e.g., engagement, persuasion, active treatment, and relapse prevention), the model recognizes that interventions should be matched to the recovery needs of the particular patient.

Other studies on treatment integration have examined matching to the particular co-occurring disorders, such as SUD and PTSD, in addition to the stages of recovery. For example, Brady et al. (2004) reported some evidence of the effectiveness of integrated treatment that attends to PTSD and SUD simultaneously, rather than individually, regardless of the patient's stage of recovery. This is in contrast to the traditional view that single-model therapies or sequential therapies (e.g., first for SUD, then for PTSD) work best. Although exposure-based PTSD therapy has been supported as effective in helping patients confront memories or situations that remind them of the trauma, until recently, exposure-based therapy was not considered beneficial for patients with PTSD and SUD due to concern about precipitating relapse for the patient.

THE ROLE OF ATTACHMENT PROCESSES IN TREATMENT

Finally, it is well known that attachment plays a major role in affect regulation, interpersonal functioning, and the structural development of the hippocampus during the first three years of life (Allen, 2001; Mikulincer & Shaver, 2007); that early attachment relationships are associated with adult attachment styles and relational patterns (Cassidy & Shaver, 2008); and that interpersonal relationships and subjective experiences affect memories, emotion, and self-regulation throughout life (Siegel, 2007, 2012). Difficulties with emotion regulation also are associated with substance abuse (Dozier, Stovall-McClough, & Albus, 2008), and Flores (2004) has called addiction an attachment disorder. Similarly, in AA, it is said that alcoholism is a disease of isolation. Although no known studies have evaluated a specific attachment-based treatment model for SUD treatment, several findings about attachment-informed treatment are relevant to this discussion (Slade, 2008).

Attachment research on adult treatment in general suggests that patients with insecure working models of attachment are more likely to form insecure specific attachments to their therapists, which can be challenging for therapists who often begin to match the style of the patient. Yet research suggests that therapists who are secure and can respond flexibly and counter to their patients' styles yield better treatment outcomes (Mikulincer & Shaver, 2007). In other words, a secure therapist ideally should use cognitive interventions when faced with an insecure anxious, preoccupied patient and use emotionally focused interventions with an insecure dismissing patient. Responding counter to the patient's insecure attachment style enables the patient to begin to establish an earned security, that is, to transition from insecure to secure attachment. Based on findings from their study on attachment and affect regulation among substance abusers, Thorberg and Lyvers (2010) suggested that a goal of SUD treatment should be to enable patients to establish earned attachment security by revising the patient's internal working model for attachment.

Finally, many scholars and clinicians (Doctors, 2008; Fonagy, 2003; Schore, 2002; Slade, 2008) have integrated attachment theory with self-psychology to inform clinical practice, and several have written about the treatment of substance use disorders through self-psychological methods of intervention. Attuned to the substance abuser's stage of recovery, self-psychologists Ulman and Paul (1989) proposed that clinicians should "make abstinence and sobriety basic treatment issues in the initial phase of therapy" (p. 131), because this emphasis is ultimately empathic to the patient's needs. In the following case discussion of a patient with AUD, we illustrate attunement to the patient's initial phase of therapy, her need for affect regulation, and the attachment processes that unfold within the therapeutic relationship. The clinical approach presented is based on a model of practice informed by attachment theory and self-psychology, as well as attunement to the patient's evolving recovery needs and the neurobiology of addictions.

APPLICATION TO CLINICAL PRACTICE

The Case of Cheryl

A 30-year-old professional, Cheryl was referred to me (P. Petrash) for psychotherapy by a counselor from her professional organization following a "Driving Under the Influence" (DUI). The counselor initially referred her to AA, but Cheryl was finding it impossible to connect with the program. Uncomfortable in AA meetings, she was unable to hear or benefit from what was being said, could not connect with people in the meetings, and would flee meetings as soon as possible. The counselor recognized that Cheryl needed additional psychotherapy to optimize her treatment of chronic AUD.

At the time of our first interview, Cheryl had been sober several months. What immediately impressed me was her overall presentation. She wore a beautiful designer suit with carefully coordinated stockings that were marred by a large hole in them. I thought to myself that it was too bad she had a "run" in her stockings, but in future meetings, she continued to wear the same stockings with an increasingly larger hole. I wondered how someone could wear such elegant, expensive suits and choose to put on torn stockings. Did she not notice? The second striking feature in her presentation was her voice. Although she spoke about her family as "okay" and described family life as "uneventful," her voice sounded as if someone was trying to strangle her. What was the source of her anxiety? Did she know she was anxious? Finally, Cheryl spoke of her graduate school accomplishments and subsequent career successes, yet she seemed unable to figure out the most basic problems of daily living. I noted the discrepancy between her considerable intelligence and intellectual accomplishments, in contrast to her lack of problem solving ability and, quite frankly, daily living skills.

Cheryl was the oldest of four children born to her mother over the course of 6 years. She described her father as "bright," mentioning his having earned a PhD. The example she gave of her mother as a "good mother" was that "she cooked us a good dinner every night." Reportedly, neither parent was alcoholic, but her mother's sister and several other relatives on her mother's side of the family were alcoholic. Her childhood was "uneventful" until she was in junior high school and the family moved from the Midwest to the West Coast. Afterwards, she felt she never fit in and became isolated. She turned to food for comfort and proceeded to gain 60 pounds, though her mother failed to notice her weight. I noted she did not mention people as a resource.

Cheryl's parents severed ties with her upon graduation from college, expecting her to be independent. Subsequently, she had her first drink following her first panic attack during the process of leaving home. Alcohol proved to be the perfect antidote to her anxiety. For the first time in her life, Cheryl felt "okay" and like "my shoulders dropped." Not surprisingly, her drinking quickly escalated. She found she had a high tolerance and was capable of out-drinking many of her peers. Using alcohol to medicate her anxiety, her functioning improved for a period of time. She was able to begin dating, complete graduate school, and start a career. However, in fewer than 10 years, her increasing tolerance led to dependence and craving. At the time of her DUI, she was drinking up to a fifth a day, in a struggle to avoid symptoms of withdrawal.

Our initial work together focused on the concrete issues of self-care and on how to relate in an AA meeting. "Do I talk or not talk?" "What do I do if someone invites me for coffee?" "Do I go to a meeting if I am going to be late?" "Have I eaten?" "Am I tired?" As a self-psychological and relationally oriented therapist, I felt drawn to an empathically oriented approach, identifying and responding to her selfobject needs. Clearly, she needed me to be an active participant who would provide her with concrete information, answers to her questions, and directions about issues of daily living—a process that has been described as a "selfobject in action, rather than one merely in thought or fantasy" (Ulman & Paul, 1992, p. 123). Eventually, someone in an AA meeting chose Cheryl as her sponsee, although a new member typically chooses her own sponsor. For Cheryl, the experience of being claimed by her sponsor was initially helpful as it bypassed her inability to ask someone for help. Her sponsor embraced the role of providing information, direction, and problem solving—also functioning as a selfobject in action. She told Cheryl which meetings to attend and then would meet her there and sit with her. Her sponsor was repeatedly reminding her of the AA slogans like "keep coming back," "one day at a time," or "go to a meeting."

With that provision from her sponsor, I broadened my responses to include understanding and mirroring her internal experiences. I was struck by the discrepancy between her facility with language in her professional capacity and her inability to put her emotional life into words. I had to take an active role, asking questions, offering my description of her experience, and clarifying if my mirroring fit for her. Cheryl gradually began to internalize these reflections with me, resulting in her increased self-regulation and self-care. She also began to feel connected to the program and several people in it. Yet eventually, as she remained sober and her sense of self began to consolidate, she came to resent the total accommodation required by her sponsor and wished to begin making some of her own decisions. Her desire for autonomy precipitated an irreparable rupture with her sponsor. At that point, her connection to me, including my mirroring of her wish for autonomy and her frustration with her sponsor, enabled her to remain in the program and to find a more appropriate, collaborative sponsor.

After her support system was solidly in place to maintain a more advanced recovery, we began to focus on her attachment issues. Several major themes emerged from our discussions, which are especially relevant to understanding her functioning and treatment needs. Minimizing her need and affect, she had presented with an avoidant attachment strategy. But, what became clear was that her experience of early developmental trauma was continuous and resulted in a pattern of disorganized attachment. She expanded her description of her mother with a casual and telling remark: "My mother never made eye contact." Although her mother performed household functions adequately, her limited caregiving responses were traumatizing, leaving Cheryl without the needed vitalizing and soothing responses necessary for the development of a coherent sense of self. As an illustration, Cheryl recalled being hospitalized at age 6 with mononucleosis, reflecting her massive depletion and exhaustion from her efforts to deny her feelings and needs. She remembered her mother visiting her in the hospital, but after seeing the terrified look in her mother's eyes, she told her mother not to visit again. Her mother complied.

As therapy continued to unfold, Cheryl explored her past development and the stressors that triggered her anxiety and alcohol abuse. After many years of treatment, she appropriately terminated her psychotherapy while remaining actively involved in AA. Eventually she also began attending Alanon, a 12-Step program that provided a forum for her to continue to learn how to function in relationships. Cheryl was able to stay sober without relapsing and eventually married someone who provided the interpersonal relationship and support she had not experienced as a child.

Discussion of Cheryl's Treatment

Although Cheryl's experiences are unique to her life course, the development of her addiction and her early recovery are common processes. We present her story to illustrate two main points about the neurobiology of addictions. First, we wish to emphasize that the etiology of SUD is complicated and multifactorial and, second, that therapeutic techniques must match the patient's stage of recovery. With that in mind, we stress that the physiological symptoms of addiction must be the primary focus of early treatment, as Cheryl's recovery demonstrates.

ETIOLOGY OF ADDICTION

Similar to many individuals with SUD, Cheryl was born into a family with a history of alcoholism, perhaps making her genetically vulnerable to developing the disorder when she discovered alcohol's capacity to soothe her anxiety. She may have been genetically predisposed to anxiety as well, and her early attachment traumas compromised the development of her self-regulatory and self-care capacities, creating significant vulnerabilities to anxiety and dysregulation. Her unfolding family narrative was replete with stories of separation and loss, loneliness and fear, and maternal indifference and abandonment. Without doubt, her mother's lack of attuned responsiveness contributed to Cheryl's difficulties, leaving her struggling to manage her internal states through dissociation. When we think about the strangled voice she had when she began therapy, we are reminded of Tronick's "Still Face" experiments (Zero to Three, 2007) of the baby's frustrated struggle and ultimate collapse in the face of a nonexpressive mother. This picture is reminiscent of Cheryl's depleted, empty self-experience and the fragmentation of being caught between protest and despair.

We also were struck by the story of the young Cheryl in the hospital. It is understandable that a mother would be frightened visiting her small sick child in the hospital. But, to not return in response to the child's reassurance that she was "okay" reflected a level of fearful anxiety associated with a caregiver who had a disorganized attachment. Cheryl's sparse, concrete language about her mother (e.g., good, because she cooked good meals) revealed interpersonal avoidance and a lack of awareness about her childhood neglect, cues of dismissing attachment. Her language was intermittently incoherent, suggesting signs of disorganized attachment as well, paralleling her mother's attachment. Indeed, the theme of a mother and child relationship marked by incoherence and disorganization was rampant in Cheryl's stories, culminating with the cut-off that a frightened Cheryl felt when she left home, triggering panic and her first use of alcohol to medicate her anxiety. She learned to cope with her anxious fear throughout life by cutting off her affect and expression of need.

In other words, the etiology of Cheryl's addiction seemed to emerge from the interaction of genetic factors that became activated by her early attachment disorganization, making her more vulnerable to stress and loss as she moved into adulthood. Although insecure attachment does not exist for all persons with SUD, the link between attachment disorganization and substance abuse appeared prevalent in Cheryl's case. Alcohol use helped her block the dysregulated affect associated with her disorganization, and she withdrew into alcohol as a means of survival. Although the neurobiological changes caused by alcohol intake are too complex to fully understand, we can assume that the pleasure from the drug-induced dopamine surges became addictive for Cheryl because the pleasure blunted her pain. It is thought that her alcohol use eventually led to decreased dopamine levels and a weakened, more sensitive stress–response system. This phenomenon in turn created increased tolerance for alcohol, uncontrollable cravings, and significant deficits in her cognitive functioning.

THERAPEUTIC MATCHING

Cheryl's story further demonstrates the importance of understanding a patient's level or stage of addiction and matching that knowledge with appropriate treatment. When she was first referred to therapy, the prefrontal cortex of her brain was severely impaired by acute alcoholism, causing damage to her executive functioning. The drug that served initially to regulate anxiety left her in a constant dysregulated state due to physiological adaptation. As a result, she had abnormally low levels of dopamine—a reaction to alcohol-induced dopamine surges—leaving her listless and tired. The effects of the early developmental trauma further compromised her executive functioning. Cheryl really did not know what to do. The hole in her stockings (matched with designer suits) was just one small example of her impaired judgment, her lack of body awareness, and even her inability to think flexibly to address a problem. She literally needed someone to tell her what to do to function on a daily level.

It was important to match Cheryl's cognitive deficits with a form of treatment that would rebuild her executive functioning and increase her cognitive skills. AA provided the necessary structure and behavioral approach that her cognitive impairments required at that time. For the first two years of recovery, she needed simple, consistent, and repetitive directions to rebuild cognitive skills she lost due to the damage to her brain. Over time, the structure and skill building that AA provided served as a secure base-safe haven for Cheryl. In terms of psychotherapy, Cheryl's cognitive impairments and limited functioning required a supportive, nonconfrontational form of treatment that complemented the messages she was receiving in AA. As Cheryl's experiences were reflected and her affect and words were mirrored, she eventually began to use the therapist as a secure base as well.

We wish to emphasize that the initial approach to treatment integrated cognitive and behavioral techniques to help Cheryl learn new coping skills for dealing with anxiety and maintaining her sobriety. This approach tended to the physiological symptoms of early sobriety and focused on increasing her executive functioning skills, such as judgment, thought processes, and impulse control. It took several years of sobriety and ongoing AA involvement for Cheryl to develop enough cognitive improvement and regulatory capacity to tolerate a more in depth exploration of her life history. The therapist could not address the underlying attachment issues that influenced Cheryl's alcohol use until she learned new ways of managing her stress and the physiological symptoms of her addiction were no longer overwhelming her daily functioning. By the time Cheryl terminated psychotherapy, she had developed a state of earned attachment security, because she had resolved the loss and trauma of her childhood and no longer needed alcohol to mask the painful memories of her past. Despite her significant therapeutic gains, however, she understood that the permanent physiological changes caused by her addiction prevented her from being able to safely drink alcohol again.

SUGGESTIONS AND CONCLUSION

This case discussion and the neurobiological research presented earlier support the value of using a multidimensional framework for understanding the etiology and treatment of substance use disorders. In addition, the context of psychotherapy—the social context and reason for referral, the patient's interpersonal capacities, the patient's acceptance of the disorder, and the quality of the therapeutic relationship—determines how best to intervene. Keeping this context in mind, we summarize our approach by suggesting the following guidelines we find beneficial for treating patients with alcohol use disorder.

1. Keeping in mind the progression of the addiction, evaluate the patient's stage of substance use and encourage a thorough medical exam. This intervention helps the nonmedical clinician discern the necessity of medication and the appropriate intensity of treatment. Initially, patients in advanced stages of addiction often require ongoing medical supervision to undergo a medically safe detoxification. This can occur in the form of hospitalization, a residential 30-day program, or a structured outpatient day treatment program.
2. Provide structured, active, and direct supportive interventions, especially in the initial stages of recovery; encourage patients to participate in a 12-Step self-help group or a formal treatment program in addition to individual psychotherapy. Based on the level of impairment, the clinician should provide the level of support required to facilitate someone attending a group meeting. If necessary, go with patients to open 12-Step meetings to help them begin the process; use multiple providers, collaborating with all who provide care; and employ multiple treatment modalities, such as group and individual treatment. Such direction and structure provides compensation for the patient's inadequate and damaged cognitive abilities, whereas group and family modalities address the importance of social context. Patients in early recovery do not have the neurocognitive capacities to engage in unstructured, interpretive dynamic treatment.
3. Assess the patient's history of substance use within the context of the patient's family development and the family's substance use, as well as the patient's historical patterns of dealing with stress. This intervention incorporates knowledge that patients often have hereditary vulnerabilities and that stress activates genetic traits. History taking helps to sensitize patients to the connection between their minds and their bodies and to become aware of triggers for relapse. For example, many patients relapse following loss, the death of a loved one, or a particularly stressful work situation, and they must learn new methods of coping with such stress.
4. Use multiple models of individual intervention (e.g., cognitive, behavioral, relational, motivational interviewing) that are interactive, focused on the present, and match what works best with the patient's particular stage of recovery and co-occurring issues. Many patients in early recovery need

clinicians to employ more structured CBT interventions to enhance their cognitive skills and to learn behavioral techniques for managing anxiety and stress. Still other patients may be sufficiently stable physiologically that they can tolerate relational methods of intervention to treat the psychosocial underpinnings of their substance use. Note, however, that no one method is appropriate for all SUD patients at all stages of recovery. When addressing co-occurring issues (e.g., trauma, depression, anxiety), maintain focus on physiological symptoms and triggers for substance use or relapse. For example, most patients are prone to distancing or dissociation when dealing with their complex trauma history, and it becomes essential to keep them focused on the present to avoid retraumatization and relapse.

5. Attend to the patient's extended social context through family or couple's interventions; group interventions; and AA, NA, and Alanon. Although difficulty in spousal or family relationships is a certainty, it is often beneficial for the family members of the patient in early recovery to engage in treatment separate from the identified patient due to the patient's cognitive impairment and reactivity. Groups for family members or Alanon can be particularly beneficial. Such interventions provide support and education for the patient and the patient's significant others and may increase the partner or family's awareness of how they sometimes trigger the patient's repeated use. It is especially important to educate patients and their families regarding the chronic nature of substance use disorders and how relapse may be prevented through awareness of personal triggers and specific methods to address them. Finally, 12-Step groups are vital because they help patients develop friendships and a sense of belonging to a social community, which lessens shame about addiction and reinforces hope that recovery is feasible. Twelve-Step groups also provide the skill building and structure that is essential for early recovery.

We believe these multidimensional guidelines attend to the complex, yet dynamic needs of patients who have SUD. Clinicians should provide treatment that is attuned to the relational needs of these patients, because they often have histories of significant loss, trauma, and disorganized attachments. Further, clinicians who are sensitively attuned to the particular environmental, behavioral, and psychosocial factors shaping patient capacities will be more likely to establish a secure base for treatment and maintain a therapeutic working alliance. However, it is essential to take note of the neurobiological factors influencing the patient's stage of addiction as well, because these factors shape the patient's cognitive abilities and capacities for treatment. With these multiple factors in mind, the unfolding therapeutic process should match the patient's functioning and level of substance use disorder—be it early recovery or long-term abstinence.

REFERENCES

Allen, J. (2001). *Traumatic relationships and serious mental disorders*. New York, NY: John Wiley & Sons.

American Psychiatric Association. (2013). *Diagnostic and statistical manual of mental disorders* (5th ed.). Arlington, VA: American Psychiatric Publishing.

Brady, K., Back, S., & Coffey, S. (2004). Substance abuse and post-traumatic stress disorder. *American Psychological Association, 13*, 206–209.

Cassidy, J., & Shaver, P. (Eds.). (2008). *Handbook of attachment: Theory, research, and clinical applications* (2nd ed.). New York, NY: Guilford Press.

Doctors, S. (2008). Notes on incorporating attachment theory and research into self psychological and intersubjective clinical work. *International Journal of Psychoanalytic Self Psychology, 3*, 34–49. doi:10.1080/15551020701743451

Dozier, M., Stovall-McClough, C., & Albus, K. (2008). Attachment and psychopathology in adulthood. In J. Cassidy & P. Shaver (Eds.), *Handbook of attachment: Theory, research, and clinical applications* (2nd ed., pp. 718–744). New York, NY: Guilford Press.

Flores, P. J. (2004). *Addiction as an attachment disorder*. New York, NY: Jason Aronson.

Fonagy, P. (2003). The development of psychopathology from infancy to adulthood: The mysterious unfolding of disturbance in time. *Infant Mental Health Journal, 24*, 212–239. doi:10.1002/imhj.10053

Kalant, H. (2009). What neurobiology cannot tell us about addiction. *Addiction, 105*, 780–789. doi:10.1111/j.1360-0443.2009.02739.x

Koob, G. (2010). The potential of neuroscience to inform treatment. *Alcohol Research & Health, 33*(1/2), 144–151.

Levy, N. (2013). Addiction is not a brain disease (and it matters). *Frontiers in Psychiatry, 4*(24), 1–7. doi:10.3389/fpsyt.2013.00024

Mikulincer, M., & Shaver, P. (2007). *Attachment in adulthood: Structure, dynamics, and change*. New York, NY: Guilford Press.

National Institute on Drug Abuse. (2009). *Drug facts: Treatment approaches for drug addiction*. Retrieved from http://www.drugabuse.gov/publications/drugfacts/treatment-approaches-drug-addiction

National Institute on Drug Abuse. (2010). *Drugs, brains, and behavior: The science of addiction* (NIH Pub No. 10-5605). Washington, DC: National Institutes of Health, U.S. Department of Health and Human Services. Retrieved from http://www.drugabuse.gov/publications/science-addiction

Niciu, M., Chan, G., Gelernter, J., Arias, A., Douglas, K., Weiss, R., . . . Kranzler, R. (2009). Subtypes of major depression in substance dependence. *Addiction, 104*, 1700–1709. doi:10.1111/j.1360-0443.2009.02672.x

Pihl, R., & Stewart, S. (2013). Substance use disorders. In L. Castonguay & T. Oltmanns (Eds.), *Psychopathology: From science to clinical practice* (pp. 241–274). New York, NY: Guilford Press.

Schore, A. (2002). Advances in neuropsychoanalysis, attachment theory, and trauma research: Implications for self psychology. *Psychoanalytic Inquiry, 22*, 433–485. doi:10.1080/07351692209348996

Shean, G. D. (2010). *Recovery from schizophrenia: Etiological and evidence-based treatments*. New York, NY: Hindawi Publishing.

Siegel, D. (2007). *The mindful brain: Reflection and attunement in the cultivation of well-being.* New York, NY: W. W. Norton.

Siegel, D. (2012). *The developing mind: How relationships and the brain interact to shape who we are* (2nd ed.). New York, NY: Guilford Press.

Silberman, Y., Bajo, M., Chappell, A., Christian, D., Cruz, M., Diaz, M., . . . Weiner, J. (2009). Neurobiological mechanisms contributing to alcohol-stress-anxiety interactions. *Alcohol, 43,* 509–519. doi:10.1016/j.alcohol.2009.01.002

Slade, A. (2008). The implications of attachment theory and research for adult psychotherapy: Research and clinical perspectives. In J. Cassidy & P. Shaver (Eds.), *Handbook of attachment: Theory, research, and clinical applications* (2nd ed., pp. 762–782). New York, NY: Guilford Press.

Substance Abuse and Mental Health Services Administration. (2013a). *About co-occurring disorders training. Motivational interviewing.* Retrieved from http://www.samhsa.gov/co-occurring/topics/training/motivational.aspx

Substance Abuse and Mental Health Services Administration. (2013b). *About co-occurring disorders training. Stage-wise treatment: A key component in an evidence-based approach to treating co-occurring disorders.* Retrieved from http://www.samhsa.gov/co-occurring/topics/training/stage-wise-treatment.aspx

Thorberg, F., & Lyvers, M. (2010). Attachment in relation to affect regulation and interpersonal functioning among substance use disorder in patients. *Addiction Research and Theory, 18,* 464–478. doi:10.3109/16066350903254783

Ulman, R., & Paul, H. (1989). The self-psychological theory and approach to treating substance abuse disorders: The "intersubjective absorption" hypothesis. In A. Goldberg (Ed.), *Dimensions of self experience: Progress in self psychology* (Vol. 5, pp. 121–141). Hillsdale, NJ: Analytic Press.

Ulman, R., & Paul, H. (1992). Dissociative anesthesia and the transitional selfobject transference in the intersubjective treatment of the addictive personality. In A. Goldberg (Ed.), *Dimensions of self experience: Progress in self psychology* (Vol. 8, pp. 109–139). Hillsdale, NJ: Analytic Press.

Weiss, R., Jaffee, W., de Menil, V., & Cogley, C. (2004). Group therapy for substance use disorders: What do we know? *Harvard Review of Psychiatry, 12*(6), 339–350. doi:10.1080/10673220490905723

Zero to Three. (2007). *Still face experiment: Dr. Edward Tronick.* Retrieved from http://www.youtube.com/watch?v=apzXGEbZht0

Trauma's Neurobiological Toll: Implications for Clinical Work With Children

KAREN ZILBERSTEIN

A Home Within, Northampton, Massachusetts, USA

Traumatic stress in childhood exacts a particularly high developmental toll. When traumatic experiences start early, continue chronically, and/or occur in conjunction with inadequate caretaking, neurobiological consequences intensify. Implicated brain regions include those mediating stress reactions, emotional arousal and regulation, attention, inhibition, impulse control, and various types of memory. To address those issues psychotherapeutically, treatment must comprehensively target underdeveloped or damaged neural networks. This article reviews current knowledge of the neurobiological and developmental affronts caused by traumatic stress during childhood and examines the various treatments and treatment implications for psychotherapeutic work with children.

INTRODUCTION

Severe and prolonged traumatic stress, experienced in childhood, often exacts a developmental toll. Trauma disrupts neurobiological maturation by provoking alterations in emotional, behavioral, interpersonal, cognitive, sensory, and biological areas of functioning (Ford, 2009). When traumatic experiences occur in conjunction with inadequate caretaking, so that the attachment figure either serves as the source of fear and/or cannot help the child cope, the disruptive, dysregulating effects increase exponentially

(Lieberman & van Horn, 2008; Lyons-Ruth, 2003; Streeck-Fischer & van der Kolk, 2000). Recent research on child development, attachment, and trauma has begun to explain when and how neurobiological domains optimally evolve and the damage they can sustain. This knowledge, in turn, is beginning to generate more refined and innovative treatments for traumatized children. However, though solid documentation now exists for children's typical and overt traumatic symptoms, as well as some of the associated and affected brain regions and neural pathways, the precise mapping of the underlying areas and understanding of causal mechanisms responsible for those symptoms remains rudimentary (H. Hart & Rubia, 2012; McCrory, DeBrito, & Viding, 2010). Open questions that continue to limit precise and targeted treatments include a better understanding of psychological change mechanisms, how the staging of interventions can best capitalize on the brain's variable plasticity, and to what extent treatment should seek to remediate or to compensate for developmental and structural damage (Cicchetti, 2013; Ford, 2009; McCrory et al., 2010; Perry, 2009; Zilberstein, 2014a). This article reviews current knowledge of the neurobiological and developmental affronts caused by adversity and maltreatment at vulnerable points in childhood and examines the various treatments and treatment implications of emerging research that guides psychotherapeutic work with children.

NEUROBIOLOGY OF CHILD DEVELOPMENT

Developmental neurobiology in part explains children's susceptibility to ongoing difficulties following chronic or severe trauma. Children's brains develop rapidly during the first 3 years of life and undergo a relatively long period of maturation. Growing in a bottom-up fashion, the lower brain matures first, with the most primitive structures already well developed by birth. Those primarily include the brain stem and midbrain, which govern autonomic, bodily functions such as respiration, digestion, and some types of visual and motor control. Postnatally, the brain continues to grow and organize as a function of age and experience. Various neurohormonal, neurotransmitter, and neuromodulator signals, which also originate in the lower brain, orchestrate this growth (Cozolino, 2002; Perry, 2009). They help form increasingly efficient pathways and communication between brain regions, especially when activated by repeated use. However, when faced with adversity, the brain favors development of some areas over others, at the expense of overall fluidity. For instance, stress causes the body to release the hormone cortisol, which provides the adrenaline rush needed to react quickly to threat. However, prolonged or frequent cortisol secretion, which occurs during chronic trauma or ongoing attachment difficulties, sensitizes and conditions the body to stress, thus contributing to recurrent and easily induced episodes of physiological and emotional dysregulation (Ford, 2009; Gunnar & Quevedo, 2007). Once established, such neurologically wired patterns of reactivity can become hard to change, particularly if they begin early in life and affect the development of other neural pathways and brain regions.

During the first few years of life, rapid growth and synchronization occurs in three primary brain areas: the limbic system, which processes emotions, coordinates self-regulation and the formation of memories; the cortical areas, which coordinate the cognitive and executive functions; and the stress response system (S. Hart, 2011; Schore, 2001). Cortical areas, such as the prefrontal cortex that mediates complex thought, executive functions, and inhibitory control over emotions take longest to develop. They do not reach full potential until early adulthood. This long interval of growth renders children's brains particularly vulnerable and sensitive to environmental factors, for better and for worse (Thompson-Schill, Ramscar, & Chrysikous, 2009). A less advanced prefrontal cortex allows youth to explore flexibly, learn rapidly, think creatively, and adapt to their surroundings (Thompson-Schill et al., 2009). However, it also reduces children's behavioral and cognitive control, making them especially at risk when their milieu does not monitor or protect them or promote optimal learning.

As is discussed further below, experiences of traumatic stress and inadequate caretaking in the early and formative years can interrupt the development of each of those brain structures in detrimental ways. The type of damage that transpires depends in part on that child's previous development and genetic make-up (Goslin, Stover, Berkowitz, & Marans, 2013). The child's age also has a tremendous effect as it determines which parts of the brain and nervous system are developing most quickly and so most likely to be thrown off course (Herringa et al., 2013; Salmon & Bryant, 2002). Because experience partly shapes and organizes the brain, especially relational and attachment experiences, earlier, more severe, and more persistent traumatic occurrences and attachment difficulties lead to more negative, enduring, and extensive consequences (Beers & DeBellis, 2002; Chae, Ogle, & Goodman, 2009; Cozolino, 2002; Streeck-Fischer & van der Kolk, 2000). This is in part because when lower brain regions and neurotransmitter systems develop suboptimally, they hamper growth of the higher, cortical regions and of efficient communication between various brain regions (Perry, 2009). This has far-reaching consequences for how children learn to regulate and attend to sensory, emotional, and social stimuli as well as for the consolidation of memory and the ability to understand and make meaning of experiences.

ATTACHMENT'S CONTRIBUTION TO CHILDREN'S OUTCOMES

The strongest predictor of psychological health and resiliency remains the quality of interpersonal relationships, particularly attachment relationships

(Bowlby, 1982; Siegel, 1999). A caregiver's attunement and sensitivity to the young child's state and reflection of that emotional understanding appear crucial to attachment and to development, in general (Ainsworth, Blehar, Waters, & Wall, 1978; Bowlby, 1982; S. Hart, 2011). Available and attuned attachment figures serve as secure bases that encourage exploration, learning, and multiple other developmental achievements (Ainsworth et al., 1978; S. Hart, 2011; Siegel, 1999). Studies of parents and infants playing together elucidate the interactive dance in which the dyad's movements and expressions become synchronized in microsecond responses (Beebe & Lachman, 2003). Early attachment patterns consolidate through these sensorimotor and emotional communications that include voice tone, touch, gestures, and vocalizations (Beebe & Lachmann, 2003; Bowlby, 1982; S. Hart, 2011). Through these experiences, children also form schemas, or internal working models, of the self, others, and relationships that help guide their behavior in times of danger or need (Bowlby, 1982).

Below the surface, these interpersonal exchanges correlate with important neurological developments. The infant's nervous system literally organizes itself through these microinteractions (S. Hart, 2011). During the same developmental period in which attachments become established and consolidated into working models, that is, during the first 3 years of life, the limbic, cortical, and stress response systems are simultaneously developing (Gunnar & Quevedo, 2007; S. Hart, 2011; Schore, 2001). Those regions govern physical arousal, regulation, and social affiliation, areas particularly affected and shaped by attachment experiences. When an infant imitates the movements, countenance, and sounds of the caregiver, that child learns to connect bodily sensations with feelings, words, and the emotional states of others, thus building important synaptic connections in regions of the brain associated with language, emotions, and sociability (Hart, 2011). As a consequence, infants of responsive and sensitive mothers show more activity in left frontal brain areas that coordinate positive emotion and affiliation (Gunnar & Quevedo, 2007; Schore, 2001).

Through those interactions, emotional and physical regulation also consolidates (Fonagy, Gergely, Jurist, & Target, 2002; S. Hart, 2011; Schore, 2001). Attuned caretakers regulate and keep tolerable a child's arousal and encourage that child to use them to soothe distress in times of need, thus further reducing anxiety. As a consequence of multiple, successful experiences of managing mild disturbances, the child's limbic and cortical regions mature and become better and better at bearing and coping with stress (Ford, 2009). Language also helps this process. Skillful attachment figures encourage reflection and discussion of emotional material, thus building understanding, toleration and regulation of mental and emotional states (Cozolino, 2002; Fonagy et al., 2002; S. Hart, 2011; Hughes, 2004; Siegel, 1999). Supportive care and secure attachments thus establish important neurologically based buffers that help children withstand future stressful events.

By the end of the first year of life, securely attached infants display resiliency, in part because of their strengthened stress response and cortical systems (Gunnar & Quevedo, 2007; Hane & Fox, 2006; S. Hart, 2011). Although negatively affected by traumatic experiences, their more advanced regulatory skills, more sophisticated coping mechanisms, and comfortable dependence on caregivers who cushion the effects of stress allow them to manage more tenaciously when faced with adversity.

On the other hand, children without secure attachments exhibit various difficulties coping with disturbing thoughts, feelings, and experiences. Whether they reveal it overtly, insecurely attached children show biological markers of apprehension when desiring care and comforting. Their heart rates and cortisol levels rise (Gunnar & Quevedo, 2007). Securely attached infants show no such elevation in cortisol levels when crying to get their parents' attention. Children with insecure and disorganized attachments also display more difficulty recognizing, regulating, and integrating various cognitive and emotional cues. Self-reflection and problem solving remain less developed as the child's attempts to cope with dsyregulation leave little space for concentrating on, utilizing, and developing higher order cortical regions and skills (Fonagy et al., 2002; Ford, 2009; S. Hart, 2011). This leaves them especially vulnerable to trauma and stress.

NEUROBIOLOGICAL EFFECTS OF TRAUMA

Trauma constitutes one of the most stressful and taxing experiences children may encounter. A number of studies have now looked at its neurobiological and long-term effects. They suggest that childhood maltreatment and adverse experiences trigger cascading physiological, hormonal, and neurochemical changes that alter brain structures and functions (Beers & DeBellis, 2002; H. Hart & Rubia, 2012; McCrory et al., 2010; Perry & Pollard, 1998). Although the results of these studies must be viewed with caution due to their small sample sizes, populations spread heterogeneously across different traumatic experiences, lack of consistent measures of maltreatment severity, limited studies on children, and difficulties separating the effects of maltreatment from psychopathology, some fairly consistent and robust findings have emerged (H. Hart & Rubia, 2012; McCrory et al., 2010). Altered or diminished structures and systems include the hypothalamic-pituitary-adrenal axis (HPA) or the stress response system, reduced volume in the corpus callosum and cerebellum, and reduced activity and functioning in certain localities of the prefrontal cortex, limbic, and paralimbic systems. Those implicated brain regions influence stress reactions, emotional arousal and regulation, attention, inhibition, impulse control, and various types of memory. Although some of those areas overlap with and perhaps exacerbate problems in children experiencing insufficient attachments—that is, the stress response and regulatory systems—others, having to do with attention, inhibition, impulse control, and memory are unique. These deficits then have far reaching influence on children's overall functioning.

Trauma affects children so severely in part because it interrupts and overwhelms developing neural pathways with stimuli and experiences that the brain is not yet equipped to manage. Before language and symbolic representation fully form, the brain encodes memories implicitly and does not integrate them with verbal centers, so that consciously remembering and making sense of traumatic experience—even later in life—becomes difficult (Salmon & Bryant, 2002; Streeck-Fischer & van der Kolk, 2000). With little prior knowledge upon which to understand experiences, young children also process new occurrences more slowly and with less detail (Perry & Pollard, 1998; Salmon & Bryant, 2002). This fragments memory, making it less available for appraisal or integration. In addition, because of the highly arousing and emotional nature of traumatic experience, the child's nascent stress response system and coping abilities become compromised and overwhelmed, leading to dysregulation on biological, emotional, and behavioral levels and further complicating efforts to remember or derive meaning out of what happened.

Trauma interferes with neurobiological domains in other ways, as well. Traumatic experiences stimulate a heightened fear response in the limbic areas of the amygdala and hippocampus and selective attention to those parts of the experience necessary for survival. This overexcites the amygdala, which mediates memory for emotional events, and weakens the hippocampus, which consolidates short-term into long-term memory (S. Hart, 2011; Herringa et al., 2013). As a consequence, individuals experience high arousal and diminished processing and integration of memories. Sensory, emotional, and cognitive reactions become dissociated so that the child can neither evaluate nor curtail the associated fear and arousal (Cozolino, 2002). In addition, because the trauma and later traumatic triggers command attention, the child directs less attention to other stimuli, at the expense of broad learning (Ford, 2009; Perry & Pollard, 1998). When such demands are made repeatedly during developmentally sensitive times, the child's emerging biology and brain become structured around hypervigilance and safety seeking (Perry & Pollard, 1998; Streeck-Fischer & van der Kolk, 2000). This conditions the child to become overly attentive and reactive to stress, as the child's stress system responds more and more quickly and efficiently to smaller and smaller stresses, thus contributing to the child's general behavioral and emotional dysregulation (Ford, 2009; Gunnar & Quevedo, 2007). The ensuing hyperarousal and misinterpretation of threat and fear further impels the child to miscue to social and other situations, contributing to problems in multiple domains (Cozolino, 2002; Zilberstein, 2014a). These states of hyperarousal, fragmentation, and restricted attention and learning then establish a weaker foundation for navigating subsequent developmental challenges.

Variations in Traumatic Stress Responses

Although chronic, adverse experiences and traumatic experiences tend to afflict specific neural regions, there remains much variation in individuals' reactions. Many factors affect a child's ability to tolerate stress. These include prior history of trauma, whether parenting has been supportive or hostile, and other genetic or learned competencies and skills (Goslin et al., 2013; Lieberman & van Horn, 2008). Temperament and inborn stress reactivity also leave an imprint (Phillips, Fox, & Gunnar, 2011). So may innate cognitive ability, though it is often hard to separate out environmental factors that decrease cognitive functioning and IQ from genetic potential (Beckett et al., 2006; Saltzman, Weems, & Carrion, 2006; Shonk & Cicchetti, 2001). Each of these pre-event factors serves either to mitigate or exacerbate a child's response and recovery and is important to understand as part of the contextual landscape that affects treatment.

Factors following traumatic exposure also influence children's adjustments. As children strive to cope with or compensate for early deficiencies, they continue to develop adaptively and maladaptively in various cognitive, emotional, and relational domains (Gerber, 2006; Sroufe, Carlson, Levy, & Egeland, 1999). New relational experiences as well as growing cognitive and self-regulatory abilities can help children gain new skills and resources that aid recovery (Raikes & Thompson, 2005). Dysregulation combined with attentional and cognitive difficulties can also lead to cascading problems such as poor peer relationships or school performance that add additional stresses (Cozolino, 2002; Zilberstein, 2014a). A child may also develop certain defensive strategies, such as avoidance, so as not to feel the intense pain, fear, and dysregulation engendered by those experiences. In addition, many other developmental and environmental factors (such as family, race, culture, and poverty) mix together to determine a child's relative response. Children's responses to trauma can thus be flexible and durable, both modified by and shaping of subsequent experiences.

RIGIDITY AND PLASTICITY IN DEVELOPMENT

Neural mechanisms and their associated patterns of thinking, feeling, and behaving sometimes rigidly persist. They influence perceptions of and reactions to future events, thus strengthening and confirming preexisting pathways, ideas, and responses (Cozolino, 2002). Studies indicate that this can occur in response to both attachment and traumatic triggers. Working models of attachment influence memory for attachment-related experiences so that insecure children recall more negative events and rejecting parental responses than securely attached children, even when given the same attachment-related scenarios (Chae et al., 2009; Rowe & Carnelley,

2003). Avoidantly attached children and adults also show less accuracy in recounting distressing or traumatic experiences, partly because they exclude and so do not reflect upon or encode information that might activate their attachment systems (Chae et al., 2009). This means that without focusing those individuals on various types of omitted and overlooked information, they are not likely to notice, process, or remember them, thus perpetuating their perceptions and belief systems.

Despite such rigidity, the brain also remains plastic throughout life. Ingrained biological, emotional, and behavioral patterns can and do change in response to new experiences and stimuli (S. Hart, 2011; Perry, 2009). In fact, the brain and nervous systems' malleability, which make them so vulnerable to damage, also render them receptive to reparation and growth. Growing evidence suggests that the children who show the most susceptibility to adverse events are also the most amenable to positive experiences (Belsky & Pluess, 2009). Highly reactive children and those with difficult temperaments develop more poorly than others when experiencing inadequate parenting but outperform peers when parenting is skillful (Belsky & Pluess, 2009). Although it is not clear whether the damage caused by severe trauma diminishes that pliability, it does suggest that some of the children most hurt by maltreatment may also retain significant ability to adjust positively when circumstances improve.

TREATMENT

An understanding of the neurobiological processes underlying childhood trauma lends itself to a few important principles when formulating treatments. First of all, individual variation in how children respond to adversity and stress depends, in part, on their unique genetics, biology, and circumstances and means that comprehensive assessments are needed (Ford, 2009; Zilberstein, 2014a). Second, research on child development, resiliency, and plasticity particularly highlight the role of caregiving in promoting positive or negative outcomes and neurological change (Cicchetti & Gunnar, 2008; Hane & Fox, 2006). Treatment of traumatized children cannot be conducted independently of the caregiving and relational environments in which they function. Third, reversing the accumulated wear and tear of traumatic experiences and insufficiently protective attachment relationships requires interventions that appropriately target underdeveloped or damaged brain regions, particularly in the areas most affected by trauma: sensory integration, self-regulatory ability, relationships, cognitive and executive functioning, and memory. To change neural networks, treatment must first activate those systems (S. Hart, 2011; Perry, 2009), though the best ways to do so remain an open question. Last, developmental considerations are important as the timing and aiming of an intervention can enhance its effectiveness. Just as the brain and nervous system endures more damage during periods of rapid brain development, those phases also provide opportunities for heightened plasticity and growth (Cicchetti & Gunnar, 2008; Herringa et al., 2013; Perry, 2009).

Comprehensive Assessment

Children vary in their response to trauma based on their genetics, temperament, history, security of attachment, the age at which the trauma occurred, and its duration and severity. A child whose immature neural systems become dysregulated by trauma before they have organized and developed will sustain more damage than children traumatized later in life (Beers & DeBellis, 2002; Chae et al., 2009; Streeck-Fischer & van der Kolk, 2000). In addition, the effects of trauma on a child or family cannot be separated from other risk or protective factors that affect that child. A variety of cultural, familial, and contextual factors affect children's responses. Other stressors, such as poverty, racism, and parental depression or supportive factors such as a caring network of adults, peers, and community also shape the child and development. Last, as development progresses, efforts to cope or compensate with the trauma and the damage it creates may adaptively or maladaptively affect the child. Those factors cannot be considered simply as accessories to the primary treatment of trauma but, in fact, mold a child's symptoms in unique and important ways that must be addressed conjointly (Zilberstein, 2014b). In this regard, assessment must broadly assess a wide spectrum of developmental, relational, and contextual factors so that interventions can be appropriately tailored to the unique needs and circumstances of each child and family (Ford, 2009; Perry, 2009). However, given what is known about the typical and most enduring neurodevelopmental impact of trauma, relational capacity and emotional dysregulation must be considered crucial concerns and considered in depth. If interventions do not target those needs, not only will they be ineffective, they could make emotional demands that exceed a person's ability to cope and thus create additional harm (Ford, 2009; Perry, 2009).

Role of Relationships and Attachments

Treatment of trauma must enhance attachment relationships. This entails helping caregivers learn to attune to and sensitively parent the child and aiding children in accurately cueing attachment needs and using relationships for support (Blaustein & Kinniburgh, 2010; Hughes, 2004; Lieberman & van Horn, 2008; Zilberstein, 2014b). Attachment-based treatments generally achieve these goals by working together with parents and children to challenge existing internal working models, develop affect regulation and reflective functioning, and repair empathic breaks through attuned responses (Berlin, Ziv, Amaya-Jackson, & Greenberg, 2005; Hughes, 2004; Lieberman & van Horn, 2008). Parents learn to reflect upon their own and their child's feelings and behavior and to match the child's affect through verbal and nonverbal means, thereby increasing positive and effective responses to that child. Most current attachment-based treatments target younger children who appear to derive the most benefit from those interventions (Berlin et al., 2005; Lieberman & van Horn, 2008; Zilberstein, 2014b). This may be partly due to the fact that children's limbic systems are growing rapidly and are most plastic in the early years, making them more open to attachment-based and regulatory learning (Perry, 2009; Schore, 2001). Young children also depend more upon attachment figures than do older individuals, encounter fewer external influences, and exhibit less rigidly formed working models, all of which boost the likelihood of successful attachment-based treatment (Zilberstein, 2014b).

As children age, their dependence on attachments shifts, yet continued attention to the caregiving environment remains important. Although other relationships, experiences, and capabilities also influence the older child, attachment figures continue to guide and affect children, even in adolescence (Allen, 2008; Raikes & Thompson, 2005). In addition, as is discussed further, children with cognitive and regulatory deficits secondary to trauma often require many repetitions of new skills to modify and reorganize the affected neural networks (Perry, 2009). Such children commonly have difficulty independently generalizing or practicing therapeutic gains in daily life. They thus show increased benefit when caregivers learn to structure the home environment in certain ways and provide opportunities to practice relational and regulatory skills (Blaustein & Kinniburgh, 2010; Hughes, 2004; Lieberman & van Horn, 2008). When a caregiver is not available or ready to provide those arrangements, the therapist may need to consider whether other milieus in which the child functions, such as schools, can provide the necessary adjunctive experiences (Perry, 2009; Warner, Koomar, Lary, & Cook, 2013).

Not just caregivers, but therapists can also provide important, curative attachment relationships. Research consistently shows that the quality of the therapeutic relationship has a strong influence on the outcome of therapy (Norcross & Wampold, 2011). Knowledge of the neurobiology of attachment can thus assist the clinician in adopting relational stances and behaviors most likely to promote change. This involves attention to those aspects of the therapeutic relationship that foster secure attachments: safety and boundaries, attunement, responsiveness, reflective functioning, verbal and nonverbal emotional communication, and repair of empathic breaks (Bowlby, 1982; Cozolino, 2002; Fonagy et al., 2002; S. Hart, 2011; Hughes, 2004).

Activation of Neural Networks

Neurobiological change occurs as a function of experience. Novel stimuli and learning opportunities engineer new connections between different brain regions that then communicate more rapidly and efficiently the more they are exercised (Cozolino, 2002; Perry, 2009; Siegel, 1999). Because the brain initially develops in a bottom-up fashion, with the lower regions helping to organize the higher ones, some clinicians suggest that treatment should replicate that sequence (Perry, 2009; Warner, Cook, Westcott, & Koomar, 2011). A few studies support this approach (Barfield, Dobson, Gaskill, & Perry, 2012; Warner et al., 2013). "Bottom-up" tactics first target somatosensory self-regulation through repeated rhythmic activities (dance, drumming, rocking, and other types of movement), then relational skills, followed by verbal and insight-oriented work. Because those lower-level brain realms show less plasticity than higher-level cognitive domains, Perry (2009) notes that altering them requires more patterned, frequent, and predictable enrichment opportunities.

It is not yet clear how these sensory interventions differ or compare to more common types of age-appropriate physical training and activities that could be used in combination with other trauma and relational treatments. Research on nontraumatized populations robustly indicates that exercise and movement, in general, decrease anxiety and increase resilience to stress (Schoenfeld, Rada, Pierunzzini, Hsueh, & Gould, 2013). Taken together, however, these theories and associated studies suggest, at the very least, an important role for structured physical and sensory activity in promoting regulatory ability in traumatized children.

Activating and regulating the lower brain regions appears to improve self-control and decrease emotional responses, thus creating a necessary platform for other types of growth. But it likely does not, in itself, remediate the many other difficulties that often accompany experiences of trauma. Research suggests, for instance, that although secure attachments formed in early childhood help inoculate children from numerous later difficulties, many of the behavioral, social, cognitive, and emotional difficulties that poor attachments and adverse experiences engender can persist even after secure attachments are eventually formed (Beckett et al., 2006; Colvert et al., 2008). Therapy must thus also specifically stimulate the neural networks governing those other processes, as well.

Traumatized children often need help acquiring coping skills, gaining social competence, and learning to attend to, think about, and process sensory, emotional, and interpersonal cues rather than allowing their stress response systems to react automatically (Blaustein & Kinniburgh, 2010; Ford, 2009). Those abilities will not necessarily develop without the therapist drawing the child's attention to them and helping her or him to reflect upon and practice the associated skills. Some of this work may take on a structured, didactic component (Blaustein & Kinniburgh, 2010), whereas other aspects can occur through relational work or play therapy.

Therapies that involve expression of and reflection on feelings, motivations, and mental states and motivations, such as found in psychodynamic and play treatments, can also enhance overall regulatory ability and provide important activation of cortical regions (Cozolino, 2002; Fonagy et al., 2002; S. Hart, 2011; Hughes, 2004; Levy, 2011). Language and the representation of experience constitute powerful tools that allow for increased self-control over emotions and better integration of thoughts with feelings (Chae et al., 2009; Cozolino, 2002; Fonagy et al., 2002; Siegel, 1999). Interactive play also aids growth of the orbital frontal cortex, which coordinates social activities (Pellis & Pellis, 2007). Such methods provide important experiences for traumatized children, who, biologically primed to react to stress and danger, often misinterpret events as threatening and respond to them as such (Ford, 2009; Gunnar & Quevedo, 2007; Herringa et al., 2013). However, some children who show high levels of dysregulation and have little ability to engage in relationships or organize their internal worlds may find that psychodynamic and play treatments do not offer enough directed attention, structure, or scaffolding to build a wide range of necessary skills (Vanheule, Verhaeghe, & Desmet, 2010; Warner et al., 2013).

Like other neural networks, memories must also be activated if they are to be integrated or changed (Dorfman & Mandler, 1994). For children who have experienced prolonged and multiple traumatic experiences, or whose traumatic experiences occurred early in life, remembering and processing that trauma is a complex endeavor (Blaustein & Kinniburgh, 2010; Herringa et al., 2013; Salmon & Bryant, 2002). Sometimes distinct episodes of trauma exist while at other times it simply pervades the overall landscape of the child's experience. However, as trauma dissociates sensory and emotional experiences from cognitive appraisals and understandings, some attention must be given to helping children integrate and make meaning from those fragmented aspects of themselves. This involves directing attention to their sensory and emotional reactions, helping them understand why and how those reactions occurred, developing a cohesive narrative about the past, and creating new meanings upon which to proceed. Careful attention must be given to the potential dysregulating effects of this work, which must be paced, dosed, and accompanied by adequate building of coping and regulatory skills (Blaustein & Kinniburgh, 2010; Cohen, Mannarino, & Deblinger, 2006; Hughes, 2004).

Developmental Considerations

Research on the effects of trauma and early adversity makes clear that such experiences interrupt and compromise development in numerous areas. Clinicians must understand the various ways children are and are not on track developmentally as well as the reasons for those discrepancies. Often development in traumatized children proceeds unevenly, with skills in some areas outpacing those in others. Children delayed or handicapped by traumatic experience generally show some natural improvements in developmental abilities as they age, even when their overall proficiency and repertoire of skills remain well below those of similarly age peers (Cicchetti, 2013). For instance, a school-age child might perform adequately in some cognitive or motor tasks, while functioning at a very young level socially and emotionally. Therapists need to understand how to meet those "younger" needs in ways that still recognize and honor the child's chronological age.

Just as the brain and nervous systems endure more damage when exposed to toxic environments during periods of rapid development, those times also provide opportunities for heightened plasticity and growth (Cicchetti & Gunnar, 2008). Interventions targeted to emerging skills during normative growth spurts are hypothesized to show increased efficacy. This means, for instance, that infants and young children will likely respond more quickly to somatosensory and physically nurturing activities than will adolescents (Perry, 2009). This also means that when nurturing and sensory activities are offered to older children, they must match the physical and cognitive capacities and interests of those ages rather than replicate activities geared toward younger children (Ford, 2009; Zilberstein, 2014b). As children mature, they also generally acquire more cognitive and regulatory proficiency, which affords them new tools for handling the dysregulating effects of trauma. Those include increased working memory, better logical thinking, improved emotional and behavioral regulation, the ability to plan and set goals, more advanced social understanding, and an ability to reflect on and monitor their own thoughts and behavior (Bumge & Wright, 2007; Raikes & Thompson, 2005; Salmon & Bryant, 2002). Adolescence, a time in which abstract representational understanding blossoms, may provide a prime opportunity for children to reappraise old beliefs and acquire new schemas of the self, others, relationships, and the world (Allen, 2008; Ford, 2009). Such gains allow for the introduction of some cognitive-behavioral techniques in the treatment of school-age and adolescent youth that can focus on conscious understanding and control of emotions, behavior, and social relatedness (Blaustein & Kinniburgh, 2010; Cohen, Mannarino, & Deblinger, 2006; Gruber, Hay, & Gross, 2014).

The variable availability of a child's budding skills and resources for therapeutic work suggests that remediation of defective or underdeveloped brain structures may not always need to follow a more normative, "bottom-up" developmental pathway. Although trauma disrupts and interrupts the acquisition of many skills, it does not necessarily derail them altogether or even uniformly (Cicchetti, 2013). Harnessing a child's particular strengths and areas of resiliency may, in fact, aid healing. Such a strategy resembles the treatment of children with learning disabilities, who also struggle with neurodevelopmental deficits. Those remedies encompass numerous techniques that could be helpful with traumatized children: specific skill training, pairing strength in one domain with weakness in another, and the use of various compensatory strategies (Dehn, 2008; Greenspan & Wieder, 2006; Zilberstein, 2014a).

CONCLUSION

Understanding how childhood trauma afflicts various neural systems can aid clinicians in selecting and utilizing those interventions most likely to affect change. Although much remains unknown about the efficacies of different approaches for various subpopulations, consensus now exists on a number of broad principles. Most treatments for trauma rightly emphasize the need for children to be anchored in secure and nurturing relationships, and the primacy of that goal as a therapeutic target (Blaustein & Kinniburgh, 2010; Fonagy et al., 2002; Ford, 2009; Hughes, 2004; Lieberman & van Horn, 2008). After all, attachment constitutes the developmental foundation and tool upon which neurobiological self-regulation grows (Schore, 2001). Interventions must also focus on helping children gain or remedy insufficient developmental capacities and do so within the child's current context and utilizing that child's developmental aptitudes and strengths. Primary among these are the building of regulatory and reflective ability that allows for the development of a range of coping skills (Blaustein & Kinniburgh, 2010; Fonagy et al., 2002; Ford, 2009; Perry, 2009). Given that the brains of traumatized children organize around survival, safety, and detecting threat, which affects numerous neural systems, treatment must also activate many different brain regions to stimulate new learning (Cozolino, 2002; S. Hart, 2011; Ford, 2009; Perry & Pollard, 1998). This may entail the use of various interventions and change components that span sensory, attachment-based, relational, and cognitive approaches as well as didactic, skill-building exercises (Berlin et al., 2005; Blaustein & Kinniburgh, 2010; Cohen et al., 2006; Cozolino, 2002; Fonagy et al., 2002; Ford, 2009; Hughes, 2004; Lieberman & van Horn, 2008; Perry, 2009; Warner et al., 2012). Whether treatment must occur in a "bottom-up" or "top-down" fashion, however, remains unclear. More likely, interventions that engage multiple networks by combining both bottom-up and top-down interventions (depending on the needs and developmental age of the child) will increase integration of dissociated networks and enhance learning.

REFERENCES

Ainsworth, M., Blehar, M., Waters, E., & Wall, S. (1978). *Patterns of attachment: A psychological study of the Strange Situation*. Hillsdale, NJ: Erlbaum.

Allen, J. (2008). The attachment system in adolescence. In J. Cassidy & P. Shaver (Eds.), *Handbook of attachment: Theory, research and clinical applications* (2nd ed., pp. 419–435). New York, NY: Guilford Press.

Barfield, S., Dobson, C., Gaskill, R., & Perry, B. (2012). Neurosequential model of therapeutics in a therapeutic preschool: Implications for work with children with complex neuropsychiatric problems. *International Journal of Play Therapy, 21*(1), 30–44.

Beckett, C., Maughan, B., Rutter, M., Castle, J., Colvert, C., Groothues, C., . . . Sonuga-Barke, E. (2006). Do the effects of early severe deprivation on cognition persist into early adolescence? Findings from the English and Romanian adoptees study. *Child Development, 77*(3), 696–711.

Beebe, B., & Lachmann, F. (2003). The relational turn in psychoanalysis: A dyadic systems view from infant research. *Contemporary Psychoanalysis, 39*(3), 379–409.

Beers, S., & De Bellis, M. (2002). Neuropsychological function in children with maltreatment-related posttraumatic stress disorder. *American Journal of Psychiatry, 159*, 483–486.

Belsky, J., & Pluess, M. (2009). The nature (and nurture?) of plasticity in early human development. *Perspectives on Psychological Science, 4*(4), 345–351.

Berlin, L., Ziv, Y., Amaya-Jackson, L., & Greenberg, M. (2005). *Enhancing early attachments: Theory, research, intervention, and policy.* New York, NY: Guilford Press.

Blaustein, M., & Kinniburgh, K. (2010). *Treating traumatic stress in children and adolescents: How to foster resilience through attachment, self-regulation, and competency.* New York, NY: Guilford Press.

Bowlby, J. (1982). *Attachment and loss: Attachment* (2nd ed.). New York, NY: Basic Books.

Bumge, S., & Wright, S. (2007). Neurodevelopmental changes in working memory and cognitive control. *Current Opinion in Neuroscience, 17*, 243–250.

Chae, Y., Ogle, C., & Goodman, G. (2009). Remembering negative childhood experiences: An attachment theory perspective. In J. Quas & R. Fivush (Eds.), *Emotion and memory in development: Biological, cognitive, and social considerations* (pp. 3–27). New York, NY: Oxford University Press.

Cicchetti, D. (2013). Research review: Resilient functioning in maltreated children—Past, present and future perspectives. *Journal of Child Psychology and Psychiatry, 54*(4), 402–422.

Cicchetti, D., & Gunnar, M. (2008). Integrating biological measures into the design and evaluation of preventative interventions. *Development and Psychopathology, 20*, 737–743.

Cohen, J., Mannarino, A., & Deblinger, E. (2006). *Treating trauma and traumatic grief in children and adolescents.* New York, NY: Guilford Press.

Colvert, E., Rutter, M., Beckett, C., Castle, J., Groothues, C., Hawkins, A., . . . Sonuga-Barke, E. (2008). Emotional difficulties in early adolescence following severe early deprivation: Findings from the English and Romanian adoptees study. *Development and Psychopathology, 20*, 547–567.

Cozolino, L. (2002). *The neuroscience of psychotherapy: Building and rebuilding the human brain.* New York, NY: W.W. Norton.

Dehn, M. (2008). *Working memory and academic learning: Assessment and intervention*. Hoboken, NJ: John Wiley & Sons.

Dorfman, J., & Mandler, G. (1994). Implicit and explicit forgetting: When is gist remembered? *Quarterly Journal of Experimental Psychology*, *47*(3), 651–672.

Fonagy, P., Gergely, G., Jurist, E., & Target, M. (2002). *Affect regulation, mentalization, and the development of the self*. New York, NY: Other Press.

Ford, J. (2009). Neurobiological and developmental research: Clinical implications. In C. Courtis & J. Ford (Eds.), *Treating complex traumatic stress disorders: An evidence-based guide* (pp. 31–58). New York, NY: Guilford Press.

Gerber, A. (2006). Attachment, resilience, and psychoanalysis: Commentary on Hauser and Allen's overcoming adversity in adolescence. *Psychoanalytic Inquiry*, *26*(4), 585–595.

Goslin, M., Stover, C., Berkowitz, S., & Marans, S. (2013). Identifying youth at risk for difficulties following a traumatic event: Pre-event factors are associated with acute symptomatic. *Journal of Traumatic Stress*, *26*, 475–482.

Greenspan, S., & Wieder, S. (2006). *Engaging autism: Using the floortime approach to help children relate, communicate, and think*. New York, NY: DaCapo Lifelong Books.

Gruber, J., Hay, A., & Gross, J. (2014). Rethinking emotion: Cognitive reappraisal is an effective positive and negative emotion regulation strategy in bipolar disorder. *Emotion*, *14*(2), 388–396.

Gunnar, M., & Quevedo, K. (2007). The neurobiology of stress and development. *Annual Review of Psychology*, *58*, 145–173.

Hane, A., & Fox, N. (2006). Ordinary variations in maternal caregiving influence human infant's stress reactivity. *Psychological Science*, *17*(6), 550–556.

Hart, H., & Rubia, K. (2012). Neuroimaging of child abuse: A critical review. *Frontiers in Human Neuroscience*, *6*(52), 1–24.

Hart, S. (2011). *The impact of attachment: Developmental neuroaffective psychology*. New York, NY: W.W. Norton.

Herringa, R., Birn, R., Ruttle, P., Burghy, C., Stodola, D., Davidson, R., & Essex, M. (2013). Childhood maltreatment is associated with altered fear circuitry and increased internalizing symptoms by late adolescence. *PNAS Early Edition*. Retrieved from http://www.pnas.org/content/early/2013/10/30/1310766110.full.pdf+html

Hughes, D. (2004). An attachment-based treatment of maltreated children and young people. *Attachment and Human Development*, *6*(3), 263–278.

Levy, A. (2011). Neurobiology and the therapeutic action of psychoanalytic play therapy with children. *Clinical Social Work Journal*, *39*(1), 50–60.

Lieberman, A., & van Horn, P. (2008). *Psychotherapy with infants and young children: Repairing the effects of stress and trauma on early attachments*. New York, NY: Guilford Press.

Lyons-Ruth, K. (2003). Dissociation and the parent-infant dialogue: A longitudinal perspective from attachment research. *Journal of the American Psychoanalytic Association*, *51*, 883–911.

McCrory, E., DeBrito, S., & Viding, E. (2010). Research review: The neurobiology and genetics of maltreatment and adversity. *Journal of Child Psychology and Psychiatry*, *51*(10), 1079–1095.

Norcross, J., & Wampold, B. (2011). Evidence-based therapy relationships, research conclusions and clinical practices. *Psychotherapy*, *48*(1), 98–102.

Pellis, S., & Pellis, V. (2007). Rough-and-tumble play and the development of the social brain. *Current Directions in Psychological Science*, *16*, 95–98.

Perry, B. (2009). Examining child maltreatment through a neurodevelopmental lens: Clinical applications of the neurosequential model of therapeutics. *Journal of Loss and Trauma*, *14*, 240–255.

Perry, B., & Pollard, R. (1998). Homeostasis, stress and adaptation: A neurodevelopmental view of childhood trauma. *Stress in Children*, *7*(1), 33–51.

Phillips, D., Fox, N., & Gunnar, M. (2011). Same place, different experiences: Bringing individual differences to research in child care. *Child Development Perspectives*, *5*(1), 44–49.

Raikes, H., & Thompson, R. (2005). Relationships past, present, and future: Reflections on attachment in middle childhood. In K. Kerns & R. Richardson (Eds.), *Attachment in middle childhood* (pp. 255–282). New York, NY: Guilford Press.

Rowe, A., & Carnelley, K. (2003). Attachment style differences in the processing of attachment-relevant information: Primed-style effects on recall, interpersonal expectations, and affect. *Personal Relationships*, *10*, 59–75.

Salmon, K., & Bryant, R. (2002). Posttraumatic stress disorder in children: The influence of developmental factors. *Clinical Psychology Review*, *22*, 163–188.

Saltzman, K., Weems, C., & Carrion, V. (2006). IQ and posttraumatic stress symptoms in children exposed to interpersonal violence. *Child Psychiatry and Human Development*, *36*(3), 261–272.

Schoenfeld, T., Rada, P., Pierunzzini, P., Hsueh, B., & Gould, E. (2013). Physical exercise prevents stress-induced activation of granule neurons and enhances local inhibitory mechanisms in the dentate gyrus. *Journal of Neuroscience*, *33*(18), 7770–7777.

Schore, A. (2001). Effects of a secure attachment relationship on right brain development, affect regulation, and infant mental health. *Infant Mental Health Journal*, *22*(1/2), 7–66.

Shonk, S., & Cicchetti, C. (2001). Maltreatment, competency deficits, and risk for academic and behavioral maladjustment. *Developmental Psychology*, *37*(1), 3–17.

Siegel, D. (1999). *The developing mind*. New York, NY: Guilford Press.

Sroufe, L., Carlson, E., Levy, A., & Egeland, B. (1999). Implications of attachment theory for developmental psychopathology. *Development and Psychopathology*, *11*(1), 1–13.

Streeck-Fischer, A., & van der Kolk, B. (2000). Down will come baby, cradle and all: Diagnostic and therapeutic implications of chronic trauma on child development. *Australian and New Zealand Journal of Psychiatry*, *34*, 903–918.

Thompson-Schill, S., Ramscar, M., & Chrysikou, E. (2009). Cognition without control: When a little lobe goes a long way. *Current Directions in Psychology Science*, *18*(5), 259–263.

Vanheule, S., Verhaeghe, P., & Desmet, M. (2010). In search of a framework for the treatment of alexithymia. *Psychology and Psychotherapy: Theory, Research and Practice*, *84*, 84–97.

Warner, E., Cook, A., Westcott, A., & Koomar, J. (2011). *Sensory motor arousal regulation treatment: A manual for therapists working with children and adolescents: A "bottom up" approach to treatment of complex trauma.* Brookline, MA: Trauma Center at Justice Resource Institute.

Warner, E., Koomar, J., Lary, B., & Cook, A. (2013). Can the body change the score? Application of sensory modulation principles in the treatment of traumatized adolescents in residential treatment. *Journal of Family Violence, 28,* 729–738.

Zilberstein, K. (2014a). Neurocognitive considerations in the treatment of attachment and complex trauma in children. *Clinical Child Psychology and Psychiatry, 19,* 336–354.

Zilberstein, K. (2014b). The use and limitations of attachment in child therapy. *Psychotherapy, 51*(1), 93–103.

Resonance in the Dissociative Field: Examining the Therapist's Internal Experience When a Patient Dissociates in Session

JACQUELINE R. STRAIT

University of Pennsylvania, Philadelphia, Pennsylvania, USA

This study employed a qualitative research design utilizing intensive interviews and written case accounts to examine the therapist's internal experience when a patient with an early-life trauma history dissociates in session. Findings support emerging theory and research from the intersecting fields of relational psychoanalysis and interpersonal neurobiology that frame the internal experience of the therapist as a pathway for empathy and understanding. The findings suggest that the therapist's willingness to enter into a patient's dissociation in session and observe one's own internal experience during the dissociation can promote states of resonance, attunement, and implicit knowing in the therapy dyad.

The constructs of dissociation and resonance stand in stark contrast to one another. *Dissociation* refers to a separation of mental contents, a splitting of oneself, whereas *resonance* describes the coupling of otherwise separate entities and the emergence of synchrony. Dissociation, in its most severe form, almost always arises from a rupture in relationship, whereas resonance implies deep connection, a feeling of being seen and held by the other. What happens, then, when dissociation enters the therapy relationship? What happens when a highly traumatized patient dissociates in the course of a therapy session? In these moments, the patient is most in need of an attuned other to promote a sense of safety and co-regulation of traumatic affect, however, dissociation intrudes upon the therapy dyad, foreclosing intersubjectivity. Emerging theory and research from the intersecting fields of interpersonal neurobiology, trauma and dissociation, and relational psychoanalysis suggest that even in a dissociative state there is a capacity for interpersonal resonance and attunement (Hopenwasser, 2008; Howell, 2011; Sands, 2010). Accordingly, the therapist's painstaking presence and willingness to enter into a patient's dissociation can promote states of resonance and understanding in the dyad, strengthening the working alliance rather than leading to withdrawal and disconnection.

There is scant empirical research that examines what happens in the therapy dyad when a patient dissociates in session. Available research accounts for only the generalized impact that engagement in trauma work has on the therapist and neglects the moment-to-moment and shifting inner experience of the therapist in session with a survivor of trauma. I engaged in a qualitative study to learn about the in-session experience of therapists that occurs when a patient with an early-life trauma history dissociates in session. I specifically explored the impact of a patient's dissociation on the therapist, queried for states of resonance or attunement that evolved in the dyad, and explored what, if anything, was shared by way of a patient's dissociation in session and by what mechanism. In the following, I briefly review the theoretical literature and empirical research that frames this inquiry.

CONCEPTUAL FRAMEWORK

Dissociation has long been understood as an adaptation to extreme trauma, wherein the mind learns to turn off or disconnect to promote survival. This is seen in psychic phenomena such as trance, experiences of numbness or blankness, depersonalization and derealization, and at an extreme, gross disconnection from self or reality. When dissociation has been relied upon relentlessly in response to early and chronic trauma, the dissociative response becomes ingrained in the experience-dependent structures of the brain; any reminder of the traumatic memory or its related affect trigger dissociation. This is particularly relevant to the work of therapy, which aims at the integration of traumatic memory and regulation of affect. As such, the work of therapy itself may activate implicit trauma memories, retriggering the psychobiological processes of hyperarousal and dissociation that were set in motion by the original trauma(s) and are now ingrained in the patient's brain (Applegate & Shapiro, 2005; Lamagna & Gleiser, 2007). When a patient enters into a dissociative state in session, there is what Howell (2005) termed a "collapse of relationality" (p. 4). The patient ceases eye contact, withdraws posturally, and falls silent. She withdraws from the interpersonal matrix of the therapy relationship and retreats to her fragmented inner world.

Dissociation in the Therapy Dyad

A patient's dissociation in session is at once absorbing and deadening. The therapist is swept into what Loewenstein (1993) named the "dissociative field"—the transitional space between patient and therapist that activates the dissociative capacities of both. Within the dissociative field, the therapist is held captive by the intoxicating and hypnotic quality of the patient's dissociation and is susceptible to concomitant shifts in states of consciousness and emotional tone that often manifest as a dissociative countertransference reaction—moments of feeling dazed or disconnected (Gill, 2010; Howell, 2005). Rappoport (2012) wrote about her internal experience in the face of a patient's dissociation, describing a sense of "psychic and physical freezing" (p. 379) and a "physical woodenness and numbing" (p. 380). Similarly, Arizmendi (2008) described his own "paralyzed retreat" subsequent to his patient "fad[ing] away into a dissociative state" in session. Perlman (2004) framed such instances of dissociative countertransference as an intersubjective phenomenon that occur frequently in work with survivors of chronic trauma; he named this phenomenon "mutual dissociation" (p. 106). Both patient and therapist retreat to an inner world to achieve distance from the horrors of trauma the patient has experienced, including the frightening traumatic affect that arises in the course of therapy (Davies & Frawley, 1991). The result of this mutual dissociation is what Ogden (1995) described as the ambience of "deadness" (p. 699). There is a subjective sense that nothing is happening, seemingly reflective of a mutual retreat by the patient and therapist from that which is overwhelming and unbearable—that which compelled the dissociation in the first place.

What comes of this experience of being alone together? Contemporary theory reformulates the therapist's dissociative countertransference as an emerging state of resonance with the patient—a reflection of her intentional presence and attunement to that which is unwelcome (Howell, 2011; Siegel, 2010). Relational analytic trauma theorists conceptualize the unwelcome and unbidden in the dissociative field as dissociated self-states, parts of the patient's (or therapist's) self that are defensively split off from the conscious day-to-day experience of oneself. Current thinking in the field of relational psychoanalysis suggests that the only way to access this dissociated content is by way of the intersubjective therapeutic relationship, and more specifically, the therapist's internal and subjective experience of the patient (Bromberg, 1998, 2003, 2011; Davies & Frawley, 1991, 1994; Howell, 2005, 2011; Levenkron, 2009; Stern, 2003, 2010). These theorists argue that dissociated aspects of the patient's self will become enacted in the therapy relationship, and then be available for symbolic formulation in the mind of the therapist as the therapist engages interpersonally with the patient. These emerging theories imply that the therapist's willingness to enter into the patient's dissociative state promotes a way of knowing—an implicit knowing that occurs nonverbally and even nonconsciously in the dissociative field (Cortina & Liotti, 2007).

Dissociative Attunement

Of the many valuable contributions from relational analytic trauma literature, Hopenwasser (2008) and Sands (2010) most clearly elucidated this process of implicit knowing from within the dissociative field. Hopenwasser used observations from clinical work with chronically traumatized patients with dissociative symptoms to define the theoretical construct of dissociative attunement—the therapist's nonconscious and psychobiological attunement to the dissociated parts of the patient's self that become manifest in the therapist's subjectivity. Hopenwasser began to parcel out the component parts of dissociative attunement, labeling "empathic attunement," "dissociative transference," and "affective resonance" as three crucial components of this process that result in a "synchronized, simultaneous awareness of knowing that is nonlinear and fully bi-directional" (p. 351). She juxtaposed this construct with that of projective identification and enactments—constructs she perceives as failing to capture the fully mutual way in which traumatized people communicate states of unbearable pain. Here, Hopenwasser likely invoked Melanie Klein's original formulation of projective identification as a unidirectional process: the patient projects in fantasy a part of self onto and into the therapist resulting in dissonant (not resonant) states between therapist and patient. Likewise in an enactment, there is no simultaneous sharing of resonant states between patient and therapist; the states in the dyad are complementary (Racker, 1957). The implicit knowing and communication that Hopenwasser described, in contrast, occurs by way of attunement, sharing states with the patient. *Attunement* refers to the state of reciprocal recognition between two people that includes a synchronicity of inner experience, with the understanding that the two people are not sharing the identical state but sharing an affective experience in a different modality or intensity (Benjamin, 1995; Siegel, 2010). This process calls upon implicit knowledge and memory systems, as well as nonverbal communication processes between people. Siegel (2010) described two components of attunement: the physical component, "the perception of signals from others that reveal their internal world," such as eye contact, tone of voice, posture and facial expressions, and the subjective component, the "authentic sense of connection, of seeing someone deeply, of taking in the essence of another person in that moment" (p. 34). Hopenwasser argued that this process of attunement occurs in the midst of a patient's dissociation. Episodes of dissociative countertransference, which often look and feel like a misattunement, can instead be understood as the result of attunement to the patient's shifting dissociated states, resulting in resonance and ultimately the sense of "seeing someone deeply" as Siegel (2010) suggested.

Dissociative Unconscious Communication

Sands (2010), using the language of dissociative unconscious communication, described a similar process of nonverbal and nonconscious attunement to traumatic affect and dissociated states of chronically traumatized patients. Sands defined this implicit communication as "a powerful and visceral resonance between patient and analyst, as something dissociated in the patient grabs hold of and enters into deep communion with something dissociated in the analyst and opens up a channel of unconscious empathy" (p. 365). Sands also integrated work from the field of traumatic stress by arguing that the process of dissociative unconscious communication must occur by way of deep engagement with traumatic images and somatosensory fragments in the patient's and analyst's dreams. Sands viewed this process of dissociative communication as an inevitable and deeply reparative part of the treatment with survivors of chronic trauma.

Both Hopenwasser's (2008) and Sand's (2010) theories of dissociative communication emphasize affective attunement in the midst of a dissociative field as a way to comprehend dissociated aspects of a patient's self. Both theories allude to this attunement becoming manifest in the therapist's subjectivity in visual images, intense affective experience, or somatic sensations. Both theories espouse a model of mutuality in which access to dissociated states occurs in moments of communion and deep synchronicity with the patient. These constructs stand in stark contrast to those of vicarious traumatization and secondary traumatic stress (Bride, Radey, & Figley, 2007; McCann & Pearlman, 1990; Pearlman & Mac Ian, 1995). They suggest that something rich and rewarding can emerge from engagement with a highly traumatized patient. They suggest that the dissociative space should not be merely managed or avoided, but instead entered into. Doing so can promote a powerful experience of connection and communication through the therapist's oscillating and careful attention to self and other.

NEUROBIOLOGY OF DISSOCIATION

Despite the theoretical support and clinical utility of this concept of dissociative communication, little empirical research exists to understand how dissociated content is communicated implicitly in the therapy dyad or how it becomes manifest in the therapist's subjectivity. The emerging fields of infancy research and interpersonal neurobiology lend insight into this phenomenon, offering a framework to understand what can be shared between patient and therapist during a patient's dissociation in session and by what mechanism this occurs.

Right-Brain Communication

Neurobiological theories of right brain-to-right brain communication eluci-date how enlivened communication can occur in the midst of the dissociative field. Allan Schore (2001, 2009b, 2010) has written prolifically about the neurobiological and clinical implications of the right brain—the hemisphere of the brain responsible for processing socioemotional information and reg-ulating affective and bodily states. The right brain, known for processing information holistically, is involved in the automatic processing of nonverbal cues in human interaction. These nonverbal cues include facial expressions, prosodic vocalizations, coordinated visual eye-to-eye messages, tactile and body gestures, posture, and tone of voice (Applegate & Shapiro, 2005). A. N. Schore (2010) asserted that humans can appraise facially expressed emo-tional cues in less than 30 milliseconds, a rate far outside conscious detection. As such, the right brain is responsible for rapidly identifying and express-ing emotions and communicating them nonverbally (A. N. Schore, 2009b). The right brain can also engage the right brain of others who are "tuned" to receive these communications (J. R. Schore & Schore, 2008). A. N. Schore (2009b) named this process right brain-to-right brain communication, defined as the "ultrarapid bodily based affective communications in patient-therapist (and infant-mother) attachment transactions [that] occur beneath levels of conscious awareness in both members of the dyad" (p. 115). In right-brain communication, the therapist tracks the nonverbal sensory cues transmitted from the patient while simultaneously attending to the sensory and somatic experiences that arise in her own inner world (Siegel, 2012).

Right-brain communication is particularly salient during moments of dissociation. Unlike the left brain, the right brain can operate at very high or very low arousal levels. When a patient dissociates in session, she moves from extraordinarily high levels of arousal (activation of the sympathetic ner-vous) to very low levels of arousal (activation of the dorsal vagal branch of the parasympathetic nervous system). In both instances, the left brain goes offline while the nonconscious functions of the right brain continue unaffected (A. N. Schore, 2009a). Functional magnetic resonance imaging (MRI) research has supported this assertion, indicating that when patients are actively dissociating, it is predominately the right hemisphere of the brain that is activated (Lanius et al., 2002).

Right-brain communication is especially apparent among patients with chronic dissociative symptoms and an early relational trauma history, espe-cially when the trauma occurred prior to the development of the left brain or the capacity for verbal language. In such instances, traumatic affect and self-states can be stored only in the implicit language of the earlier-developing right brain (A. N. Schore, 2010). The implicit memory system is thought to exist from birth (Fosshage, 2010). This memory system requires neither con-scious thought nor the involvement of the hippocampus in the encoding of memories. As a result, preverbal experiences are retained as memories in the right brain but are dissociated from language. This is further supported by recent advances in the understanding of traumatic memory. During a traumatic experience, intense affect is registered in the amygdala, but such unusually high levels of activation of the amygdala hamper hipppocampal functioning (Applegate & Shapiro, 2005). Without the functioning of the hippocampus to provide a coherent and verbal narrative, trauma memories are affective and sensory based, experienced in the raw sense perceptions associated with the right brain (van der Kolk & Fisler, 1995; van der Kolk, Hopper, & Osterman, 2001). For some traumatized people, there may be no explicit, left-brain recall of the traumatic memory whatsoever; the memory may be stored only an implicit level. Fragments of such memory can only be communicated in the capacity in which they were stored: by way of the right brain.

Mirror Neuron System

Right-brain communication enables the therapist to tune in to nonverbal, sensory cues transmitted by the patient in the midst of a dissociative state (A. N. Schore, 2009b, 2010). When the therapist opens her own right brain and body to the communications of the patient, the result is a state of resonance (Siegel, 2012). This resonance is an affective resonance and a neurobiological resonance, as the therapist's autonomic nervous system synchronizes with the patient's autonomic nervous system (A. N. Schore, 2009b). A new class of premotor neurons called mirror neurons, discovered in the early 1990s, can account for these emerging states of resonance in the dyad (Gallese, Fadiga, Fogassi, & Rizzolatti, 1996). Early research on mirror neurons suggests that we mimic, neurobiologically, actions and emotional states that we observe (Gallese, 2009; Iacoboni, 2008). This mirroring includes emotional expression, tone of voice, gestures, and facial expressions that offer a way to understand the internal experience of another (Bloom & Farragher, 2011). Further evidence suggests that observing an emotion and experiencing an emotion activates the identical neural structure, that is, we internally simulate the observed emotion and its related behavior (Gallese, 2009; Gallese, Eagle, & Migone, 2007). Gallese et al. (2007) named this process "embodied simulation." This process is what enables the therapist to observe the nonverbal cues transmitted by the patient and then resonate, subcortically, with what she sees. The therapist maps his patient's actions, emotions, and sensations onto his own somatosensory and motor representations, such that he can make sense of his patient's internal experiences by sorting through his own (Gallese, 2009; Siegel, 2010). Gallese et al. (2007) described the outcome of this embodied simulation for the therapy dyad, explaining, "It is possible that the patient's emotional tone and expressions trigger in the therapist an automatic simulation and consequently the experience of at least a small dose of an emotion similar to the one experienced by the patient" (p. 148). Although research on the activation of the mirror neuron system has not been conducted specifically as it relates to a patient's dissociation in session, the findings reported here suggest that this automatic process of simulation occurs so long as the patient displays some subtle but observable cue to her internal state. The therapist's intentional attention to these cues allows for the patient's internal world to be transmitted both to and through the therapist's own senses (Siegel, 2012, p. 136).

RESEARCH

I have been impressed by the rich theoretical literature and neurobiological research that cites the importance of the therapist's use of self as a way of knowing, especially in cases where a patient has been severely traumatized in early life. Despite this, there is limited empirical research that explores the in-session experience of therapists working with traumatized patients to support these claims. To address this gap in research, I developed a qualitative study using constructivist grounded theory (Charmaz, 2006) to learn about the in-session inner experience of therapists that occurs when patients who have histories of early-life trauma dissociate in session. My research examined what kind of attunement might occur in the dissociative field and what potential this attunement holds to communicate dissociated images, affect, or somatosensory experience that otherwise cannot be spoken about.

Recruitment and Sample

I obtained participants through convenience and snowball sampling. The sample comprised 11 psychotherapists, each of whom had worked with an adult patient reporting an early and severe trauma history and active symptoms of dissociation, had the experience of this patient dissociating in session, and were willing to recount their internal and private response to this dissociation in great detail. Ten of the 11 participants were female. Five participants were doctoral-level psychotherapists and six participants were masters-level psychotherapists. Participants' experience level ranged from 3 to 31 years, with a mean of 18 years. Eight participants identified their primary practice location as private practice, whereas two identified college counseling centers and one an outpatient mental health agency. The participants each endorsed multiple and varying theoretical orientations: six participants espoused a psychodynamic theoretical orientation, three identified a cognitive behavioral orientation, and four identified an interpersonal or relational orientation. Each participant was assigned a pseudonym to ensure anonymity.

Data Collection

In keeping with the constructivist approach of this research, my primary method of data collection was the face-to-face interview. I relied upon a semistructured interview guide and adhered to this guide in a loose way, allowing for discussion of themes that each participant found meaningful. Interviewees provided written consent to be interviewed and audio-recorded, using a form approved by the University's Institutional Review Board. The interviews lasted between 61 and 93 minutes, with a mean interview time of 73 minutes. Participants were compensated $30 for participation in the interview.

To triangulate the data, procure a longer period of engagement, and to obtain more experience-near data, I asked each participant to complete a written account subsequent to the interview detailing a follow-up experience of a patient dissociating in session. Participants were compensated an additional $20 for completion of the written account. I received a total of nine written case accounts.

Data Analysis

The audio-recorded interviews were transcribed verbatim and then analyzed with line-by-ling coding of five initial interviews to examine all possible interpretations of the data. A fellow researcher engaged in open coding of one randomly selected transcript to compare codes. After adjustments to several codes, we reached a concordance rate of 87.6%. I simultaneously engaged in memoing to develop preliminary hypotheses about emerging categories, themes, and overarching theory. Line-by-line coding of the five initial interviews generated 1,690 open codes. I then began to compare these open codes to one another through a process of focused coding until review of transcripts yielded no additional focused codes. I moved to a loose form of axial coding to recontextualize emergent themes as they existed in the data, to develop subcategories and to show the associations between categories (Charmaz, 2006).

FINDINGS

A complete account of the findings of this study are outside the scope of this article. I present a select portion of the findings below that implicate the neurobiological basis of implicit communication and resonance in the dissociative field. For a more comprehensive review of the findings, see Strait (2013).

Mirroring of States

The clinicians I interviewed were reflectively able to describe how a patient's dissociative experience in the room affected them as a clinician and as a human being. There was a sequential process that the participants described moving through as they became aware that a patient was dissociating in session, which included a subjective experience of anxiety, doom, or dread; states of hyperarousal; a feeling of being left or abandoned; and states of mutual dissociation. The participants described these affective and physiological states as entirely internal and sometimes idiosyncratic reactions to a patient's dissociation. Taken in aggregate, however, the therapist's sequence of responses to a patient's dissociation in session represented a consistent and reliable phenomenon across participant accounts. This sequence of participant responses suggests that the internal experience of the therapist in the face of a patient's dissociation mirrors the human psychobiological response pattern to trauma: hyperarousal and then dissociation (Perry, Pollard, Blakely, Baker, & Vigilante, 1995; A. N. Schore, 2001). Extrapolation of this finding implies that the therapist's internal experience in the face of a patient's dissociation in session reflects a mirror of the patient's internal experience in the face of the original trauma and the reactivation of these states, stored in the experience-dependent structures of the brain, in the course of a therapy session. As such, the therapist's internal experience can offer an entry into the internal world of the patient in the dissociative space. I highlight several participant accounts below to elaborate on these findings.

THERAPIST ANXIETY

Each of the 11 participants described fear or anxiety in response to their patient's dissociation, making this a ubiquitous aspect of contending with a patient's dissociation in session. There were four unique manifestations of therapist anxiety. The first was worry about having caused the patient's dissociation. Nine participants lamented over whether they had done something to hurt the patient and cause the dissociation, unintentionally replicating cycles of harm that followed the patient throughout her life. The participants asked themselves a litany of questions to determine their level of responsibility and grapple with feelings of guilt. Kaitlyn, for instance, wondered, "Crap, did I do this?" Catherine asked herself, "Am I doing something that's hurtful? Something that's painful?" These questions reflect the participants' most basic fear that the patient's dissociation was their fault.

Seven participants reported a related manifestation of anxiety: doubts about one's own competency. Darlene clearly articulated this fear when she admitting to wondering, "Was I competent enough? Why didn't I see that [the dissociation in session was coming]? Should I have seen it? I would doubt myself and I would feel like I let her down somehow." Several other participants fantasized about referring the client to a more experienced clinician or bringing a supervisor in for a consultation while the patient was dissociated. This anxiety about one's own competency was more salient among novice therapists or between therapist–patient pairs that were just beginning their treatment relationship.

A third type of anxiety, more salient for experienced clinicians or more experienced patient–clinician dyads, was a primordial sense of dread and doom. Seven participants spoke of a guttural sense that, "This is bad" or "Something bad is going to happen" when a patient dissociated in session. In some cases, it was an inchoate doom that remained nameless and formless. Marcy, for instance, endorsed a "tightening in my stomach and a sense of kind of dread." She explained, "I call it a minefield [laughs]. Like if I misstep then something is going to blow up. And I never ever know, I don't know where the mines are." For other participants, the doom focused on a particular calamity, for instance being sued by the patient, which was particularly salient when the patient was dissociated. These worries reflect the participants' unease and paranoia in the dissociative gap.

The final type of fear that participants described was a fear of losing track of one's own sanity in the midst of the patient's dissociation in the room. The participants described this very self-focused fear as incredibly threatening and inducing a temptation to withdraw from the patient. Four participants reported this fear, alternately describing it as "being afraid of being drawn into their [the patient's] craziness" and as contemplating how to "not get sucked into" a "population living on the brink." Elise spoke most candidly about this fear of losing the tenuous connection to her own sanity in the face of her patient's dissociation. She explained, "I'm talking to someone and they're not there, and then, where does that put me?" She described the felt experience of this as "threatening." She continued, "I think it's one sanity that gets threatened . . . One's own sanity gets, like, yanked." Like several other participants, Elise identified the patient's withdrawal from relationship as promoting her intense anxiety, leaving her with a compelling pull into the patient's "craziness."

The manifestation of anxiety varied among participants, but each reported gripping fear as one of the first responses to a patient's dissociation in session. These fears reflect a parallel of those articulated by survivors of interpersonal trauma, namely, fear about having caused or somehow "asked for" the abusive treatment, doubt about one's agency to manage the threat or protect oneself, a persistent sense of dread, and fear of going crazy or losing one's mind.

THERAPIST HYPERAROUSAL

In addition to the affective experience of anxiety, participants also reported a physiological state of hyperarousal and hypervigilance when a patient dissociated in session. Seven participants noted somatic signs of hyper-arousal, including increased heart rate and perspiration as well as a sharp focus on their patient and a state of hypervigilance. Stephanie explained that when her patient dissociated, she was "watching her very closely . . . really focusing on any cues I was getting from her body and her expression and energy level." She described this as a "laser -attention" and "watching her like a hawk." Nancy likewise described a state of hyperfocused attention when her patient dissociated. She explained she was:

> Paying attention to him, aware of the stillness in the room, aware of whether or not I was moving in my chair, aware of keeping my eye on him, aware of the silence . . . . Aware of the kind of the length of time . . . . Very present. It was almost like when he dropped out of us, I picked up, which was interesting.

This particular kind of hyperfocus described by participants represents a parallel experience to a typical response pattern to a major trauma, focusing in on narrow details but losing the larger perceptual picture. Darlene described this as being "hyperpresent but not in a relaxed way." She went on to explain:

> I wasn't thinking about anything else in the world other than what do I do right now. So I was very present, but I wasn't like attending to anything else in the room . . . . I wasn't attending to anything except for what was happening with her and what I should be doing about it.

Darlene's experience of hyperarousal and hyperfocus on her patient precluded her from awareness of other sensory perceptions or her own internal experience. Elise had a similar understanding of her hypervigilance in the face of her patient's dissociation. She said, "It's not hyperfocused in a particularly helpful way. It's more hyperfocused like, 'Oh my god. What's going on? What am I going to do?' . . . I'm not clear. I'm all feeling at that moment." She likened this to the experience of whipping around and realizing there was a fire. Her account highlights the perception of danger associated with a patient's dissociation, and the anxiety and physiological manifestation of hyperarousal it sets off in its wake.

ALONENESS

The participant's hyperfocus on the patient ultimately led to a perception of nonresponsiveness from the patient, a feeling of being left alone in the room, and a pervasive sense of disconnection. Nine participants reported a peculiar sensation of feeling alone while in the presence of the patient, her body there but her person gone. Darlene likened this to the experience of a cell-phone call dropping out, and Jeff described his urge to wave his hands in front of his patient's face to rouse her. Catherine described her sense of disconnection when her patient dissociated as "almost like a prison gate slamming closed." This left her with "a feeling of being in the room with no one." Being without this connection in the dyad, oftentimes when the therapist desired so desperately to be helpful to her patient, left the therapist feeling left, or as Jeff described it, "abandoned." The participants' responses to this experience of feeling left and alone in most cases led to a retreat into their own inner world while the patient was dissociating. In some cases, this manifested as self-focused worry, in others it appeared as unrelated reveries about shopping or mental to-do lists. In the face of the patient's withdrawal of her subjectivity, the participants retreated into their own.

Mutual dissociation

Nine participants described an extreme withdrawal and retreat in the face of a patient's dissociation which I characterize as states of mutual dissociation. These states varied from momentary blankness, losing track of time or place, experiential feelings of fogginess, to total blank-outs themselves. Marcy described a particularly powerful state of mutual dissociation, comparing her internal experience during the patient's dissociation to that of being under a "spell." She experienced a "heavy cloud of fatigue" that made it "hard to stay in the room." She continued, "It was almost a physical feeling of not being present . . . I would either feel really like I could not keep my eyes open, or my mind would just go elsewhere. And I wasn't at all present . . . . It was almost a physical sensation of like this fog of tiredness." The participants described these sensations of tiredness, disorientation, and fogginess as mild states of dissociation resonant with their patient's more extreme dissociation.

The participants made sense of these states of mutual dissociation as a result of contagion, not emerging from vicarious traumatization or their own idiosyncratic internal processes. They described their own dissociative states as projected or co-constructed experiences with the patient. Elise explained this as "shar[ing] in the feeling of disorientation, confusion, not being aware of time or space or place." Rather than keeping herself at a place of "horror or distance," Elise entered into her patient's dissociative state in session. Elise's explanation reveals a common theme amongst participants of the importance of accepting both the patient's dissociation and one's own counter-dissociative processes. Rather than experiencing her patient's and her own dissociation as disturbing, she understood it as entirely necessary and even mundane, noting, "Oh well. We'll find our way back." Elise's words capture her acceptance of the utter normality of dissociation. She puts herself on a continuum with her patients, humanizing them, by acknowledging and even welcoming her own dissociative process. Still, the participants identified the importance of navigating the precarious line between entering the patient's dissociation while staying grounded enough to be helpful to the patient. Anna described this as "keep[ing] myself kind of here, but not so here that I can't experience a little of it, because I think it helps her." Elise likewise maintained this distinction between the patient's dissociation and her own by reminding herself, "I better hold onto my sanity as best I can, while allowing myself to go a little insane." The participants who endorsed states of mutual dissociation were able to toggle back and forth between immersion in the dissociative field and remaining far enough outside of it to offer containment and regulation to the patient.

The participants' reports of moving from fear to hyperarousal, to a recognition of nonresponsiveness from the patient, to ultimately entering a state of dissociation represent a curious mirror of a patient's sequential experience in the face of a traumatic encounter, and likely the repeated response to stressors that have been stored in the experience-dependent pathways of the brain. As such, the patient's dissociation in session holds the capacity to bring the internal state of the therapist into resonance with the patient's experienced or dissociated state.

Induced Feeling

Six of the participants understood their internal experience as reflective of or parallel to the patient's state, resulting in what Ruth called a "shared experience" during the dissociation in session. Tasha introduced the language of "induced feeling" to describe how she believed her internal experience represented an induced, modulated version of the patient's state—offering both a pathway for empathy and understanding. Several participants described this *as feeling the patient's feeling*, not in its original form or intensity, but in a modulated or mild way. Marcy, for instance, understood the combination of her feeling of fogginess and anger as induced by the patient. She explained,

> She'll sort of look down and she'll go completely silent . . . . The feeling is so conflictual for her and I think it's her rage that is so hard for her to stay with and so that I feel the anger, umm . . . I feel her anger at those times.

Marcy then took pains to differentiate this induced feeling from that of projective identification. She said that it feels similar to projective identification, but her grasp of the induced feeling occurred entirely outside of language. "There's no talking," she explained. "But I feel really angry and then I realize that it's probably her anger that I'm feeling." Marcy understood the anger as a result of her efforts at attunement and the subsequent synchrony of feeling that developed in the pair.

Catherine likewise reflected on her internal experience as an attenuated version of her patient's unexpressed feeling that prompted the dissociation. She explained that her feelings of uncertainty, loneliness, and doubts about her competency that arose in the midst of the patient's dissociation "might be some of what she's experiencing." She clarified her sense that the patient was anticipating "that something harsh and hurtful and critical is going to come my way and I'm all alone and I need to protect myself." She saw her own anticipation of harm and experience of loneliness as a result of coming into contact with the patient's feeling state during the dissociation. Catherine identified these resonant states as a result of her efforts to "reconnect" and "be present" with the patient through the dissociation.

In addition to contact with an induced feeling, six participants described an experience of oneself as being the "placeholder" for the patient's states when she was dissociating. Catherine introduced the language of "placeholder" to describe her willingness to step in and "hold" the patient's feelings when the patient couldn't, taking on the patient's subjectivity in the midst of her absence. Ruth elaborated on the experience of herself as "the keeper" of the patient's affective experience and historical memory during the dissociation. She explained:

> She's dissociating, she's checked out. In a way I'm the one who is holding all of the stuff. I am holding the history of our work together . . . that's all there for me, and because I'm being thoughtful and aware of what it is that we had been talking about, and how that might be impacting her . . . . I'm the keeper of that . . . . It's like this was so unbelievably painful for her . . . . so I was able to experience it for her in a way.

Ruth described holding the patient's affective state that the patient could not tolerate, while also holding a cognitive understanding of the patient and her history. Ruth served as the "keeper" by being able to feel her way through the patient's state and think about it in context.

The participants described these induced feelings as holding an important function in the dyad, bringing the patient and therapist into a state of resonance and ultimately conferring understanding. Tasha described her induced feeling during the patient's dissociation as "information that I'm getting . . . I get a feeling of 'Oh, okay *that's what it is*.'" In many cases, the participants relied on a left-brain process of verbal and cognitive understanding to "get" the induced feeling, translating somatic and affective experience into a thinkable one. The participants' willingness to enter into the patient's dissociation and serve as a "placeholder" for the patient's feelings and thoughts enabled a bridge between self and other, promoting understanding and connection in spite of (or because of) the patient's dissociation in session. Ruth's words best capture this emergence of connection through the patient's dissociation. She explained, "She was checked out, I was by her side there. Literally, I mean."

DISCUSSION

Findings of this study suggest that a patient's dissociation in session holds a powerful impact on the observing or participating clinician. Rather than conceptualizing this impact in terms of only treatment deficit or vicarious traumatization, the findings of this study suggest that the internal experience of the therapist can offer entry into the patient's internal world. The findings reported here imply that the therapist's internal experience in the face of the patient's dissociation is in attunement and resonance with the patient. Participants experienced within themselves a mild or modulated version of what they believed reflected the patients' state during the session or the patient's split-off affective experience related to the original trauma. These findings provide support for the relational analytic stance that the therapist's internal experience constitutes an important way of knowing, especially in work with patients traumatized in early life. This perspective further supports Hopenwasser's (2008) and Sands' (2010) constructs of dissociative attunement and dissociative unconscious communication, that a kind of implicit, nonconscious and psychobiological knowing occurs in the midst of the patient's dissociation in session. This knowing is an experience of resonance and communion between therapist and patient in the midst of the withdrawal of one or both parties. It is an experience of understanding and "getting it" in the midst of mental confusion. It is the resonance of internal experience such that the therapist holds onto a feeling induced by the patient or acts as the placeholder for her thoughts and experiences, while also maintaining the inherent separateness of the two and the distinctness of roles in the dyad. Finally, this kind of knowing requires a special kind of listening that demands catlike perception of nonverbal cues while also maintaining a simultaneous awareness of one's internal experience. This listening requires that the therapist be both here and there, inside and outside, all at the same time. It is a kind of knowing while feeling like you don't know anything at all.

These findings also provide support for the neurobiological understanding of dissociation and interpersonal resonance. The participants reported a sequence of affective and behavioral states during the patient's dissociation that reflect a mirror of the psychobiological response pattern to trauma: anxiety, hyperarousal, and dissociation. Neurobiologically, this response consists first of activation of the sympathetic nervous system (the fight–flight response) that responds to danger by increasing heart rate, releasing catecholamines, and activating the HPA axis, resulting in increases in the stress hormone cortisol (Porges, 2009). When these preparations to fight or flee from danger are not successful, the parasympathetic nervous system steps in to conserve energy and protect the self by freezing or feigning death. It is this parasympathetic system that is thought to be responsible for the profound detachment of dissociation (A. N. Schore, 2009b). When a patient dissociates in a therapy session, there is likely sympathetic arousal in response to triggering material and then a rapid and almost automatic activation of the parasympathetic nervous system, which manifests as a dissociative response. Findings from this study suggest that there is a reciprocal activation of the therapist's sympathetic and then parasympathetic nervous system in session, as evidenced by participant reports of anxiety, physiological states of hyperarousal, and then mild dissociation. According to A. N. Schore (2009b), this matching of patient and therapist autonomic nervous systems results in an amplification of states. A. N. Schore (2009b) explained, "this increased arousal (metabolic energy) allows hypoaroused dissociated affect to be intensified and then experienced in consciousness as a subjective emotional state" (p. 136). The therapist's autonomic nervous system is brought into resonance with the patient's, allowing her to understand the patient's internal experience and, according to A. N. Schore (2009b), to intensify the dissociated state such that it can be become a subjective and ultimately intersubjective phenomenon.

The neurobiological resonance that is achieved between patient and therapist in the dissociative field can be understood as the result of the mirror neuron system and process of embodied simulation between patient and therapist. This process hinges upon the expression and recognition of nonverbal cues. Participants consistently reported close attention to the nonverbal cues transmitted by the patient, described by one participant as "watching [the patient] like a hawk." According to research on the mirror neuron system, it is this direct observation of a person experiencing an emotion that elicits the activation of identical neural pathways in the observer (Gallese et al., 2007). This process is distinct from that of so-called simulation theory—where the observer has to rely on introspection to imagine herself experiencing the emotion of another. Simulation and introspection allow the observer to capture the affective quality of an other's feeling, but not its basic sensory qualities or related neurobiological properties. Direct observation of another person experiencing a feeling, on the other hand, allows the observer to simulate, within his own body, the identical affective state which then becomes a "shared body state" (Gallese et al., 2007, p. 144). Findings of this study suggest that the participants were directly observing the physiological and behavioral cues expressing the patient's affective states of fear and ultimately dissociation. This observation allowed the participants to embody a resonant state both affectively and physiologically.

The findings of this study also suggest that while there was a resonance of states between patient and therapist during the dissociation, there was a distinction of degree. Catherine, for instance, noted feeling fearful during her patient's dissociation and understood this as "some of what she's experiencing." She described this resonance as "very light," explaining that "there was no real danger and there was no threat to my core self," whereas for the patient the danger was real and severe. Her own sense of fear was resonant with "but *to no degree* what she [the patient] was feeling." Likewise, other participants described feeling anxious but not panicked; afraid but not afraid for their lives; foggy but not gone entirely from the room; and disoriented but still aware of their core identity. This finding dovetails with research in the mirror neuron field that suggests varying degrees of activation of the same neural structure between observer and observed. For instance, a study by Blakemore, Bristow, Bird, Frith, and Ward (2005) found that when a person witnesses another person being touched, the same neural pathway is activated in the observer as if he were touched himself, however there is a lower degree of activation that allows the observer to differentiate who is being touched. This finding is especially relevant for the therapy dyad. The lower degree of resonance protects the therapist from falling into a counter-dissociative state in session that is neither modulated nor therapeutic.

The distinction of degree in mirrored states is an important concept that acts as a hinge between mirroring in a neurobiological sense and mirroring in a psychoanalytic sense. The neurobiological processes of mirroring and embodied simulation suggest that the observer experiences an exact replica of what she sees. For the therapist, this would mean she experiences an identical state of fear, hyperarousal, or dissociation in the midst of a patient's dissociation in session. However, the findings from this study suggest that patient and therapist were able to share in these states while feeling the separateness of their experiences. The participants reported parallel or induced feelings from the patient, but only "mild" or "light" versions. The participants also described holding onto a sense of the distinctness of their role and responsibility to the patient that enabled them to resist being swept up by the tide of affective resonance. Ruth described this as an intentional resistance of a state of pure resonance. She noted, "Maybe at moments I would have like, started to go there [to dissociate], but I bring myself back. That's the responsibility piece. That's how we are different. That's why I'm in this seat and you're over there." All 11 participants identified a feeling of responsibility for their patient that distinguished the distinct roles in the dyad. This differentiation of roles and maintenance of responsibility for the patient's well-being was important in forestalling a merger of experience.

Gallese et al. (2007) argued that the mirror neuron system and process of embodied simulation lie at the basis of these therapeutic exchanges of attunement. He explained, "a person's observation of another's behavior elicits automatic simulation of that behavior, and it is this mechanism that enables empathic understanding, which can eventually lead to complementary or modulating responses" (Gallese et al., 2007, p. 151). These processes are especially important in the mirroring of a patient's state during a dissociative episode. The therapist's ability to resonate with the fear, hyper-arousal, and dissociation, but from within a different intensity or modality, keeps her autonomic reactivity in a more moderate range and allows the hippocampus and functions of the left brain to stay online. The therapist can then formulate a therapeutic response—one that arises out of a state of resonance, but is not an exact replica of the patient's state.

IMPLICATIONS AND CONCLUSION

This research is limited in its small sample size and its reliance upon clin-icians' retrospective recall of their internal experiences in the face of a patient's dissociation in session. The most marked limitation of this study is the neglect of patients' experiences of dissociating in session. To truly deter-mine states of resonance, we need research on the simultaneous experiences of patient and therapist in the midst of the dissociative field.

Despite these limitations, this research has far-reaching implications in the treatment of patients who dissociate in session. The findings call us to consider dissociative defenses not only as a symptom to eradicate, but also as an interpersonal phenomenon that holds the potential to communicate crucial information about the patient and the treatment. They prompt the therapist to neither avoid nor short-circuit a patient's dissociation in ses-sion but instead to accept the patient's dissociation, enter into it, and accept one's own counter-dissociative processes. Further, these findings offer a clin-ically relevant application of interpersonal neurobiology. We can understand emerging states of dissociative countertransference and induced feelings as evolving from processes of neuronal mirroring and right-brain com-munication that occur rapidly and outside of conscious detection. Finally, there is a suggestion that these states of resonance that emerge during a patient's dissociation in session can be therapeutic. Processes of mirroring and embodied simulation can work in both directions. The patient can res-onate affectively and neurobiologically with the therapist's more modulated and ultimately changed state of hyperarousal or dissociation and simulate that within oneself. Through this ongoing dynamic dance of resonance and simulation between patient and therapist, the pair can co-regulate the trau-matic affect and reinitiate a state of intersubjectivity, repairing the disjunction put in place by the dissociative defense (Siegel, 2010, p. 55).

Evidence from this study and the emerging literature cited in this article suggest that resonance and attunement can occur in the dissociative field. These processes are automatic and nonconscious but can also be inten-tionally reflected upon and therapeutically used. They offer the therapist a guidepost in the midst of the dizzying and disorienting dissociative field and a way to understand and know from the inside out.

REFERENCES

Applegate, J. S., & Shapiro, J. R. (2005). *Neurobiology for clinical social work: Theory and practice*. New York, NY: Norton.

Arizmendi, T. G. (2008). Nonverbal communication in the context of dissociative processes. *Psychoanalytic Psychology, 25*(3), 443–457.

Benjamin, J. (1995). *Like subjects, love objects: Essays on recognition and sexual difference*. New Haven, CT: Yale University Press.

Blakemore, S. J., Bristow, D., Bird, G., Frith, C., & Ward, J. (2005). Somatosensory activations during the observation of touch and a case of vision-touch synaesthesia. *Brain, 128*, 1571–1583.

Bloom, S. L., & Farragher, B. (2011). *Destroying sanctuary: The crisis in human service delivery systems*. New York, NY: Oxford University Press.

Bride, B. E., Radey, M. E., & Figley, C. R. (2007). Measuring compassion fatigue. *Clinical Social Work Journal, 35*, 155–163.

Bromberg, P. M. (1998) *Standing in the spaces: Essays on clinical process trauma and dissociation*. Hillsdale, NJ: Analytic Press.

Bromberg, P. M. (2003). Something wicked this way comes: Trauma, dissociation, and conflict: The space where psychoanalysis, cognitive science and neuroscience overlap. *Psychoanalytic Psychology, 20*(3), 558–574.

Bromberg, P. M. (2011) *Awakening the dreamer: Clinical journeys*. New York, NY: Routledge, Taylor & Francis Group.

Charmaz, K. (2006). *Constructing grounded theory: A practical guide through qualitative analysis*. Thousand Oaks, CA: Sage.

Cortina, M., & Liotti, G. (2007). New approaches to understanding unconscious processes: Implicit and explicit memory systems. *International Forum of Psychoanalysis, 16*, 204–212.

Davies, J. M., & Frawley, M. G. (1991). Dissociative processes and transference-countertransference paradigms in the psychoanalytically oriented treatment of adult survivors of childhood sexual abuse. In S. A. Mitchell & L. Aron (Eds.), *Relational psychoanalysis the emergence of a tradition* (pp. 269–304). New York, NY: Routledge.

Davies, J. M., & Frawley, M. G. (1994). *Treating the adult survivor of childhood sexual abuse: A psychoanalytic perspective*. New York, NY: Basic Books.

Fosshage, J. L. (2010. Implicit and explicit pathways to psychoanalytic change. In J. Petrucelli (Ed.), *Knowing, not-knowing and sort-of-knowing: Psychoanalysis and the experience of uncertainty* (pp. 215–224). London, UK: Karnac Books.

Gallese, V. (2009). Mirror neurons, embodied simulation, and the neural basis of social identification. *Psychoanalytic Dialogues, 19*, 519–536.

Gallese, V., Eagle, M. N., & Migone, P. (2007). Intentional attunement: Mirror neurons and the neural underpinnings of interpersonal relations. *Journal of the American Psychoanalytic Association, 55*, 131–176.

Gallese, V., Fadiga, L., Fogassi, L., & Rizzolatti, G. (1996). Action recognition in the premotor cortex. *Brain, 119*(2), 593–609.

Gill, S. (2010). The therapist as psychobiological regulator: Dissociation, affect attunement and clinical process. *Clinical Social Work Journal, 38*, 260–268.

Hopenwasser, K. (2008). Being in rhythm: Dissociative attunement in therapeutic process. *Journal of Trauma & Dissociation, 9*(3), 349–367.

Howell, E. (2005). *The dissociative mind*. New York, NY: Routledge, Taylor & Francis Group.

Howell, E. (2011). *Understanding and treatment dissociative identity disorder: A relational approach*. New York, NY: Routledge, Taylor & Francis Group.

Iacoboni, M. (2008). *Mirroring people: The new science of how we connect with others*. New York, NY: Farrar, Straus and Giroux.

Lamagna, J., & Gleiser, K. A. (2007). Building a secure internal attachment: An intra-relational approach to ego strengthening and emotional processing with chronically traumatized clients. *Journal of Trauma & Dissociation, 8*(1), 25–52.

Lanius, R. A., Williamson, P. C., Boksman, K., Densmore, M., Gupta, M., Neufeld, R. W. J., . . . Menon, R. S. (2002). Brain activation during script-driven imagery induced dissociative responses in PTSD: A functional magnetic resonance imaging investigation. *Biological Psychiatry, 52*, 305–311.

Levenkron, H. (2009). Engaging the implicit: Meeting points between the Boston Change Process Study Group and relational psychoanalysis. *Contemporary Psychoanalysis, 45*(2), 179–217.

Loewenstein, R. J. (1993). Post-traumatic and dissociative aspects of transference and countertransference in the treatment of multiple personality disorder. In R. P. Kluft & C. O. Fine (Eds.), *Clinical perspective on multiple personality disorder* (pp. 51–85). Washington, DC: American Psychiatric Press.

McCann, I. L., & Pearlman, L. A. (1990). Vicarious traumatization: A framework for understanding the psychological effects of working with victims. *Journal of Traumatic Stress, 3*, 131–149.

Ogden, T. H. (1995). Analysing forms of aliveness and deadness of the transference-countertransference. *International Journal of Psycho-Analysis, 76*, 695–709.

Pearlman, L. A., & Mac Ian, P. S. (1995). Vicarious traumatization: An empirical study of the effects of trauma work on trauma therapists. *Professional Psychology: Research and Practice, 26*(6), 558–565.

Perlman, S. D. (2004). Who dissociates? Incest survivor or therapist? In W. J. Coburn (Ed.), *Transformations in self psychology: Progress in self psychology: Volume 20* (pp. 95–108). Hillsdale, NJ: Analytic Press.

Perry, B. D., Pollard, R. A., Blakely, T. L., Baker, W. L., & Vigilante, D. (1995). Childhood trauma, the neurobiology of adaptation and use-dependent development of the brain: How states become traits. *Infant Mental Health Journal, 16*, 271–291.

Porges, S. W. (2009). Reciprocal influences between body and brain in the perception and expression of affect: A polyvagal perspective. In D. Fosha, D. J. Siegel, & M. Solomon (Eds.), *The healing power of emotion: Affective neuroscience, development, and clinical practice* (pp. 27–54). New York, NY: W. W. Norton.

Racker, H. (1957). The meanings and uses of countertransference. *Psychoanalytic Quarterly, 26*, 303–357.

Rappoport, E. (2012). Creating the umbilical cord. Relational knowing and the somatic third. *Psychoanalytic Dialogues, 22*, 375–388.

Sands, S. (2010). On the royal road together: The analytic function of dreams in activating dissociative unconscious communication. *Psychoanalytic Dialogues, 20*, 357–373.

Schore, A. N. (2001). The effects of early relational trauma on right brain develop-ment, affect regulation and infant mental health. *Infant Mental Health Journal*, *22*(1/2), 201–269.

Schore, A. N. (2009a). Attachment trauma and the developing right brain: Origins of pathological dissociation. In P. F. Dell & J. A. O'Neil (Eds.), *Dissociation and the dissociative disorders: DSM-V and beyond* (pp. 107–144). New York, NY: Routledge.

Schore, A. N. (2009b). Right brain affect regulation: An essential mechanism of devel-opment, trauma, dissociation, and psychotherapy. In D. Fosha, D. J. Siegel, & M. Solomon (Eds.), *The healing power of emotion: Affective neuroscience, development, and clinical practice* (pp. 112–144). New York, NY: W. W. Norton.

Schore, A. N. (2010). The right brain implicit self: A central mechanism of the psychotherapy change process. In J. Petrucelli (Ed.), *Knowing, not-knowing and sort-of-knowing: Psychoanalysis and the experience of uncertainty* (pp. 177–202). London, UK: Karnac Books.

Schore, J. R., & Schore, A. N. (2008). Modern attachment theory: The central role of affect regulation in development and treatment. *Clinical Social Work Journal*, *36*, 9–20.

Siegel, D. J. (2010). *The mindful therapist: A clinician's guide to mindsight and neural integration*. New York, NY: W. W. Norton.

Siegel, D. J. (2012). *Pocket guide to interpersonal neurobiology: An integrative handbook of the mind*. New York, NY: W. W. Norton.

Stern, D. B. (2003). *Unformulated experience: From dissociation to imagination in psychoanalysis*. New York, NY: Routledge, Taylor & Francis Group.

Stern, D. B. (2010). *Partners in thought: Working with unformulated experience, dissociation, and enactment*. New York, NY: Routledge, Taylor & Francis Group.

Strait, J. R. (2013). *Do you know what I know? Examining the therapist's internal experience when a client dissociates in session* (Doctoral dissertation). Retrieved from http://repository.upenn.edu/edissertations_sp2/36/

van der Kolk, B. A., & Fisler, R. (1995). Dissociation and the fragmentary nature of traumatic memories: An overview and exploratory study. *Journal of Traumatic Stress*, *8*, 505–525.

van der Kolk, B. A., Hopper, J. W., & Osterman, J. E. (2001). Exploring the nature of traumatic memory: Combining clinical knowledge with laboratory methods. In J. J. Freyd & A. P. DePrice (Eds.), *Trauma and cognitive science: A meeting of minds, science and human experience* (pp. 9–32). Binghamton, NY: Haworth Press.

Beneath the Surface: An Exploration of Neurobiological Alterations in Therapists Working With Trauma

BRIAN RASMUSSEN

School of Social Work, University of British Columbia, Okanagan Campus, Kelowna, British Columbia, Canada; Smith College School for Social Work, Northampton, Massachusetts, USA

SUSAN BLISS

Department of Social Work, Molloy College, Rockville Centre, New York, USA

This article explores the potential neurobiological alterations in clinicians who are exposed to the traumatic experiences of their clients. The authors speculate on the role of mirror neurons, the autonomic nervous system, the sympathetic and parasympathetic systems, the amygdala, the hypothalamus-pituitary-adrenal axis, memory, and the left and right hemispheres. A view of these neurobiological processes is integrated with psychodynamic psychotherapy processes, and current conceptions of vicarious or secondary trauma. Implications for understanding the differential effects of trauma treatment on the therapist are explored.

The past few decades have witnessed a burgeoning body of literature on the neurobiology of trauma (Levine, 2010; Perry, Pollard, Blakely, Baker, & Vigilante, 1995; A. N. Schore, 2012; J. R. Schore, 2012: van der Kolk, 1994). Over this same period, an ever-expanding literature has emerged on the negative effects of working with traumatized people (Figley, 1999; Pearlman & Saakvitne, 1995; Stamm, 2002; Tosone, Nuttman-Shwartz, & Stephens, 2012). These effects have been variously described as vicarious trauma (VT), secondary traumatic stress (STS), compassion fatigue (CF), shared trauma (ST), and burnout. However, scarce attention has been paid to understanding these potential adverse effects from a neurobiological perspective. This article begins to fill that gap. Here we speculate about neurobiological processes at the heart of therapeutic encounters for the clinician who is treating traumatized people.

We begin with a brief review of the conceptual and empirical literature on VT, STS, CF, ST, and burnout, highlighting the central distinguishing features of each construct for what it contributes to our understanding, followed by a review of research findings. Next, we examine select neurobiological features that appear central to understanding what is happening in the brain and body of the clinician while engaged in trauma treatment. In particular, the role of mirror neurons, the amygdala, the sympathetic and parasympathetic systems, the hypothalamus-pituitary-adrenal (HPA) axis, and the left and right hemispheres are explored. Further, we integrate this neurobiological perspective with theoretical ideas drawn from psychoanalytic literature that include attachment, affect regulation, psychological defenses, the holding environment, containment, and "lending an ego." Our goal is to hold the complexity of a mind–brain–body perspective, drawing on interdisciplinary literature. A brief case example is used to highlight these dynamics. Finally, we explore the implications of a neurobiological perspective for understanding the potential effects of trauma treatment on the therapist.

VICARIOUS TRAUMA: CONCEPTUAL LITERATURE AND RELATED CONSTRUCTS

Since McCann and Pearlman (1990) coined the term "vicarious trauma" there has been growing interest in the effects of trauma treatment on therapists. Important to understanding the construct of VT is holding the idea that direct therapeutic work with survivors of trauma can have transformational effects on the clinician. The increasing recognition of the potential negative effects of working with trauma is reflected in revisions to the *Diagnostic and Statistical Manual for Mental Disorders* (*DSM-5*; American Psychiatric Association, 2013b) criteria for post-traumatic stress disorder (PTSD). The new criteria specify that exposure to trauma can be direct, or can include "experiencing repeated or extreme *exposure* to aversive details of the traumatic event(s)" (American Psychiatric Association, 2013a, p. 143, italics added). Thus, unlike previous *DSM* editions, the new manual recognizes that helping professionals may develop symptoms of PTSD through indirect exposure to trauma.

Pearlman and Saakvitne (1995) define *vicarious trauma* as "the transformation in the inner experience of the therapist that comes about as a result of empathic engagement with client's trauma material . . . . It includes being a helpless witness to past events and sometimes present reenactments" (p. 31). They further suggest that therapists engage in cognitive empathy to understand the meaning and effects of the traumatic experience as well as affective empathy in which the therapist actually feels the client's pain (Pearlman & Saakvitne, 1995). Such exposure to other people's trauma challenges the therapist's own cognitive structures, or schemas. Affected is the therapist's frame of reference, self-soothing capacities, ego resources, psychological needs, and finally, disturbances to the sensory system.

The related ideas of burnout and countertransference interact with VT and STS. *Burnout* refers to the experience of exhaustion, depletion, and disengagement that can come as a consequence of high workloads and organizational demands (Maslach, 1982; Maslach, Jackson, & Leiter, 1996). Although the effects of burnout are not considered to be necessarily long lasting, all clinicians who work in settings with heavy caseloads are potentially at risk. Figley (1995) proposed the idea of STS (often used interchangeably with CF) as a syndrome with symptoms that mirror PTSD. Figley (1995) defined STS as "the natural consequent behaviors and emotions resulting from knowing about a traumatizing event experienced by a significant other—the stress resulting from helping or wanting to help a traumatized or suffering person" (p. 7). Such symptoms include intrusive thoughts or imagery, distressing emotions, hyperarousal, and impairment in functioning. STS can be differentiated from VT in that it does not affect the therapist's cognitive schemas. STS or CF can be differentiated from countertransference in that countertransference is continually experienced by therapists in their therapeutic work and is not unique to working with trauma (Berzoff & Kita, 2010).

VICARIOUS TRAUMA–EMPIRICAL LITERATURE

Not surprisingly, given the conceptual diversity and inter-relatedness of the ideas of burnout, VT, CF, STS, ST, and countertransference, the empirical literature is correspondingly diverse and sometimes contradictory. Chouliara, Hutchison, and Karatzias (2009) summed up the recent state of affairs by suggesting that, "while the concept of vicarious traumatization appears to have been enthusiastically embraced by practitioners, the empirical research remains fragmented and inconsistent and does not yet represent a coherent body of work" (p. 48). Similarly, Kadambi and Ennis (2004) raised important conceptual and empirical concerns:

> The field has not, however, reached a consensus on the identification of a single descriptor that accurately reflects the uniqueness and range of responses to providing trauma therapy. Furthermore, theorists have not yet arrived at an agreed upon explanation that accounts for how and why these professionals may be affected by their work. (pp. 4–5)

Although there is consistent support for the experience of VT from qualitative studies, results from quantitative studies have offered more mixed results (Devilly, Wright, & Varker, 2009). Although it is beyond the scope of this article to delve deeper into this controversy, it is reasonable at this time to hold the position that some, but not all, clinicians will be adversely affected by direct therapeutic exposure to people who have suffered trauma.

From their review of the literature, Baird and Kracen (2006) suggest that there is persuasive evidence that a clinician's personal history of trauma is linked to the development of VT. In addition, Tosone, McTighe, Bauwens, and Naturale (2011) studied the long-term effect of shared trauma in a sample of social workers post-9/11, and also found that greater exposure to traumatic life events influenced the development of ST stress. These researchers noted that insecure attachment influenced the development of traumatic stress in therapists, suggesting that attachment may be a mediating factor in the relationship between trauma history and the development of VT or STS. Other risk factors for vicarious trauma may include professional inexperience (Michalopoulos & Aparicio, 2012; Pearlman & Mac Ian, 1995) and lack of supervision (Baird & Kracen, 2006).

Although overall, the empirical literature is inconsistent, several studies have documented the negative consequences of this work for social workers (Bride, 2007; Cunningham, 2003). And though the boundaries between concepts such as VT, STS, and CF may be difficult to delineate, for the purpose of this article, we seek to understand the mechanisms by which the deleterious effects of this work emerge, rather than to categorize its varied outcomes. We are interested in speculating about the neurobiological processes that may underlie the experiences of practitioners who are treating trauma survivors. It is our hope that this exploration will go beyond the current state of conceptual uncertainty to offer a unifying understanding of what lies beneath the experience of working with trauma. We will begin with a case example, one that is a composite with disguised material.

CASE STUDY

Jessica, 28, has always rooted for the underdog. She was raised by a single mother who struggled with depression when Jessica was a toddler, but her mother succeeded in providing a stable life for her daughter. Academically strong, Jessica graduated from a MSW program $2\frac{1}{2}$ years ago. She was happy to find a medical social work position straight out of school. For 2 years she worked on units with varied medical specialties, gaining much experience along the way with short-term interventions. When a permanent position in outpatient psychiatry became available, she made the transition to a more psychotherapeutic setting. Her clinical work, which she described as a "huge learning curve," was varied and challenging. On some days,

Jessica acknowledged being "in over my head." But with strong relational skills, hard work, and supervision, she felt confident that she would gain the necessary clinical skills.

Jessica is surprised, however, to discover how much trauma is revealed in the lives of her clients, irrespective of diagnosis. On this particular day, Jessica was working with Anne, a 40-year-old mother of two girls age 4 and 6. Anne was diagnosed with depression and had been showing some signs of improvement on medication.

However, during her outpatient assessment, Anne revealed a history of sexual abuse by her alcoholic father. It began at age 6 and ended with his suicide when she was 12. The secret of her sexual abuse had now become the focus of treatment. However, current life circumstances served to complicate matters. In the midst of this current depression, Phil, Anne's husband of 10 years, had just left her to relocate to a nearby state. At the same time, Anne had serious concerns that Phil was sexually abusing the children. Anne arrived to the session appearing disheveled and overwhelmed.

Therapist: [somewhat alarmed by her appearance] How have you been doing?

Anne: I'm a mess. I haven't slept for days.

Therapist: [feeling anxious] What's been happening?

Anne: [begins to cry] I don't even think I can talk about it . . . it is so awful what is happening, I CAN'T believe it. I am so bloody angry . . . I just can't believe this is happening. [her voice trails off as she stares off in the distance]

Therapist: [pauses . . .] I can see that you are really upset. What do you mean you "can't believe *this* is happening"? What is this?

Anne: He wants the kids next week for spring break. He had his lawyer contact me—says I have to. Can you believe it! I hung up on him and then just started screaming at the top of my lungs like some crazy woman. Maybe I am crazy—that's what he says! Oh yeah, and if I don't send the kids off I will be in contempt of court! And then Phil says—if I deny him the kids he will kill himself! Can you believe it! [Anne is literally shaking at this point.]

Therapist: [Feeling overwhelmed, a tightness in her chest and unsure what to say. She imagines what Anne is going through. There is a long silence.] Have you spoken to *your* lawyer?

Anne: He's on holidays and his partner hasn't returned my call. This is a nightmare. . . . What do I do? I can't send those kids off to him. I can't! I feel nauseous like I want to throw up. [In the previous session Anne reported specific concerns about the sexualized behavior of her children and initiated a call to the child protection authorities. But it would be weeks before they could begin an investigation]

Therapist: [recalls those specific allegations from the previous session and at the same time is beginning to feel helpless and angry. Another pause, this time because of confusion. She waits for Anne to speak.]

Anne: You know this is strange . . . but I have to tell you . . . All week I kept thinking back to when my Dad was saying that he'd kill himself if I told anyone. And back then I had been threatening to tell others—but I hadn't. That whole scene about how I found out about him shooting himself just kept coming back . . . and I couldn't sleep.

Therapist: Wow, this is really hitting you at so many different levels.

[At this moment in the interview Anne appears to dissociate and changes the subject to something mundane. But as the interview progresses, Jessica becomes more and more agitated, anxious and confused. By the end of the interview she is exhausted.]

NEUROBIOLOGY AND THE THERAPIST EXPERIENCE

Clinicians listen intently to the client's trauma story, imagining what the experience was (is) like for the client, striving to provide a holding environment and containment for strong feelings (Applegate & Shapiro, 2005; Winnicott, 1965). In understanding their experience from a neurobiological perspective, we are speculating that when the therapist is empathically engaged with the trauma experience of the client, many of the neurobiological processes occurring in the client are similarly activated in the therapist. Although holding a relational and intersubjective perspective, we speculate on these potential neurological processes, and later, apply these dynamics to the above case study. We begin with the mirror neuron system and the role of the amygdala.

Mirror Neuron System

Recent research suggests that we may understand the thoughts, emotions, and sensations of others by simulating them in ourselves as if we were experiencing similar mental states, emotions, or sensations (Buccino & Amore, 2008; Corradini & Antonietti, 2013; Iacoboni, 2008). Research has indicated that the area of the brain that is normally activated by one's own emotion is also active when one looks at another individual feeling the same sensation or emotion (Corradini & Antonietti, 2013). For example, Hutchison, Davis, Lozano, Tasker, and Dostrovsky (1999) demonstrated that neurons in the anterior cingulate cortex that responded to painful stimuli applied to a participant's hand, also responded when the participant observed someone else being stimulated by the painful stimulus. Researchers have called these neurons that are triggered in response to observing the actions or emotions of others "mirror neurons." Buccino and Amore (2008) concluded, "that a mirror mechanism may occur not only when we judge other's actions, but also when we process others' experience, sensations or emotions" (p. 283). Thus, the mirror neurons may have crucial implications for understanding concepts such as VT and STS. If the therapist is indeed somatically experiencing some of the same emotions as the client through the mirror neuron system, this may explain why therapists can develop symptoms of PTSD similar to those of their clients. It also may give us some insight into potential risk factors for VT. Gazzola, Aziz-Zadeh, and Keysers (2006) found that those with higher scores in perspective taking had stronger auditory mirror neuron systems. This leads us to speculate that some individuals with stronger mirror neuron systems and empathic abilities may be more susceptible to literally experiencing the client's emotions, thus rendering them more susceptible to VT. Although research on the mirror neuron system is in its infancy, it does offer promising avenues for understanding the development of VT and STS.

Amygdala

Central to understanding the activation of fear, the amygdala provides information to the hypothalamus, which triggers neuroendocrine and autonomic responses such as increased heart rate, blood pressure, and defensive reactions (Cozolino, 2010). This limbic appraisal system bypasses cortical thinking and instead allows for rapid, instinctive emergency responses (van der Kolk, 2003). Cozolino (2010) noted that "..when we are frightened and our amygdala is activated . . . we have a difficult time being rational, logical, and in control of our thoughts" (p. 231). In a therapeutic context, the lack of cognitive processing in this stress response may lead to enactments and/or countertransference reactions that have also been identified as problematic sequelae of VT. Additionally, an overactive amygdala has been associated with symptoms of hyperarousal such as irritability, anger, and general hypervigilance (Montgomery, 2013), symptoms that have been identified as central to VT (McCann & Pearlman, 1990; Pearlman & Saakvitne, 1995) and STS (Figley, 1995).

Autonomic Nervous System

The autonomic nervous system regulates the internal state of the body to maintain homeostasis and promote survival. The two systems involved in this homeostasis are the sympathetic nervous system (SNS) and the parasympathetic nervous system (PNS). The sympathetic system is activated by the amygdala under conditions of stress to increase energy output to respond to external threat (Cozolino, 2010). On the other hand, the parasympathetic branch inhibits or "down-regulates" the system. These two branches of the ANS tend to work together so that when one is activated, the other is suppressed (Montgomery, 2013). Ideally, the optimal functioning of this system is like a teeter-totter, working in a smooth oscillation.

Sympathetic Nervous System

When listening to the client's trauma material, the clinician's SNS is activated. This frequent hyperarousal, over time, may lead to shorter-term symptoms of STS such as hypervigilence. In addition, the SNS may activate the "fight" (aggression) or "flight" (fear/avoidance) responses in the clinician in response to processing painful trauma material. In the case of a "fight" response, the clinician might take a critical, hostile, or punitive approach to a client. Alternatively, if the "flight" response is activated, the worker may delay decision-making processes and avoid difficult issues (Tyler, 2012). Thus, the response of the SNS may help us to understand short-term symptoms of STS as well as possible countertransference reactions of clinicians working with trauma survivors.

The Parasympathetic Nervous System

The PNS regulates emotional and behavioral responses to stress by inhibiting the SNS with rapid decreases in metabolic output (van der Kolk, 2003). It has been proposed that the PNS is also responsible for the "freeze" or dissociative responses that are seen in individuals who have experienced trauma (Tyler, 2012). Tyler (2012) suggested that the PNS "freeze" response may account for workers engaging in their work in a "superficial or procedural" manner, a commonly cited symptom of VT. We speculate that this response may also underlie the sense of detachment evident in burnout. In addition, the freeze response may lead to workers dissociating from important painful aspects of a case, such as ignoring evidence of child abuse.

Clearly, the autonomic nervous system plays a crucial role in understanding the affect regulation problems that are often seen in trauma, and it may also be central to understanding VT. On one hand, clinicians can become over-aroused (SNS)—but on the other hand they can become overly regulated to the point of dissociation (PNS) when faced with traumatic material. Behaviorally, A. N. Schore (2003) suggested that the simultaneous arousal of the sympathetic and parasympathetic systems is like "riding the gas and the brake at the same time," and the activation of hyperexcitation and hyperinhibition can result in the "freeze response" (p. 213). Presumably, the nervous system was not designed for this kind of stress over long periods of time. In addition to contributing to the freeze response, we wonder whether this dynamic also accounts for some of the extreme fatigue clinicians can feel at the end of trauma-focused sessions.

Memory

The hippocampus is important in processing information, explicit memory, and the transfer of information to the prefrontal cortex (Coates, 2010; Miehls, 2011; Montgomery, 2013). However, the hippocampus is also vulnerable to stress hormones, such as norepinephrine and cortisol, which interfere with its functioning. Although in the short-term neurohormones such as norepinephrine can potentiate the strength of a memory, van der Kolk (1994) asserted that the heightened release of these hormones interferes with hippocampal functioning, inhibiting cognitive evaluation of experience and interfering with memory storage. Under conditions of stress, memories are then stored as somatic sensations and visual images (Applegate & Shapiro, 2005; Cozolino, 2010; Miehls, 2011). Although the client's memory processing may potentially be impaired due to stress, so too may the therapist's. Commonly, trauma therapists will report blanking out on a client's story or "forgetting" large chunks of a client's history. Further, as Pearlman and Saakvitne (1995) argue, the client's trauma story may "reawaken the therapist's own memories and consequent strong feelings" (p. 310). This makes sense when we grasp the idea of implicit memory and the intersubjective context of psychotherapy (Rasmussen, 2005). Implicit memory, or nondeclarative memory, though revealed in our patterns of behavior, is mostly inaccessible to conscious awareness, constituting a vast structure beneath the surface (Cozolino, 2010). A. N. Schore (2012) wrote that "spontaneous nonverbal transference-countertransference interactions at a preconscious level represent implicit right brain-to-right brain nonverbal communications of fast-acting, automatic, regulated and especially dysregulated bodily based stressful emotional states between patient and therapist" (p. 128).

McCann and Pearlman (1990) noted that the imagery system of memory is most likely to be altered in vicarious trauma and offer examples of therapists who reexperience a client's memory as a flashback or an intrusive imagery of a client's trauma. Iliffe and Steed (2000) reported that almost all of the participants in a study on vicarious trauma reported having experienced visual imagery of their client's traumatic experiences, and almost all felt that this imagery would stay with them forever.

Hypothalamus-Pituitary-Adrenal Axis

The HPA axis plays a critical role in the stress response cycle as the "stress regulator." The hypothalamus releases corticotropin-releasing hormone (CRH) in response to stress. CRH then stimulates the release of beta-endorphin and adrenocorticotrophic hormone (ACTH) from the pituitary gland (Keeshin, Cronholm, & Strawn, 2012). Beta-endorphin produces analgesia and may reduce the physical or emotional pain associated with trauma (Weiss, 2007). This increased use of the opioid system may also partially explain symptoms of avoidance and numbing seen in VT and STS.

When the pituitary gland stimulates the adrenal gland, the adrenal gland releases cortisol, the body's primary stress hormone. When the brain is exposed to high levels of cortisol, the nervous system can become sensitized to psychologically threatening stimuli. Over time, this can lead to "kindling" whereby individuals who have experienced trauma are more likely to respond with greater intensely and speed to perceived threats (Mead, Beauchaine, & Shannon, 2010; Weiss, 2007). We can theorize that this process of kindling may be important in understanding the finding that individuals who have experienced previous trauma are also more susceptible to VT or STS.

Increased cortisol levels have also been associated with the improvement of emotionally relevant memories. According to Weiss (2007) this increased memory for traumatic events may also affect the appraisal of future events. This process may be adaptive in the sense of allowing an individual to remember, and thus potentially avoid, threatening situations. On the other hand, vivid memories may lead to overgeneralization of negative experience to situations that others might judge as nonthreatening. It may be that this process contributes to the changes in cognitive schema (such as perceptions of the self, others, and the world) often seen in trauma therapists who experience VT.

There is also evidence that persistent, overactivation of cortisol may lead to a negative feedback loop in the HPA axis, resulting in a suppression of cortisol (hypocortisolism). This may be the brain's way of protecting itself from chronic hyperarousal. However, excessive suppression of cortisol may potentiate dissociative or numbing responses that may lead to stressful events being kept out of awareness (Mead et al., 2012). Such self-protective strategies may ultimately be problematic for the trauma worker as, without conscious access to the painful material, she is less able to cognitively process raw affects. These "unprocessed" affects may then leave the worker more vulnerable to developing symptoms such as intrusive thoughts or images about the client.

Left and Right Brain

Focusing more broadly on basic brain structure, neurobiologists often refer to the left brain as having a leading role in conscious logic, linearity and language, whereas the right tends to process more of the unconscious social and emotional information (Miehls, 2011; Montgomery, 2002). A. N. Schore (2012) underscores the importance of the right hemisphere saying,

> [T]his right-lateralized emotional brain is deeply connected into the body and the autonomic nervous system (ANS), and it has a different anatomy, physiology, and biochemistry than the later-forming left hemisphere. The

right hemisphere processes not only emotion but more precisely, unconscious emotion and is the locus of an implicit procedural memory system.
(p. 31)

Optimal functioning depends on the "horizontal integration" of left- and
right-brain functions, which occurs through the connecting tissue, the corpus
callosum (Miehls, 2011). In clients with trauma, this hemispheric integration
is compromised. That is, clients may find themselves experiencing either raw
emotion without the benefit of cognitive mediation, or a dissociated state of
logic without the benefit of emotional awareness. Accordingly, A. N. Schore
(2012) noted that in the treatment of individuals with trauma, the "right
brain to right brain communication" is essential. The therapist then experiences the intense affects connected with these relational patterns through the
countertransference. The therapist not only listens to traumatic material, but
through the right brain tracks, at a preconscious level, the patient's affective
states and his or her own bodily responses. The consistent containment of
these communications may well contribute to some of the potential negative
effects of working with trauma.

Defenses

Given the nature of trauma work, both the conscious processing of painful
material, and the experiential unconscious "right-brain" processing of affect,
it is natural that therapists unconsciously use defense to regulate affect. These
defensive strategies may contribute to a number of the symptoms of STS
and VT and can also have a negative effect on the ability of the therapist
to contain the client's experiences. As clinicians, our awareness of the bodily sensations and emotions associated with distress is key. Levine (2010)
cautioned that,

> It is important to understand that when therapists perceive that they
> must protect themselves from their clients' sensations and emotion,
> they unconsciously block those clients from therapeutically experiencing
> them. By distancing ourselves from their anguish, we distance ourselves
> from them and from the fears they are struggling with. To take a self-
> protective stance is to abandon our clients precipitately. At the same time,
> we also greatly increase the likelihood of their exposure to secondary or
> vicarious traumatization and burnout. (p. 42)

When feelings are too overwhelming to integrate, the therapist may
use denial or emotional numbing to manage his or her affect (McCann
& Pearlman, 1990). Neurologically speaking, denial and dissociation are
parasympathetically driven defenses that are used to attempt to lower the
level of stimulation when an individual is overwhelmed (Montgomery, 2013).

Although temporarily adaptive for the client, when employed by the therapist over time, this ongoing "down-regulation" of the PNS might also lead to the therapist's disengagement. Montgomery (2013) suggested that more adaptive defenses do not preferentially utilize the SNS or the PNS but allow the therapist to regulate affect while at the same time staying connected to the client.

Adams and Riggs (2008) found that 54 trainees with an adaptive defense style (including the use of suppression, sublimation, and humor) consistently reported the lowest level of VT symptoms. Interestingly, they also found that a self-sacrificing defensive style was a risk factor for VT. The authors concluded that one's defensive style may play a moderating role in the relationship between personal history and VT. Individuals using a self-sacrificing defensive style need to maintain an image of the self as kind, helpful, and never angry, often accomplished through the use of reaction formation and pseudoaltruism. We posit that it may be that this defensive style interferes with the ability of the worker to be aware of, or process, his or her own affective experiences in treating individuals with trauma. Because the therapist needs to keep these affects unconscious, left–right brain integration is compromised and the individual may be more susceptible to negative effects of trauma treatment.

Attachment

Central to our discussion is the role of affect regulation and its relationship to attachment. Numerous studies have suggested that infants learn to regulate affects in mirroring interactions with their primary caregivers (Shapiro & Applegate, 2000; Siegel, 2003, 2007). Neurobiologists have outlined the ways in which the early emotional availability of the caretaker influences brain development and the individual's subsequent capacity for regulating socioemotional functioning (A. N. Schore, 2012; Shapiro & Applegate, 2000). For example, there is evidence that the number of neuronal connections in the child's brain correlates with the quality of parental stimulation (Shapiro & Applegate, 2000). Given the importance of the early attachment relationship, a clinician's capacity to manage a client's traumatic material is potentially mediated by his or her own attachment pattern and style of affect regulation. In fact, Brandon (as cited in Canfield, 2005) found evidence that mental health professionals who had secure attachment styles reported having fewer symptoms of VT. Attachment style also has implications for the clinician's use of colleagues and supervisors to mitigate negative effects of working with trauma. For instance, a clinician who leans toward an avoidant attachment style may be less inclined to seek out the support of others when overwhelmed, preferring instead to withdraw to a private space.

CASE STUDY DISCUSSION

It is apparent that Jessica is empathically engaged with her client Anne, resonating with many of her verbal and nonverbal, bodily based affects including fear, horror, and anger. Her mirror neuron system is activated as she experiences many of the same emotional states as her client. Given some of the parallels with her early development, it is possible that Jessica overidentifies with Anne and her vulnerable and powerless state thus accentuating this response. Undoubtedly, Jessica's amygdala is activated. The physical signs of tightness in her chest, increased heart rate, and muscular tension suggest the heightened activation of the sympathetic nervous system. Jessica is also flooded with affect. Outside her awareness, her psychological defenses and parasympathetic nervous system attempt to down regulate this highly aroused state and preserve cognitive performance. A dysregulated state affects Jessica's capacity to fully engage her frontal cortex, potentially interfering with higher level cognitive functioning, while she attempts, in ego psychology terms, to "lend an ego." However, at times she feels lost. Unable to flee or fight, Jessica struggles to self-regulate and maintain empathic emotional contact with her client with implicit right-brain activity.

Further, we can speculate that Jessica holds visual memories of Anne's reported child sexual abuse and also may have generated visual images of the children's anticipated trip to visit the father. For the clinician, these memories and images may linger on long after the session is over. In the case of Jessica, we are presenting a single slice of one session. But we have to imagine the cumulative impact over the course of this therapy and across her caseload, day in, day out.

Implications

Neurobiology offers important insights with respect to the negative effects of trauma treatment on the clinician. Briefly summarized, we have speculated the following. A clinician's mirror neurons fire in response to the client's affective states when empathically immersed in the client's trauma story. The amygdala, sensing danger, signals the autonomic nervous system to respond in a fight, flight, or freeze manner. However, when sustaining empathic connection, the clinician's SNS and PNS may work simultaneously at odds with each other. The client's dysregulated bodily based emotional state is communicated nonverbally from right brain to right brain, potentially amplifying a dysregulated state for the clinician and producing disturbing visual memories or inhibiting memory. High levels of cortisol may further intensify this affective response. The clinician draws on his or her affect regulation capacity, developed early in life as a consequence of attachment experiences, to maintain equilibrium. Defensively, the therapist may alternatively draw on major protective measures like denial and dissociation to cope with the affective overload.

Researchers and scholars in the field agree that empathy is the main conduit for developing VT and STS, thus presumably putting all clinicians who work with trauma at risk. Although this may be true, it seems reasonable to speculate that the interaction of a number of factors exerts a variable impact. Some of the factors include being younger and/or new to the profession, insufficiently trained, highly cognitively and affectively empathic; and/or having a personal history of trauma without the benefit of therapy, an anxious attachment style, a self-sacrificing interpersonal style, inadequate supervision, an unsupportive work environment, and a heavy caseload with high trauma acuity. These factors, put together in any number of permutations, serve to create the conditions under which the negative effects of trauma treatment may take hold.

Some of the factors mentioned above have significant organizational implications (beyond our focus here), whereas others point to neurobiological links, in particular affect regulation. This function, as A. N. Schore (2003, 2012) has convincingly argued, is closely related to the nature and quality of early attachments, and is clearly affected by early relational trauma. In this regard, clinical supervisors, beyond providing basic support and guidance, must be mindful of the therapist's defensive style and affect regulation needs.

Further, it seems evident that differences in one's neurological development potentially play an important role in understanding resilience and vulnerability in the face of traumatic experiences, direct and indirect. This leads to the yet unanswered question as to whether some clinicians may be better suited for this work than others, or at least bring to the work additional protective factors. Nonetheless, even for the clinicians well suited for this work, the desire to help, rescue, or heal, may exceed one's neurobiological capacity over time. These points reinforce the importance of self-reflection, self-care, clinical supervision, and organizational responsiveness in responding effectively to clinicians' ongoing needs. These neurological differences may also be helpful in explaining some of the conflicting research findings regarding risk factors for developing VT and STS. It may be that one's neurobiological capacity to regulate affect interacts with other risk factors such as years of experience, previous trauma, and organizational support, to lead to VT and STS. Further research is needed to continue to clarify the role of neurobiological factors in the development of VT, and to develop best practices for protecting clinicians who engage in this important and challenging work.

CONCLUSION

It is important to keep in mind that though we have drawn on solid inter-disciplinary knowledge about the brain, much of our work here should be considered speculative. The challenges to knowing with certainty the relative influences of various neurobiological processes require additional research methodologies beyond the expertise of most clinicians. Nonetheless, this article addresses a gap in the literature with respect to a neurobiological understanding of the negative effects of trauma treatment on the therapist. In so doing, we have explored how this understanding can add to our current knowledge of the mechanisms by which the negative effects of trauma work affect the therapist, and of the differential effects of trauma treatment. It is our hope that the awareness of neurological processes may help clinicians gain a better appreciation for the biological reactions to affectively laden client material, that which lies beneath the surface. Such knowledge may lead to the development of effective protective strategies to manage affect, minimize potential harm, and enhance therapeutic effectiveness.

REFERENCES

Adams, S. A., & Riggs, S. A. (2008). An exploratory study of vicarious trauma among therapist trainees. *Training and Education in Professional Psychology, 2*(1), 26–34.

American Psychiatric Association. (2013a). *Desk reference to the diagnostic criteria from DSM-5*. Washington, DC: Author.

American Psychiatric Association. (2013b). *Diagnostic and statistical manual of mental disorders* (5th ed.). Arlington, VA: American Psychiatric Publishing.

Applegate, J. S., & Shapiro, J. R. (2005). Cognitive neuroscience, neurobiology and affect regulation: Implications for clinical social work. *Clinical Social Work Journal, 28*, 9–21.

Baird, K., & Kracen, A. C. (2006). Vicarious traumatization and secondary traumatic stress: A research synthesis. *Counselling Psychology Quarterly, 19*(2), 181–188.

Berzoff, J., & Kita, E. (2010). Compassion fatigue and countertransference: Two different concepts. *Clinical Social Work Journal, 38*, 341–349.

Bride, B. E. (2007). Prevalence of secondary traumatic stress among social workers. *Social Work, 52*, 63–70.

Buccino, G., & Amore, M. (2008). Mirror neurons and the understanding of behavioral symptoms in psychiatric disorders. *Current Opinion in Psychiatry, 21*(3), 281–285.

Canfield, J. (2005). Secondary traumatization, burnout, and vicarious traumatization: A review of the literature as it relates to therapists who treat trauma. *Smith College Studies in Social Work, 75*, 81–101.

Chouliara, Z., Hutchison, C., & Karatzias, T. (2009). Vicarious traumatisation in practitioners who work with adult survivors of sexual violence and child sexual abuse: Literature review and directions for future research. *Counseling and Psychotherapy Research, 9*(1), 47–56.

Coates, D. (2010). Impact of child abuse: Biopsychosocial pathways through which adult mental health is compromised. *Australian Social Work, 63*, 391–403.

Corradini, A., & Antonietti, A. (2013). Mirror neurons and their function in cognitively understood empathy. *Consciousness and Cognition, 22*(3), 1152–1161.

Cozolino, L. (2010). *The neuroscience of psychotherapy: Healing the social brain* (2nd ed.). New York, NY: W. W. Norton.

Cunningham, M. (2003). Impact of trauma work on social work clinicians: Empirical findings. *Social Work, 48*, 451–459.

Devilly, G. J., Wright, R., & Varker, T. (2009). Vicarious trauma, secondary traumatic stress or simply burnout? Effect of trauma therapy on mental health professionals. *Australian and New Zealand Journal of Psychiatry, 43*, 373–385.

Figley, C. (Ed.). (1995). *Compassion fatigue: Coping with secondary traumatic stress disorder in those who treat the traumatized*. New York, NY: Brunner/Mazel.

Figley, C. R. (1999). Compassion fatigue: Toward a new understanding of the costs of caring. In B. H. Stamm (Ed.), *Secondary traumatic stress: Self-care issues for clinicians, researchers, and educators* (pp. 3–28). Lutherville, MD: Sidran Press.

Gazzola, V., Aziz-Zadeh, L., & Keysers, C. (2006). Empathy and the somatotopic auditory mirror system in humans. *Current Biology, 16*, 1824–1829.

Hutchison, W., Davis, K., Lozano, A., Tasker, R., & Dostrovsky, J. (1999). Pain related neurons in the human cingulate cortex. *Nature Neuroscience, 2*, 403–405.

Iacoboni, M. (2008). *The new science of how we connect with others: Mirroring people*. New York, NY: Farrar, Straus and Giroux.

Iliffe, G., & Steed, L. G. (2000). Exploring the counselor's experience of working with perpetrators and survivors of domestic violence. *Journal of Interpersonal Violence, 15*, 393–412.

Kadambi, M., & Ennis, L. (2004). Reconsidering vicarious trauma: A review of the literature and its limitations. *Journal of Trauma Practice, 3*(2), 1–21.

Keeshin, B. R., Cronholm, P. F., & Strawn, J. R. (2012). Physiologic changes associated with violence and abuse exposure: An examination of related medical conditions. *Trauma, Violence, & Abuse, 13*, 41–56.

Levine, P. A. (2010). *In an unspoken voice: How the body releases trauma and restores goodness*. Berkeley, CA: North Atlantic Books.

Maslach, C. (1982). *Burnout, the cost of caring*. Englewood Cliffs, NJ: Prentice Hall.

Maslach, C., Jackson, S. E., & Leiter, M. P. (1996). *Maslach Burnout Inventory manual*. Palo Alto, CA: Consulting Psychologists Press.

McCann, I. L., & Pearlman, L. A. (1990). Vicarious traumatization: A framework for understand the psychological effects of working with victims. *Journal of Traumatic Stress, 3*, 131–149.

Mead, H. K., Beauchaine, T. P., & Shannon, K. E. (2010). Neurobiological adaptations to violence across development. *Development and Psychopathology, 22*, 1–22.

Michalopoulos, L. M., & Aparicio, E. (2012). Vicarious trauma in social workers: The role of trauma history, social support, and years of experience. *Journal of Aggression, Maltreatment & Trauma, 21*, 646–664.

Miehls, D. (2011). Neurobiology and clinical social work. In J. R. Brandell (Ed.), *Theory and practice in clinical social work* (2nd ed., pp. 81–98). Thousand Oaks, CA: Sage.

Montgomery, A. (2002). Converging perspectives of dynamic theory and evolving neurobiological knowledge. *Smith College Studies in Social Work*, 72, 177–196.

Montgomery, A. (2013). *Neurobiology essentials for clinicians: What every therapist needs to know*. New York, NY: W. W. Norton.

Pearlman, L. A., & Mac Ian, P. S. (1995). Vicarious traumatization: An empirical study of the effects of trauma work on the trauma therapists. *Professional Psychology: Research and Practice*, 26, 558–565.

Pearlman, L. A., & Saakvitne, K. W. (1995). *Trauma and the therapist: Counter-transference and vicarious traumatization in psychotherapy with incest survivors*. New York, NY: W. W. Norton.

Perry, B., Pollard, R., Blakely, T., Baker, W., & Vigilante, D. (1995). Childhood trauma, the neurobiology of adaptation, and "use-dependent" development of the brain: How "states" become "traits." *Infant Mental Health Journal*, 16(4), 271–289.

Rasmussen, B. (2005). An intersubjective perspective on vicarious trauma and its impact on the clinical process. *Journal of Social Work Practice*, 19(1), 19–30.

Schore, A. N. (2003). *Affect regulation and the repair of the self*. New York, NY: W. W. Norton.

Schore, A. N. (2012). *The science of the art of psychotherapy*. New York, NY: W. W. Norton.

Schore, J. R. (2012). Using concepts from interpersonal neurobiology in revisiting psychodynamic theory. *Smith College Studies in Social Work*, 82, 90–111.

Shapiro, J. R., & Applegate, J. S. (2000). Cognitive neuroscience, neurobiology and affect regulation: Implications for clinical social work. *Clinical Social Work Journal*, 28, 9–21.

Siegel, D. J. (2003). Toward an interpersonal neurobiology of the developing mind: Attachment, mindsight, and neural integration. *Infant Mental Health Journal*, 22, 67–94.

Siegel, D. J. (2007). *The mindful brain: Reflection and attunement in the cultivation of well-being*. New York, NY: Norton.

Stamm, B. H. (2002). Measuring compassion satisfaction as well as fatigue: Developmental history of the Compassion Satisfaction and Fatigue Test. In C. R. Figley (Ed.), *Treating compassion fatigue* (pp. 107–119). New York, NY: Brunner-Routledge.

Tosone, C., McTighe, J. P., Bauwens, J., & Naturale, A. (2011). Shared traumatic stress and the long-term impact of 9/11 on Manhattan clinicians. *Journal of Traumatic Stress*, 24, 546–552.

Tosone, C., Nuttman-Shwartz, O., & Stephens, T. (2012). Shared trauma: When the professional is personal. *Clinical Social Work Journal*, 40(2), 231–239.

Tyler, T. A. (2012). The limbic model of systemic trauma. *Journal of Social Work Practice*, 26(1), 125–138.

van der Kolk, B. A. (1994). The body keeps the score: Memory and the evolving psychobiology of posttraumatic stress. *Harvard Review of Psychiatry*, 1, 253–265.

van der Kolk, B. A. (2003). The neurobiology of childhood trauma and abuse. *Child and Adolescent Psychiatric Clinics*, 12, 293–317.

Weiss, S. J. (2007). Neurobiological alterations associated with traumatic stress. *Perspectives in Psychiatric Care, 43*, 114–122.

Winnicott, D. W. (1965). *The maturational process and the facilitating environment*. New York, NY: International Universities Press.

Casting Light on the Shadow: Clinical Implications of Contextualizing Racial Experience Within a Neurobiological Framework

YVETTE M. ESPREY

University of the Witwatersrand, Johannesburg, South Africa

Neurobiological findings indicate that the right brain houses implicit relational templates that contain the individual's earliest experiences of the social world, transmitted through the unconscious communications of caregivers. These templates have the potential to influence the sense of self, other, and world throughout the life span, often in insidious and unidentifiable ways. This article explores the implications of this for the development of racial experience and identity and for the intergenerational transmission of racial trauma, looking at how earliest experiences of identity potentially affect the clinical space, and the intersubjectivity between client and therapist.

This article focuses on the racialized subjectivities of therapist and client, which it suggests have the potential to insidiously influence the psychotherapeutic encounter. It explores the neurobiological origins of race-based schemas within the context of early attachment relationships and emphasizes the importance of bringing into conscious awareness the workings of race in any clinical relationship. The article aims to underscore the imperative that clinicians face to actively interrogate and examine their own racial identity and history in the service of reducing the possibility of racially based enactments. The clinical implications of not doing so are significant and can compromise the workings of the therapeutic process. Neurobiology offers a viable rationale for consciously thinking about race in an unfolding therapeutic relationship and gives insights into how such a relationship can be a vehicle for change in relation to unconscious racial dynamics. The article links relational psychoanalytic and attachment theory with current neurobiological findings that support the proposition that deeply embedded racial schemas have their origin in early brain development.

The assumption that subjectivity develops within a particular social, political, and historical context (Lobban, 2013) means that race, as an aspect of subjectivity making its way into the clinical encounter, needs to be contextually considered. As such, though the clinical implications of race described in this article are pertinent to any racialized society in which psychotherapy is practiced, the subjectivity and context of the author cannot be separated from that which is written. I am writing this article from the vantage point afforded me by my particular historical and personal context, as a White, educated, middle-class woman, born in 1970s South Africa, at the height of Apartheid. This is not a neutral position—it is a position which, because of my Whiteness, is implicitly one of power and which, as suggested by Suchet (2007), can never be separated from privilege.

The subjective nature of the topic brings with it particular dynamics within the writing of it. Although striving to maintain the academic rigor which is a cornerstone of sound authorship, there is also the pull to position myself in relation to what is being described. This particular dynamic is one that Msebele and Brown (2011) identified as a dilemma that is intrinsic to writing about race. They warned against resorting to "the proud but calcified (third person [my addition]) language of the academy" (Morrison, as cited in Msebele & Brown, 2011, p. 454) that risks obscuring "the influence of the personal and subjective" (Msebele & Brown, 2011, p. 454). As such, I am aware of the slippage between the multiplicity of selves (Bromberg, 1996) which contribute to this paper's authorship—at times the writing is that of an academic, at others I am the clinician and then the individual, for whom race has deeply personal meaning.

Current neurobiological research tells us that in the first 18 months of life the right brain develops in response to the particular attachment environment in which the individual is raised (Miehls, 2011). Relational psychoanalytic writers suggest that this early attachment environment extends beyond the direct familial milieu to include the broader social context such that social and cultural conditions will affect the texture of the "familial and cultural enclaves of love and hate" (Layton, 2006, p. 264) in which we are raised. This suggests that traces of the prevailing social discourses including assumptions, prejudices, and stereotypes are embedded in right-brain templates developed in infancy—these infiltrate the conscious and implicit communications of our caregivers. This proposition has important and startling implications if we begin to consider the particular patterns of social discourse, specifically around identity, that exist within society at any given time. Social discourses around race, for example, then begin to shape not only societal norms, but also the relational templates that we internalize from birth as part of implicit memory. These same relational templates accompany our clients and us, as clinicians, as we enter the consulting room.

RACE IS IN THE ROOM

The relevance of race in clinical contexts has received increasing attention in contemporary relational psychoanalytic writing, specifically in the last three decades (see Altman, 2000; Leary, 1997; Morgan, 2008; Straker, 2004; Suchet, 2007; Young, 1987). This intensity of engagement around race is in stark contrast to the paucity of race-related theorizing and clinical writing prior to the 1990s; an omission that has been strongly criticized by current writers (Suchet, 2007).

In her seminal text on trauma, Judith Herman (1992) described the study of psychological trauma as having a "curious history—one of episodic amnesia. Periods of active investigation have alternated with periods of oblivion" (p. 7). She posits an explanation for this episodic amnesia in suggesting that the study of trauma brings with it the recognition of the potential for human cruelty and evil, and for the potential of human beings to do damage to themselves and others (Herman, 1992). As such, studying it is too personally implicating and calls us to bear witness to the phenomenon of trauma in a very subjective way. I would suggest that a similar dynamic may have contributed to the relative absence of race as a subject of focus in psychoanalytic writing. Race, on the face of it, is an empty construct (Rustin, as cited in Morgan, 2002), and yet it is one that operates as a receptacle for powerful social constructions and is inextricably linked to trauma (Leary, 1997). It too is a reminder of the capacity for human cruelty, for othering, discrimination, and persecution. It is not possible to think, write about, or study race without taking ourselves as objects of scrutiny.

In spite of the burgeoning of experience-near writing that documents the shape of race in the clinical space, it remains "one of the most vulnerable of social discourses" (Leary, 2000, p. 639). Leary (2000) asserted that the most common enactment around race is the relative silence about racial issues, in the therapy room, and within the therapeutic community. In the author's context, that of post-Apartheid South Africa, even though cross-cultural issues in psychotherapy are discussed, and cultural sensitivity is taught in the training of clinicians (Eagle, 2005), the issue of race remains one that is not readily spoken about within the clinical community, even though psychotherapy in

South Africa occurs in the context of a society that is saturated currently and historically with powerful discourses around race. There is a conspiratorial silence around race, and a tendency toward color-blindness (Esprey, 2013).

Loya (2011, 2012) made a similar observation in her U.S.-based research that looked at color-blind attitudes in White social work students (Loya, 2011), and racial attitudes in White social workers (Loya, 2012). She found that even though cultural competency and cultural sensitivity are prerequisites in clinical social work training, many White social workers express feeling discomfort when working with culturally diverse populations, and if they had the choice, would choose not to do so (Loya, 2012). She found too that frequently White social workers express a "color-blind" stance, indicating that they do not consider the race of the other to be of relevance in contemporary America. Loya (2012) quoted Bonilla-Silva in saying that color-blindness is the new form of racism, where discrimination along racial lines continues to be entrenched in society.

And yet, race is inextricably part of identity and subjectivity (Suchet, 2007) and as such cannot but be present in the consulting room. Writers such as Leary (1997), Altman (2000), Suchet (2004), and Smith (2006) contend that because race as an aspect of identity carries such powerful social meaning, it will always be present, in some way, in any clinical encounter irrespective of the particular configuration of the dyad. This article aims to contribute further to discussions around the clinical context of race and in so doing to increase illumination through dialogue and to further nudge racial experience into the foreground of clinical consciousness.

THE DEVELOPMENTAL ORIGINS OF RACIAL SUBJECTIVITY

Mama (as cited in Lobban, 2013), defined *subjectivity* as "the conscious, unconscious thoughts and emotions of the individual, her sense of herself and her ways of understanding her relation to the world" (p. 58). This subjectivity is created by a confluence of psychodynamic and societal influences and includes a sense of one's racial self (Lobban, 2013). Identity and subjectivity, though developing within individual contexts, can never be separated from sociohistorical conditions (Mama, as cited in Lobban, 2013). This proposition is in keeping with the suggestion made by current relational psychoanalytic writers (Dimen, 2011; Layton, 2006) that individual psychic development is not only a product of what occurs within the nuclearity of the immediate attachment environment, but that the psyche develops also in response to the broader social, cultural, and political context into which an individual is born. This assertion signifies a fundamental shift in psychoanalytic thinking and writing toward a position that suggests that the psyche is affected not exclusively by the immediate object relational environment, but also by forces which lie beyond the familial realm, that it is political and social and cultural (Dimen, 2011). Contrary to earlier psychoanalytic conceptualizations, this suggests that racial subjectivity affects directly on the psychic realm, and on the unconscious.

The Normative Unconscious

Outlining her concept of a normative unconscious, Layton (2006) asserted that race cannot be avoided in clinical contexts, and that it is always present, in some form, in the clinical dyad. Whether we are consciously aware of it, there is always the potential for the enactment of deeply internalized social norms—organized around aspects of identity, such as race—that were communicated to us within our relational "enclaves of love and hate" (Layton, 2006, p. 264).

Normative unconscious processes result from the osmotic internalization of prevailing ideologies and norms that define a culture and serve to maintain societal equilibrium. Layton (2006) asserted that intergroup comparison exists in every society, and that individual identities are forged relative to the dominant ideology. She explains the process by which the normative unconscious splits and organizes particular attributes along lines of identity such as gender, race, and class:

> Power hierarchies create and sustain differences that mark out what is high and low, good and bad, pure and impure, and there is certainly a tendency for those not in power to internalize the denigrating attributions that come at them. (Layton, 2006, p. 240)

In this way, for example, Whiteness becomes synonymous with purity and goodness, and Blackness is imbued with badness and impurity. As a consequence, individuals project and introject the split-off attributes that are assigned to their particular racial identity.

Interpellation

The notion of interpellation—"the mechanism through which ideology takes hold of the individual" (Guralnik & Simeon, 2010)—is relevant here. Through this "the voice of the State recognizes the individual and hails him into social existence" (p. 407), Black and White individuals begin to "live" their racial identity in circumscribed ways. Interpellation, then, becomes the gateway to recognition and affirmation (Guralnik & Simeon, 2010), even though it simultaneously attacks identity. One of the consequences of this is the potential for racial melancholia—for the denouncing and splitting off of one's own cultural and racial identity to adopt the dominant norms and ideals of a society (Eng & Hahn, 2000). This tendency was identified through research into the experiences of immigrants who, by necessity, became acculturated into American society (Eng & Hahn, 2000).

Lobban (2013), Swartz (2007), and Layton (2006) warned against the potential for the enactment of unconscious processes in the process of psychotherapy. Clinicians are equally at risk of being interpellated, and of manifesting the normative unconscious through the enactment of racist stereotypes and assumptions, even if we consciously disavow racism, or assume a nonracist position. The implications of this for clinical work are significant. Layton suggested that as clinicians we need to be aware of the shape and texture of the normative unconscious that we bring into our work, and of the patterns of social norms that therapist and client will be drawn in to enacting, albeit unconsciously. Writing with the context of the United States, Layton highlighted the dominance of racialized ideology in recent American history and warned against the impact of this on developing psyches, and on the shared normative unconscious of American society.

Pretransference

In one of a few earlier psychoanalytic papers that focused on race (Msebele & Brown, 2011), Curry (1964), a Black psychoanalyst, introduced the term "pretransference" to describe the thoughts and feelings based on race, which predate the therapeutic encounter and that are brought to bear in the room. Curry wrote specifically about the response that a White client may have when sitting with a Black therapist, highlighting the potential for the splitting and projection defined by Layton's (2006) notion of the normative unconscious:

> But when the therapist does possess characteristics—such as "black skin"—which can motivate symbolic processes, fantasies, fears and counterphobic reactions, we must not confuse this with transference reactions. For these responses are certainly something other; they are archaic, mythological responses which will have crucial effects upon the manifestation of the transference, which occurs later in time. These symbolic processes appear to be dramas to be played out—they can take very definite shape, being not only irrational but "mythic". And, from the logic of these, the Negro therapist becomes "the black psychotherapist"—recalling the symbolic "meaning" of black, this becomes a contradiction to whom the client must somehow relate! (Curry, 1964, p. 10)

Relational psychoanalytic thinking, having evolved since the writing of Curry's (1964) article, emphasizes the subjectivity of the therapist (Harris, 2011), and therefore the potential for this pretransference to exist too in the mind of the therapist, which then shapes the assumptions, stereotypes, and projections that are present in the clinical encounter before it has even begun. There is a tendency among clinicians to claim that we do not carry prejudice or stereotypes into the room, and to deny the potential workings of our own racial identity (Esprey, 2013; Loya, 2011; Morgan, 2008). Pertinent to this is Hook's (2005) warning about the dangers of the disavowal of racism. He commented on the common paradox of expressing racial tolerance and nonracism that is then coupled with behavior which is undeniably racist. By disavowing or denying holding racist feelings, racially motivated behavior that may be harbored unconsciously is tolerated or excused, or rendered invisible (Smith, 2006). In this way racism cannot be challenged. As clinicians, it is tempting for us to hide behind the analytic myth of therapeutic neutrality in saying that we repudiate racism and do not allow it to contaminate the therapeutic space. In this, we ignore the deeply unconscious workings of prejudice, and run the risk of falling into the trap about which Hook warned us.

Prejudice as Pervasive

In similar vein, Fonagy (2005), an attachment theorist, suggested that prejudice is ubiquitous and needs to be understood as being part of the human condition. He summarizes psychoanalytic renderings on prejudice as being based on the assumption that prejudice restores internal equilibrium in the face of conflict or threat, and as such it plays an essential psychic function (Fonagy, 2005). The tendency to "other" therefore is an adaptive one. He offered an attachment-based perspective on the development of what he termed normal prejudice, which he differentiates from malignant, ego-syntonic prejudice, which is psychopathic (Fonagy, 2005).

Fonagy (2005) grounded his theory of prejudice within the context of secure versus insecure attachment. He suggests that ordinary prejudice arises from early experiences outside of the immediate attachment environment that activate an insecure working model. When caregivers, who are mostly able to provide a secure attachment environment, encounter interpersonal situations that create anxiety, this anxiety is consequently communicated to the receptive infant, creating an insecure working model, and prompting an identification with the caregiver, and a disidentification with the threatening other (Fonagy, 2005). Early identifications begin to be organized along lines of "us and them" to regulate internal equilibrium and to restore a secure base. To heighten a sense of identification and therefore security, characteristics belonging to the self become homogenized, and the differences belonging to the other become exaggerated. One of the consequences of this is that the racial other becomes seen as wholly different, as alien. The other is stripped of any characteristics and attributes that would render them familiar or similar, resulting in the dehumanizing splitting which Shakespeare's

(1989) genius captures poignantly in Shylock's monologue, which surfaces the absurdity of racism:

> I am a Jew. Hath a Jew not eyes? Hath a Jew not hands, organs, dimensions, senses, affections, passions? Fed with the same food, hurt with the same weapons, subject to the same diseases, healed by the same means, warmed by the same winter and summer as a Christian is? If you prick us, do we not bleed? If you tickle us, do we not laugh? If you poison us, do we not die? And if you wrong us, shall we not revenge? If we are like you in rest, we will resemble you in that. (*Merchant of Venice*, Act 3, Scene 1, lines 58–69)

Fonagy (2005) suggested that prejudice is a function of normal neuro-cognitive social functioning, the strength of which is directly related to the quality of early attachment. In situations of disorganized attachment, where a sense of mistrust and threat functions as an intrinsic weave in the attachment environment, there is the potential for the development of malignant, pernicious prejudice. But for most people, early secure attachment environments create the context for the growth of ordinary prejudice.

As a function of internalized experiences of self and other, attachments throughout life are more readily created among individuals who share characteristics of identity. Fonagy (2005) suggests that it is easier to mentalize—to attribute mental phenomena such as intentions, desires, and goal (Byeon, 2011)—about the internal worlds of others with whom we share common attributes. This proposal implies that mentalization across difference requires more psychic work, and, as indicated in neuro-cognitive studies (Byeon, 2011; Mitchell, Macrae, & Banaji, 2006) the tendency to mechanize—the attribution of behavior based on physical descriptors (Byeon, 2011)—asserts itself when faced with difference. Normal prejudice, then, involves the temporary relinquishing of mentalization (Fonagy, 2005).

The implications of this arrest of mentalization within the clinical sphere are crucial, particularly when there are clear differences of identity, such as race, in the clinical dyad. Client and therapist, then, are strangers to one another at the deepest level of identification, and the task of mentalizing becomes something that needs to be consciously motivated. Successful mentalization is based on finding points of intersection, and a resonance of alikeness (Swartz, 2007) that will allow for the oscillation between two subjectivities (Teicholz, as cited in Swartz, 2011) that is the foundation of empathy.

The notion that prejudice is an inherent human tendency has roots too in the philosophical tradition. Heidegger (as cited in Fonagy, 2005) wrote that the communal web into which we are born is interwoven by historical, cultural, and relational circumstances that create a preverbal infrastructure upon which conscious and verbally-mediated experience is constructed. Similarly, Bourdieu's concept of *habitus*, described as a structural concept that concerns the way in which individuals inhabit the world, constitutes a kind of "grammar of social action and interaction" (Straker, 2006, p. 731) that organizes inclusion and exclusion and communicates social hierarchy and position. *Habitus* precedes a conscious awareness of the world. Gadamer (as cited in Fonagy, 2005) too asserted that prejudice emerges from "fore-meanings" that are not available to conscious articulation.

A NEUROBIOLOGICAL EXPLANATION

The idea that prejudice develops in a preverbal realm and is therefore out of the reach of conscious observation, suggests that racial experience may be thought about as "unformulated experience" (Stern, as cited in Leary, 2000) that is "experience that is not yet reflected on or linguistically coded but which remains part of our everyday psychic grammar" (p. 640). Stern (1989) describes unformulated experience further as:

> Experience which has never been articulated clearly enough to allow application of the traditional defensive operations. One can forget or distort only those experiences which are formed with a certain degree of clarity in the first place. The unformulated has not reached the level of differentiation at which terms like memory and distortion are meaningful. (p. 9)

Current and emerging findings in the field of neurobiology provide a means of locating these concepts—the normative unconscious, pretransferences, prejudice—within a biological substrate, making it possible to identify how the brain may be implicated in the formation and maintenance of racially based schemas about self and other that remain largely unconscious and therefore intransigent. Considering racial experience in these terms suggests that it constitutes psychic material that resides in that "unconscious subjective internal world that is instrumental in guiding the individual's moment to moment interactions with the external environment" (Schore, 2003, p. 206), that is, in the dynamic unconscious. Developments in neuropsychoanalytic research have located the "emotion processing right mind in the neurobiological substrate of Freud's dynamic unconscious" (Schore, 2003, p. 207), directly linking the right brain to unconscious processes. It is in the right brain that the earliest socioemotional experiences begin to be processed (Miehls, 2011), locating it as the foundation of social understanding that affects the processing of socially related information for the rest of life (Schore, 2003).

Badenoch (2008) shed light on how these experiences find leverage in right-brain functioning. She described how the first 18 months of life provide a fertile platform for the development of internal mental models and attachment styles which become imprinted in the right brain. These working models parallel those of caregivers, internalized via right brain-to-right brain transmission that is largely unconscious. In these crucial first months, implicit memory is created and clustered into mental models based on repeated experience of the internal and external world. These experiences are nuanced by affective experience, perceptions, sensations, and images and prompt processes in the amygdala that then create:

> generalized, non-verbal conclusions about the way life works—the essence of mental model. These conclusions create *anticipations* of how life will unfold and remain largely below the level of conscious awareness, guiding our ongoing perceptions and actions in ways that tend to reinforce foregone conclusions. (Badenoch, 2008, p. 24)

These foregone conclusions are experienced as "The Truth of the Way Things Are" (Badenoch, 2008, p. 25). In the subsequent development of the left brain, when verbal capacity comes to the fore, words are then found for these "truths" that consequently become articulated as absolute realities. Memories that are created implicitly are not linked to any sense of temporality, which means that when implicit memories are activated through daily experience, the consequent feelings, perceptions, and sensations are experienced as if they are in direct response to current experience, rather than being memories of infantile experience, reinforcing the validity of the emotional response. In this way, earliest memories create generalizations about the reality of things that are then carried through life (Badenoch, 2008).

The implications of this for the development of a relational matrix, and for an understanding of how the social world works, are important. If we consider, as is proposed in relational theory, that the earliest attachment environments expand beyond the familial to include influences from broader society (Dimen, 2011), then we can assume that these influences will become part of what shapes internal working models. This understanding of the link between right-brain development and the context of the external social world substantiates the argument for:

> a neurobiological model (which holds) that the affective events that occur in the early postnatal stages of maturation of the emotional brain are critical to the development of systems that process socio-emotional information at levels beneath awareness and regulate affective and motivational states for the rest of the lifespan. (Schore, 2003, p. 216)

The earliest messages given by caregivers, at a nonverbal and deeply unconscious level, essentially groom the receptive right brain for functioning in the social world. This suggests that the sociopolitical milieu of child-hood becomes stamped, prescriptively, in the unconscious, ever-ready for expression in response to external triggers. These neurobiological findings substantiate the relational assertion that the psyche is political (Dimen, 2011) and evidence a biological substrate for the normative unconscious. They also support the suggestion that racial experience and identity become encoded in the unconscious, to be retrieved as a generalization or stereotype later in life.

In Apartheid South Africa, for example, where society was landscaped according to racial identity, where Blackness was assigned an inferior status and Whites held a superior one, the meaning of race would have been internalized by caregivers and subsequently transferred implicitly into the right-brain knowledge bank of infants. For many White South Africans, Black people were to be feared, avoided, and split off as "Other." For Black South Africans, Whites too were to be feared, envied, idealized, hated. Attributes of goodness and badness, purity and impurity were split racially and internalized then as part of "the way things are," establishing a context-specific, normative unconscious (Layton, 2006), and entrenching prejudice and racism. In this way the color of a person's skin became an unconscious trigger for emotional expression at a very primitive level. In South Africa a Black man signaled fear, anxiety, and mistrust for Whites, as the ideology of Apartheid propaganda seeped into familial spaces. For Black people, White skin too signaled fear and anxiety, and mistrust. And so the message of Apartheid became neurobiologically encoded.

CLINICAL IMPLICATIONS

If we consider that the earliest messages that are internalized by infants and children are influenced by dominant social discourse, which are then encoded biologically and driven into the unconscious imprint as the brain develops its unique individuality (Miehls, 2011), then we must assume that race as an aspect of identity will always be a factor to consider when mind meets mind in the intersubjective context of psychotherapy. Relational psychoanalysis, in its emphasis on the intersubjective, brings into stark relief the subjectivity of the therapist as it affects the clinical relationship (Harris, 2011), reminding us that it is not only the racialized self of the client which we need to consider, but that too of the therapist. As neurobiologically encoded relational templates are unconsciously activated by external cues (Miehls, 2011) so the therapeutic endeavor runs the risk of being shaped and limited by unconscious blueprints that prescribe the social world.

What are the clinical implications of this? Bromberg (1996) proposed that we all carry within a multiplicity of selves that are more or less dissociated from one another. If clinicians do not actively turn attention toward the racialized self that we all carry, this part of self remains unintegrated, and its presence in the consulting room is not recognized. As a consequence, the "ubiquitous, haunting presence of racial trauma" (Harris, as cited in Suchet, 2004, p. 433) remains unmetabolized in the clinical encounter. This opens up the possibility for enactment around race, particularly if, at a conscious level, there is the disavowal of any feelings or experiences of prejudice or racism.

Racial enactments, defined by Leary (2000) as "interactive sequences embodying the actualization in the clinical situation of cultural attitudes toward race and racial difference" (p. 639), potentially manifest in the therapeutic encounter in a number of ways. These include the avoidance of race altogether and the manifestation of color-blindness, the dominance of left-over right-brain processing, a reduction in mentalization strategies, and an increase in mechanistic thinking about the other, and acting on pretransferences. Suchet (2004), in referring to the disavowal and avoidance of race in clinical settings, asserts that if race continues to inhabit "a melancholic structure" (Suchet, 2004, p. 432), it becomes the potential site for projections and introjections.

Badenoch (as cited in Miehls, 2011) described how, if the therapist is not in touch with her own right-brain (unconscious) messages, the client will detect these cues and react to them unconsciously, affecting the therapy, and on the client's ability to bring her multiplicity of selves (Bromberg, 1996) into the room. In addition, ignoring the messages emanating from the right-brain templates pushes the therapeutic process into the "cold cognition" (Schore, 2003) of left-brain processing, and reducing the clinician's ability to hear the right-brain cues coming from the client. In the case of race then, the racially based, right-brain messages emanating from client and therapist are banished from the room and are left with the option of invading it only through unconscious, and potentially debilitating racial enactments.

Does this indicate that race, as an important facet of a clinical exchange, should be actively introduced at the outset of a therapy? A number of writers (Morgan, 2008; Swartz, 2007) suggested that race should be foregrounded early on in the therapy, to open up the space for discussion. This article argues that doing so may in fact have the opposite impact of closing down the space. By naming race as a conscious fact, the clinician pushes the exchange into left-brain cognition, and the shape of the therapeutic encounter becomes immediately strait-jacketed and circumscribed. The ordinary progression of a therapeutic journey becomes truncated.

An example of this comes from my work with a young Black woman who initiated therapy following a relationship break-up.[1] In preparing for our first meeting I decided that I would bring up the fact of our biracial relationship at the outset, to make her aware of my sensitivity to it, and hopefully to open up the possibility of relevant discussion. This, I did toward the end of our first session. Mary responded to my intervention by saying that it felt like all that I saw in her was a Black woman, when what she needed help with was her broken heart, which had nothing to do with race. I had formulaically foregounded something that was not yet in the material, and as such the space between us closed down. It took a while for us to recover from this enactment, which I recognized in retrospect as an intervention motivated by my left-brain processing that resorted to what I cognitively assumed would be important and culturally competent, rather than waiting to hear through intuitive right brain-to-right brain resonance, what she needed of me. I realized too that resorting to left-brain processing was also defensive on my part, protecting me from the discomfort of sitting with the not knowing of what might emerge in the relational space between us.

Miehls (2011) suggested that the only way in which to illuminate the unconscious workings of right-brain templates is to consciously focus on our own right-brain cues. Not doing so results in an inability to accurately receive information about the client's right-brain activity, restricting the work of psychotherapy to that which is consciously perceived. Furthermore, the client becomes aware of the therapist's implicit right-brain communication, responding unconsciously to its messages. Therapy remains at a superficial level of cognitive relating, and the deep work that occurs when right-brain meets right-brain (Schore, 2003) cannot evolve. The pathway to achieving a greater self-awareness is through active engagement with one's racialized self.

A common racial enactment, for White clinicians, is to deny and thereby ignore the fact of Whiteness as racially significant (Suchet, 2007). The result of this is to enact the precise racial dynamics that are often present in racialized society, where Whiteness stands as the norm and notions of race are applied only to people of color. For many White clinicians, the concept of a racial identity is unfamiliar (Loya, 2011). Suchet (2007) wrote about the invisibility of Whiteness, about how it represents an "uninterrogated space, as if it has no color" (p. 867). Typically writings about race focus on people of color, and Whiteness as a race remains invisible (Suchet, 2007). And yet it is precisely this invisibility which needs to be challenged in ourselves if we are to gain ground in the understanding of how race affects our work.

Whiteness studies suggest that it is only in "unraveling" our own Whiteness that we can begin to understand how race affects our practice as clinicians and indeed in our lives (Suchet, 2007). Miehls (2001) called for training clinicians to focus deliberately on their own racial development. He suggests that the "White gaze" acts as a powerful symbol of superiority, rendering as different the racial other in the clinical exchange. It is only in engaging in racial self-awareness that a dimensionality of self can be achieved, freeing the clinical space for reciprocity of dialogue. An absence of dialogue entrenches "us–them" binary thinking that has the potential to paralyze the development of a therapeutic relationship. Miehls (2001) suggested that, "practitioners with a highly developed sense of racial identity will be more prepared to experience the multiplicity of selves within themselves and the other" (p. 238).

And yet Gadamer (as cited in Fonagy, 2005) held the belief that prejudice could not be entirely corrected, that there will always remain a limitation to understanding. Although Whites may appreciate a Black person's point, they will never understand their "point of view" because the lens of perspective is always subjectively skewed. And vice versa. Gadamer (as cited in Fonagy, 2005) asserted that we allow ourselves to believe, erroneously, that we know about a person with whom we interact, when there are always blind spots, and more so, across difference. A White person, for example, can never understand or know how being Black pervades every aspect of life; how the experience of being Black is "a grid upon which every aspect of psychic development is constructed" (Thompson, as cited in Suchet, 2004, p. 426). It is possible, however, to become increasingly aware of prejudice, and of the workings of the normative unconscious such that we can be on guard for moments of enactment.

Holding Race in Mind

Neurobiological insights reinforce the importance of relationship development in the context of clinical work. Badenoch (2008) held that the nurturing of a relationship based on reciprocal right-brain resonance is crucial to the therapeutic endeavor. If the neurobiology of client and therapist is held in mind, the emphasis in the relationship will be to "recognize, accept, and actively construct relationships with clients that are secure and consistent" (Miehls, 2011, p. 88). The intrinsic plasticity of the brain promises that even the most deeply imprinted, right-brain relational templates can be remodeled in the context of a secure relationship. The implication for this in the healing around issues of race is powerful. Through the development of such a relationship, therapist and client have the opportunity to identify underlying schemas, to recognize how they affect subjectivity, to uncover ways in which they have been interpellated by race, or how race presents itself in pretransferences and a normative unconscious.

I have such an opportunity in my therapy with John. A Black man in his forties, he sought therapy after a relationship break-up in which his girlfriend told him that he is unable to show his feelings. Bothered by this assertion, and generally puzzled by his feeling world, John agreed to begin a process with me. I am acutely aware when sitting with John of the ways in which I am pulled to respond to him. Although his English is good, it is not his mother tongue, and we struggle at times to understand one another. In the past I suspect that I would have been tempted to work cognitively with John, to help him in a problem-solving kind of way, to avoid the sense of helpless not knowing when he tells me about aspects of his history and culture that are so very foreign. To avoid also the sense of guilt that I feel when John recounts a childhood characterized by trauma, loss, and deprivation directly linked to his status as a second-class citizen in our shared country.

Instead, I try in each session to sit with whatever emerges. I follow Swartz's (2007) suggestion that I be curious about his world, and that I be not ashamed to ask him questions when I do not understand. In the past, asking such questions would have felt threatening as they would have foregrounded my White ignorance, and his Black unfamiliarity, highlighting the differences between us. John asks me questions too, and rather than reverting to my tried-and-tested analytic stance of neutrality, I tell him things about myself, aware that we are trying to find bridges to a resonance of alikeness, and to successful mentalization. I work hard in these sessions, as I tackle my internal unconscious impulses, and my conscious clinician's voice; as I commit, each moment to being aware of what might be happening in the intersubjective space between, knowing that we are, indeed, learning from one another (Casement, 1992).

Swartz (2007) asserted that it is in encounters with the Other that unconscious templates will be aroused, and as such when working with conscious self-awareness in cross-racial dyads "we have an unparalleled opportunity to understand better what lives inside us, unconsciously" (p. 181). Self-awareness becomes the archaeologist's brush that has the potential to surface the detail of our embedded right-brain relational templates. As I hold in mind the insights provided by theory, and I marry these with my own self-observation, I begin to understand how my particular history and context have shaped my implicit relational blueprints. I recognize increasingly not only the importance of interrogating the subjectivity of race, but also of how crucial it is to the integrity of our clinical work. For me, as the racialized individual penning this article, this means encountering the pain of Whiteness, and being able to tolerate bearing witness to the pain of Blackness that I see in my clients and colleagues. Now, as I walk into a room, and shake my client's hand for the first time, I open myself up to the complex multiplicity of selves greeting one another. And in my mind's eye I hold the image of a kaleidoscope of subjectivities that settle into the chairs and embark on this unique therapeutic journey.

NOTE

1. Case material referred to in this article comprises composite and heavily disguised client detail that is unidentifiable.

REFERENCES

Altman, N. (2000). Black and white thinking: A psychoanalyst reconsiders race. *Psychoanalytic Dialogues*, *10*, 589–605.

Badenoch, B. (2008). *Being a brain-wise therapist. A practical guide to interpersonal neurobiology*. New York, NY: W.W. Norton.

Bromberg, P. (1996). Standing in the spaces: The multiplicity of self and the psychoanalytic relationship. *Contemporary Psychoanalysis, 32*, 509–535.

Byeon, H. (2011). *What is an out-group? Asian American and Caucasian Americans racial versus other identification with others* (Unpublished dissertation). Georgetown University, Washington, DC.

Casement, P. (1992). *Learning from the patient*. New York, NY: Guilford Press.

Curry, A. (1964). Myth, transference and the black psychotherapist. *Psychoanalytic Review, 51*, 7–14.

Dimen, M. (2011). Introduction. In M. Dimen (Ed.), *With culture in mind* (pp. 1–10). New York, NY: Routledge.

Eagle, G. (2005). "Cultured clinicians": The rhetoric of culture in clinical psychology training. *Psychology in Society, 32*, 41–64.

Eng, D., & Han, S. (2000). A dialogue on racial melancholia. *Psychoanalyic Dialogues, 10*, 667–700.

Esprey, Y. (2013). Raising the colour bar: Exploring issues of race, racism and racialised identities in the South African therapeutic context. In C. L. Smith (Ed.), *Psychodynamic psychotherapy in South Africa. Contexts, theories and applications* (pp. 31–53). Johannesburg, South Africa: Wits University Press.

Fonagy, P. (2005, December). *The development of prejudice: An attachment theory hypothesis explaining its ubiquity*. Paper presented at the International Conference on Prejudice, Salt Lake City, UT.

Guralnik, O., & Simeon, D. (2010). Depersonalisation: Standing in the spaces between recognition and interpellation. *Psychoanalytic Dialogues, 20*, 400–416.

Harris, A. (2011). The relational paradigm: Landscape and canon. *Journal of the American Psychoanalytic Association, 59*, 701–735.

Herman, J. (1992). *Trauma and recovery. From domestic abuse to political terror*. London, UK: Harper Collins.

Hook, D. (2005). The racial stereotype, colonial discourse, fetishism, and racism. *Psychoanalyic Review, 92*, 701–734.

Layton, L. (2006). Racial identities, racial enactments and normative unconscious processes. *Psychoanalytic Quarterly, 75*, 237–269.

Leary, K. (1997). Race in psychoanalytic space. *Gender and Psychoanalysis, 2*, 157–172.

Leary, K. (2000). Racial enactments in dynamic treatment. *Psychoanalytic Dialogues, 10*, 639–653.

Lobban, G. (2013). Subjectivity and identity in South Africa today. In C. L. Smith (Ed.), *Psychodynamic psychotherapy in South Africa. Contexts, theories and applications* (pp. 54–73). Johannesburg, South Africa: Wits University Press.

Loya, M. (2011). Color-blind racial attitudes in White social workers: A cross-sectional study. *Smith College Studies in Social Work, 81*, 201–217.

Loya, M. (2012). Racial attitudes in White social workers: Implications for culturally sensitive practice. *Politics, Bureaucracy and Justice, 3*(1), 23–31.

Miehls, D. (2001). The interface of racial identity development with identity complexity in clinical social work student practitioners. *Clinical Social Work Journal, 29*(3), 229–244.

Miehls, D. (2011). Neurobiology and clinical social work. In J. Brandell (Ed.), *Theory and practice in clinical social work* (2nd ed., pp. 81–98). Thousand Oaks, CA: Sage.

Mitchell, J. M., Macrae, C. N., & Banaji, M. R. (2006). Dissociable medial pre-frontal contributions to judgements of similar and dissimilar others. *Neuron, 50*, 655–663.

Morgan, H. (2002). Exploring racism. *Journal of Analytical Psychology, 47*(4), 567–581.

Morgan, H. (2008). Issues of 'race' in psychoanalytic psychotherapy. *British Journal of Psychotherapy, 24*(1), 34–49.

Msebele, N., & Brown, H. (2011). Racism in the consulting room: Myth or reality. *Psychoanalytic Review, 98*(4), 451–492.

Schore, A. (2003). *Affect regulation and the repair of the self.* New York, NY: W.W. Norton.

Shakespeare, W. (1989). *The Merchant of Venice.* In *The unabridged William Shakespeare.* Baltimore, MD: Running Press.

Smith, H. (2006). Invisible racism. *Psychoanalytic Quarterly, 75*, 3–19.

Stern, D. (1989). The analyst's unformulated experience of the patient. *Contemporary Psychoanalysis, 25*, 1–33.

Straker, G. (2004). Race for cover: Castrated whiteness, perverse consequences. *Psychoanalytic Dialogues, 14*, 405–422.

Straker, G. (2006). The anti-analytic third. *Psychoanalytic Review, 93*, 729–753.

Suchet, M. (2004). A relational encounter with race. *Psychoanalytic Dialogues, 14*, 423–438.

Suchet, M. (2007). Unravelling whiteness. *Psychoanalyic Dialogues, 17*, 867–886.

Swartz, S. (2007). The power to name: South African intersubjective psychoanalytic psychotherapy and the negotation of racialized histories. *Eurpoean Journal of Psychotherapy and Counselling, 9*(2), 177–190.

Swartz, S. (2011). *The broken mirror: Difference and shame in South African psychotherapy.* Paper presented at The International Self-Psychology Conference, Cape Town, South Africa.

Young, R. M. (1987, October). *Psychoanalysis and racism: A loud silence.* Paper presented at the Association of Child Psychotherapists Conference on Psychoanalysis and Racism, London, UK.

Neuroscience Insights That Inform Clinical Supervision

DENNIS MIEHLS

Smith College School for Social Work, Northampton, Massachusetts, USA

This article makes links between neuroscience literature that helps to inform a clinical supervision relationship. There has been a beginning, but limited, application of neuroscience to clinical supervision; this article offers vignettes of supervisory dyads that illustrate how understanding right-hemisphere communications between the supervisor and supervisee can further a more complex understanding of the clinical processes that are being discussed in supervision. The article draws from supervision theory that has been conceptualized using relational theory and trauma theory. The article encourages supervisor and supervisee to pay heed to their bodily reactions when discussing clinical material. Individuals expose their right-hemisphere reactions to the content of the therapy and/or supervisory sessions through a variety of well-known behavioral manifestations, including facial expression, tone, and prosody of the voice; bodily manifestations of anxiety or "tightness" in the chest or stomach; and averted eye glance, to name a few. The vignettes describe supervisory dyads that deconstruct supervisee reactions in the face of working with neo-natal intensive care infants, suicidality, and trauma.

INTRODUCTION

This article applies contemporary literature in neuroscience to the clinical supervisory relationship. There has been limited application of the concepts of neurobiology to the clinical supervisory process in spite of the increasing literature that integrates a range of neurobiological theory with clinical processes (Applegate & Shapiro, 2005; Chapman, 2014; Cozolino, 2010; DeKoven Fishbane, 2013; Miehls, 2014; A. N. Schore, 2012). Later, I summarize the beginning literature that more directly links neurobiology to supervision (Binder, 1999; Montgomery, 2013; Wilkinson, 2010); this article furthers this literature as its purpose is to offer a number of illustrations of supervisor–supervisee dyads that are conceptualized as being influenced by largely based right-hemisphere interactions between the supervisory dyad. As such, I emphasize how understanding the meaning and significance of implicit communication between the supervisory dyad sheds light on the clinical process issues that are the foci of the supervision hours. The conceptual tenets of this article are framed in neuroscience literature that underscores that individuals communicate through language (left-hemisphere activities) and nonverbal implicit communication (right-hemisphere activities). Consistent with many other articles in this special issue of *Smith Studies*, we emphasize that working dyads, in this instance, the supervisory relationship, can be strengthened when the supervisee and the supervisor utilize bodily sensations, nonverbal communication, intuition, points of rupture, and dissociative experiences during the supervision (to name a few) as sources of data that help to explain and unearth the rich dynamic interplay of factors between the client–supervisee dyad and the supervisee–supervisor dyad. Individuals expose their right-hemisphere reactions to the content of the therapy and/or supervisory sessions through a variety of well-known behavioral manifestations including facial expression, tone and prosody of the voice, bodily manifestations of anxiety or "tightness" in the chest or stomach, and averted eye glance, to name a few.

PREVIOUS RELEVANT LITERATURE

Some supervision literature can be conceptualized as a precursor to utilizing neuroscience to understand supervisory processes. For example, some of the principles of relational supervision foreshadowed the application of neurobiological literature to clinical supervision. In addition, supervision theory that is conceptualized with trauma theory principles also provides some scaffolding to the use of neurobiological literature in the supervision relationship. Supervision theory that is broadly framed in relational theory and trauma theory emphasize the intersubjectivity of the supervisory dyad (the supervisor and the supervisee) and/or the supervisory triad (the supervisor, the supervisee, the client). The tenets of relational supervision underscore that the supervisory relationship is cocreated and that each person has mutual influence on the other (Frawley-O'Dea, 2003; Ganzer & Ornstein, 2004; Lindy, 2012; Miehls, 2010; Schamess, 2006a, 2006b, 2012). In addition, supervision that is framed in relational theory also understands that each participant will bring unconscious relationship templates to the supervisory relationship that will be enacted between the two, often most notable at times of conflict. For example, Bennett and Holtz Deal (2012) reviewed a comprehensive literature that suggests that the attachment styles of the supervisee and supervisor inform transference and countertransference responses in the supervisory relationship. They suggest that understanding attachment styles of the two can provide understanding about problematic dynamics (p. 199). Miehls (2010) suggested that "supervision can be most helpful when supervisors and supervisees engage in an ongoing dialogue that explores difficulties and/or mutual transferences that occur during the supervision" (p. 372). These mutual transferences may be first detected when either participant experiences some "free-floating" anxiety or some bodily responses that are difficult to explain—however, exploration of the unconscious or nonconscious interactions between the two may lead to fruitful discoveries that will contribute to the resolution of conflict between the supervisory dyad.

Sarnat (2012) discussed the supervisory experience from a relational psychodynamic model emphasizing the centrality of relationships in forming the structures of the mind. She said, "Patient, therapist, and supervisor are viewed as co-creators of two reciprocally influential dyads. Exploration of the supervisory relationship, as it relates to the clinical relationship, is considered central to accomplishing the tasks of supervision" (p. 153). She noted that attending to disruptions in the supervisory relationship is an important teaching tool that not only builds the learning alliance but also models to the supervisee how the deconstruction and working through of conflict in the treatment relationship is an important clinical process to master and utilize in clinical work. The supervisor who is influenced by neurobiology will pay attention to ruptures in the supervisory relationship utilizing body responses as the diagnostic indicator that something is amiss in the supervisee response to her client—I demonstrate this in more detail later in the article. Frawley-O'Dea (2003) went further toward using neuroscience literature in her supervisory relationships as she suggests that a relational supervisor can be "open to considering primary process material delivered into the supervision by dreams, somatic states, fantasies, and dissociative experiences" (p. 360). Here too, some of these sources of data may be most readily experienced by paying attention to implicit communication that is conveyed through right-hemisphere interactions.

Contributions From Trauma Theory

The influence of trauma theory on the supervision literature is also useful in considering how neuroscience findings are filtering their way into the supervisory relationship. Frawley-O'Dea (1997) made some interesting observations in her article "Who's Doing What to Whom? Supervision and Sexual Abuse." She noted that supervision addressing clients with traumatic histories can become troubling encounters when the supervisory dyad enacts parts of the dyadic constellations of trauma identity in a "kaleidoscopically shifting pattern" (p. 12). She emphasized that a main defense of traumatized clients may be dissociation. These dissociative processes can leak into the supervisory process and leave the supervisory dyad somewhat in a "fog." In these instances, it is instructive for the supervisory dyad to understand the dissociative defense is being used to guard the supervisory dyad from the potentially overwhelming feelings that would be stimulated while integrating the horror of the abuse that the client may have experienced. A later example illustrates a supervisory exchange that typifies this process.

Similarly, Sarnat (2012) offered an interesting example of supervision in which dissociative defenses dominated the supervision and the clinical treatment that was being supervised. She recounted that the client was a severely traumatized woman who used dissociation as her main defense. This defensive posture caused the supervisee to feel anxious and uncertain in the work; this uncertainty led to the supervisor (Sarnat, 2012) also feeling overwhelmed. Sarnat informed her supervisee that she had received consultation from a group of colleagues about her perceived "stuckness" in the supervision. The consultation helped her to feel more confident, and she went to the next supervisory hour having a better understanding of the clinical situation. The consultation and new insights gained during the consultation freed the supervisor enough to forge a reconnection with the supervisee that was able to move beyond the "fog" that was clouding their interactions. This disclosure modeled to the supervisee that even experienced analysts/supervisors need to consult with others at times. Sarnat reported,

> I told my supervisee about the consultation, and about my understanding of what had happened to us all, (and) her dissociative fog began to lift as well. In that moment my supervisee "got" the value of using another mind to process overwhelming affect. (p. 155)

Miehls (2010) reported that supervisory dyads may unconsciously start to enact the trauma triangle of "victim/victimizer/bystander" in their supervisory relationship. Clinicians who work with survivors of childhood trauma well recognize that clients have internalized all three aspects of this trauma triangle. It is common in treatment that the client uses projective identification as a defensive action that positions and compels the clinician to take on one of the three aspects of the trauma triangle. In other words, powerful unconscious messages are manifest in the treatment relationship. As an example, Miehls (2010) suggested that a "client who was victimized by a parent may try to have the clinician victimize them" (p. 373). Of relevance to this discussion, it is likely that the supervisory hour may be characterized by examples of the supervisor, supervisee, and client being positioned in the various aspects of the trauma triangle of the victim/victimizer/bystander dynamic. Paying attention to the visceral and often uncomfortable bodily sensations that the supervisor or supervisee is experiencing during the supervision hour can help the supervisory dyad to develop reflective capacities and insight to move the clinical process away from these intransigent projective identification traps. However, the supervisory dyad might not be able to move to these left-hemisphere activities until they understand and deconstruct the powerful unconscious implicit communication that is organized through the defensive postures stimulated in right-hemisphere trauma responses of the supervisory dyad. In sum, Sarnat (2012) suggested that "Supervisors are most effective when they take seriously the importance of attending to the relationship and the nonverbal, affective, unconscious-to-unconscious bond between supervisee and supervisor" (p. 156).

Literature That Links Neuroscience and Supervision

As noted above, there is a beginning literature that links neuroscience to the supervisory process. Years ago, Binder (1999) identified the process of developing skills in psychotherapy as fluid and one that evolves with experience and with supervision. He noted that therapists initially approach clients with declarative knowledge that is "acquired through didactic course work and through supervision to the extent that the supervisor takes a directive, authoritative approach" (p. 711). Of relevance to this article, he suggested that utilization of declarative knowledge matures into the utilization of procedural knowledge—a form of tacit knowledge. He suggested that more seasoned clinicians are able to draw upon their experience and begin to use procedural knowledge that "becomes increasingly nonconscious and automatized with practice" (p. 712). This is an important factor to recognize as this author suggested that the clinician may be intervening with clients increasingly without full conscious awareness of her actions. Thus, it is vital that the supervisor be able to find ways to help the supervisee become more conscious of what motivates her interpretations, for example. It is quite likely that paying attention to implicit communication between the supervisor–supervisee dyad in these instances will reveal useful explanatory material. For example, the supervisor may have an increasing sense of anxiety when hearing the details of the supervisee's formulation of a troubled client. It would be important for the supervisor to trust her affective response as a sign that perhaps the supervisee is missing some aspects of the client's dynamics (see Clinical Vignette #2 below).

In her chapter "Mirroring, Resonance, and Empathy in the Supervisory Process," Margaret Wilkinson (2010) extrapolates concepts of neurobiologically informed psychotherapy to the supervisory relationship. She agrees with many authors (Gallese, 2007; Lyons-Ruth, 1998; J. R. Schore & Schore, 2008) who suggested that our interactions with others are not only explicit but that there is another level of interaction that is reflex-like and automatic. She noted,

> In supervision as in therapy, the right-hemisphere to right hemisphere resonance that arises from the nonverbal aspects of communication, such as tone of voice, gesture, and posture, as well as the fast-acting communications that often occur below levels of conscious awareness will underpin the work. (p. 163)

She suggests that such communications "arise from the earliest experience of right-hemispheric bodily, facial, and gestural communication between mother and child, out of which the capacity to relate and the development of communicative language gradually emerge" (p. 164). Her suggestion is that this process applies to the supervisory relationship as well—that is, that initially the supervisory partners in the dyad form impressions of each other at this nonconscious level and that this is gradually influenced and modified by mutual conscious awareness of each other.

Wilkinson (2010) emphasized that those supervisors who have the capacity to generate in one's own mind the mental activities and processes of the other will develop key aspects of supervisory functions that utilize neurobiological concepts. She explained that this is more than having an empathic stance with one's supervisee—rather, she quoted Decety and Chaminade (2003) who refer to this as "unconscious imagination, that is, a generating of neural experiencing at an unconscious level of similar activities and processes in oneself" (p. 582). She suggested that the effective supervisor allows herself to "receive communications concerning underlying feeling states, via what might well be described as the 'gut reaction', which may be one aspect of an empathic response to distress in the patient" (p. 165). Additionally, she suggested that effective supervisors have the capacity to capture "fleeting emotions in others" (p. 165). And last, as noted above, Wilkinson said effective supervisors will have "a capacity for unconscious imagination, that is, an experiencing at an unconscious level in oneself the feelings experienced by the other" (p. 165).

Montgomery (2013) commented that there are many opportunities to teach and supervise treatment theories, techniques, and strategies utilizing left-hemisphere functions of language, linearity, and logic. However, noting that some clinicians experience strong affective responses to their clients, she commented that "concerns arise about the felt experience of the supervisee with the client and the often-resulting confusion and consternation, a right-hemisphere experience" (p. 255). She suggested that there is often some crisis of confidence in the supervisor if the clinician appears somewhat dys-regulated in the clinical work that likely challenges the therapeutic alliance between the client and clinician. She argued that it is commonplace for a clinician to experience bodily reactions to the "imagery, affects, or thoughts that have been induced nonconsciously by the client" (p. 256). She went on to say that "recognition of the physical responses and wondering about their meaning is an important skill to learn for any clinician—and not easy to accomplish, revealed only by doing something clinically useful with the information" (p. 256).

Rather than suggesting that new clinicians are "overidentified" with their clients or that they are taking "empathy too far" or that the clinician needs their own therapy (p. 256), Montgomery (2013) suggested that the clinician's responses could be considered a source of data about the client. She recognizes that internal responses of the clinician are not necessarily countertransference responses that are impeding the clinical work—rather, as said, these reactions can be utilized to try and understand the client's right-hemisphere attempts to communicate poignant aspects of her internal world to the clinician. The effective supervisor, who understands the likelihood of right brain-to-right brain communication between client and clinician can normalize these responses and help the clinician learn to tolerate, if not even welcome, these physical manifestations in her own body.

As summarized, there is a beginning literature that applies some concepts of neuroscience to the supervisory relationship. Following are three vignettes of supervisory experiences that give exemplars of how understanding neuroscience can assist supervisors to become more effective with their supervisees. The following vignettes are composite illustrations of supervisory processes, disguised to protect the confidentiality and anonymity of the supervisees and their clients. These supervisory vignettes reflect an accurate representation of supervisory processes that I have offered over the last many years. More recently, my understanding of the supervisory relationship is informed by neuroscience literature. Each vignette will demonstrate aspects of neurobiologically informed interventions in the supervision process.

VIGNETTE #1

Many years ago, I supervised a number of medical social workers in a large urban teaching hospital. I supervised social workers who worked in the emergency room of the hospital, an HIV clinic, in-patient and out-patient psychiatry and a neonatal intensive care unit, to name a few. I did not have the benefit of the knowledge base of neurobiology at the time, but in retrospect, I think my intuition about one worker's difficulties in certain clinical situations speaks to the implicit communication patterns that occurred between the two of us.

Social work in a neonatal intensive care unit is multifaceted, difficult, and rewarding. Social workers assist couples dealing with neonatal death, premature birth and extensive medical attention for the neonate, and often referral to child protective services in those instances when the neonate is unable to be cared for by her birth mother. The work requires social workers to be flexible in their approach to couples and their fledgling children. One of my supervisees, Grace, was a talented young worker who seemed to operate with grace (like her name) and authenticity—even in the most painful situations, her ease with families was remarkable and she helped many families deal with grief on many levels.

I began to notice, however, that Grace was beginning to show some signs of distress when babies were surviving in the neonatal intensive care unit at increasingly younger and younger gestational ages. The technology in the field was rapidly improving and many neonates who were previously considered "nonviable" were being kept alive and nursed to eventual health in the unit. For example, neonates who had only 24 or so gestational weeks of development were increasingly surviving in the neonatal intensive care unit. Although most of the social workers and other staff were excited by the advanced technology, Grace began to express her concerns about what "we were all doing to these poor children." In her supervision, she began to talk with me about her conviction that these young neonates would have abnormalities later in childhood; she was convinced that the babies saved with this technology would never "survive." I was curious about this response as there was increasing data to suggest the opposite, and I decided to see how this unfolded with Grace. My gut feeling or hunch told me that these "miracle babies" (as they were being termed then) were disturbing Grace's world view in a way that I did not understand.

Grace came into a subsequent supervisory hour in an angry and uncharacteristically agitated manner. She shouted at me that the doctors were trying to "SAVE A 23-WEEK OLD NEONATE—WHERE WAS THIS GOING TO STOP?" She was clearly experiencing shortness of breath, some tears, and she had a panicked look on her face. She was not her usual calm and "graceful" self. I tried to engage her question in a rational manner (left-hemisphere response). I tried to appeal to her with logic and reason. To my surprise, Grace seemed to shut down completely—she became mute and she seemed dissociated. She was sitting in my office with a blank look and would occasionally say something like "oh" or "umh." I tried to engage her two or three times with language, and she was virtually immobilized and unable to attach words to her experience.

I was not aware of neuroscience during this exchange but thankfully, but I had a gut feeling that I needed to tell Grace that I was feeling intense discomfort as we were talking. I told her that I felt like I could not understand what was going on and that I was somewhat frightened for her. She seemed to begin to hear me and slowly engaged in direct eye contact with me. With tears, she asked, "Do you think they (the doctors and other team members) will be able to save a fetus of 14 weeks (gestation)?" I said I didn't know but I thought that was highly unlikely.

Her next statement was so powerful—she said "Oh, I guess I didn't murder a viable child then"—she remained quiet for a long time and finally said, "I had an abortion when I was a teenager and the baby was 14 weeks." I simply said "I am sorry" and I can't imagine how difficult it must have been for her to think of herself in that way, that is, as a child murderer. We shed a few tears, and I told her how much I respected her and her work. She wondered if she should transfer to another unit, and I said that we could defer that conversation to another time but that I thought she did fine work with so many families in her current assignment.

Understanding the Vignette From a Neuroscience Perspective

As noted, I did not know anything about neuroscience when I was supervising Grace (mid-1980s). However, in retrospect, I can understand that Grace was increasingly experiencing the advanced technology that could keep younger and younger neonates alive as a type of traumatic experience. Grace's defensive structure was being directly challenged with each "success story" on the unit. I knew "in my gut" that something was off with Grace when she began to suggest that these younger survivors would develop later developmental difficulties. As she dissociated (a response of the right hemisphere while experiencing a traumatic event) and when she was mute during our supervision (in times of trauma one's brain function of the Broca's area is shut down, rendering the individual speechless), I recognized that something very powerful was going on inside of her. I also felt immobilized for some time, and I felt a tremendous connection with her. I could feel the intensity of her inner struggle (likely as a result of mirror neurons that enhanced my empathic connection), and I was thus able to sit with her distress until she was ready to reconnect with language. It is unlikely that she would have disclosed her abortion to me had she not felt the resonance between the two of us in our right-hemisphere connection—a connection that was mixed with terror, sadness, empathy, and caring.

VIGNETTE #2

I recently had the experience of assisting a supervisee to recognize the increasing minimization of the suicidality of her client's presentation. I know the therapist to be an astute clinician who is skilled at tracking her client's affect, even in the most difficult and labile clinician situations. The super-visee's current work with a 55-year-old man, Mr. A., seemed to be stalled; and in fact, the client seemed to be regressing to a state of despair that was concerning to me. The client was a divorced, angry man who was diagnosed with a major depressive disorder and some features of a narcissistic person-ality disorder. I became somewhat didactic in the supervisory hour noting to my supervisee that this client was in a high-risk demographic group for sui-cidality. She intellectually agreed with my observation and reported that she would do a more formal mental status exam, including a suicide assessment, in her next appointment with her client.

In between our weekly supervision time, I was aware of being some-what preoccupied with this supervisee and her depressed client. I had a disturbing dream that seemed to be related to Mr. A.'s increasing despair. In spite of these factors, I had refrained from calling the supervisee to check in with her about Mr. A. The supervisee came to the following supervisory time and suggested that she wanted to shift her focus in supervision to a new client. She had met with this new client in consultation during the previous week. I acknowledged that we could do so but that I thought we should first discuss Mr. A., her depressed client. My supervisee became agitated in our interaction; she said she was tired of talking about Mr. A. and she thought he was fine and simply going through a "low period." It was startling that my supervisee seemed to be unaware that she was talking in a high pitched and rapid voice. She was also unaware that she seemed to be having some difficulty breathing; she had tears in her eyes as she told me that Mr. A. would probably feel better soon as his psychiatrist had increased the dosage of his antidepressant medication. I was aware of my increasing anxiety and certainly felt tension throughout my own body. I was experiencing some tightness in my chest and also was experiencing my heart racing—clearly my body was reacting to my supervisee's implicit communication.

Her words had a logic and coherence to them. However, her automatic right-hemisphere communication was exhibiting a message of panic and dis-orientation. My supervisee adopted a stance of shame in the room—she averted her glance from me, hung her head, and slumped her shoulders. Again, she seemed unaware of her behavior and she said something to the effect that Mr. A. was not her favorite client and she wished he would termi-nate the therapy as she did not feel that she could be helpful to him. I asked the supervisee if she had completed a suicide assessment of Mr. A. in the last session and she simply said "no" and "I don't know why you keep pres-suring me about this." She increasingly seemed to be alternating between "hyperarousal" behaviors (tears, rapid breathing) and "numbing" behaviors (a bodily-based defense against shame). As far as Mr. A. was concerned, I recognized that I was not going to be able to "reason" with my supervisee at this time. I also recognized that Mr. A. was likely at increased risk for suicide, especially if he was sensing that my supervisee was emotionally disengaging from him in the treatment relationship.

I firmly spoke my supervisee's name—she gave me eye contact for the first time in about 10 minutes in our supervisory session. I repeated her name again and commented that I could see that she was quite distraught. I noted her tears, her rapid breathing, and that her body language seemed to be demonstrating that she felt some sense of shame. Hahn (2001) cautioned supervisors from directly commenting to supervisees about witnessing a shame reaction in them, saying that bringing attention to shame in the supervisee is often subjectively experienced as a humiliation and embarrassment and is certainly often experienced as a painful confrontation. However, he suggested that "supervisors may consider confronting supervisee's shameful reactions when it is damaging to the supervisees' patients" (p. 281). In this instance, I made a decision that I needed to bring the behaviors of the supervisee to her attention. My supervisee seemed to settle quickly with my labeling her behavior. Her breathing slowed and her tears were lessening. She also apologized and said that she was unsure why she was reacting so strongly to Mr. A. Although I recognize that supervision is not therapy, there are some instances in which the boundary between the two processes does need to be challenged (Ganzer & Ornstein, 2004; Hahn, 2001; Schamess, 2012). I asked my supervisee what personal experiences she had had with suicide, perhaps especially with suicidal men.

She became obviously reflective and with some tears reported that indeed her father had committed suicide when she was a young adolescent. She went on to say that she had been worried about his safety and that she had been aware of his increasing depression and withdrawal from her and the rest of the family. She did not give voice to her concerns but rather suppressed her feelings of concern. She also talked about her great guilt and shame for not having tried to "help" her father. She exclaimed to me "oh, poor Mr. A.—I am doing the same thing to him." I commended her for coming to these realizations, and we proceeded to develop a safety plan for Mr. A., including a plan that my supervisee would call Mr. A. to arrange for an extra session. This proved to be a turning point in their treatment relationship and my supervisee went on to work with him over a longer term therapy. The treatment was not easy for her, but she was able to work through some of her own guilt and shame in her own therapy.

Understanding the Vignette From a Neuroscience Perspective

As supervisor, I had some conscious awareness of my increasing discomfort with the supervisee's treatment process with Mr. A. Additionally, I realized that my preoccupation with the supervisee and her case, my dream about the dyad, and my increased tension in my body during the supervisory session were all signals that the supervisee was having a difficult time maintaining a treatment alliance with her client. The supervisee clearly was getting flooded by affect that was related to her father's suicide. Indeed, beyond conscious awareness, the right hemisphere processes information in a rapid fashion; the right brain processes traumatic emotional responses based upon past experiences. As such, the supervisee was getting overstimulated (the agitation of her voice and tears) and simultaneously shutting the emotion down (the shame posture). The supervisee was immobilized when her parasympathetic and sympathetic nervous systems were simultaneously activated. As supervisor, I needed to lend some of my left hemisphere functions to the supervisee—indeed, the supervisee was able to respond to my insistence that she regulate her affect (when I deliberately used her name and also pointed out her implicit communication during the supervisory session). This freed the supervisee up to begin to attach some insight (left hemisphere function) to her work with Mr. A., and she became less emotionally flooded as a plan of action was formulated in concert with me. In essence, in that moment I was able to become a secure attachment figure for her who could help to regulate her affect that was stimulated in this highly charged clinical situation.

VIGNETTE #3

Susan, my supervisee, was an experienced MSW who was working as a private practitioner in an urban setting. She primarily worked with individuals in long-term therapy, and many of her clients were survivors of childhood trauma. I supervised Susan's caseload in her private practice, and we had discussed a number of her clinical experiences over a number of months. I knew her to be open to feedback; she generally showed good capacity for reflection, and I thought of her as a skilled clinician.

Susan seemed to be increasingly confused about a therapy that she was conducting with a young lesbian-identified client (Jane) who had been sexually abused by her father over a protracted time period from age 8 to 13. Jane had started therapy with Susan when she began to become immobilized with a number of post-traumatic stress disorder (PTSD) symptoms. At the beginning of treatment, the client was experiencing a number of "hyperarousal" symptoms including nightmares, flashbacks, intrusive thoughts and images of the abuse, and tremendous difficulty sleeping. She was having trouble functioning in her employment as a nursing assistant at a rehabilitation center. Susan's early work with the client was, as typical, Phase I trauma work (Basham & Miehls, 2004). Susan was assisting the client to become stabilized through a variety of interventions including supportive therapy techniques, a referral for pharmacological assistance to moderate some of her more intense symptoms, developing a structured routine that offered consistency and safety to her days, and some psychoeducation about PTSD and complex posttraumatic syndrome. The client did well in Phase I work, and Susan I agreed that Jane was ready to move to Phase II work that would include a recounting of the trauma, and a restorying of the events. Such interventions are often designed to assist the survivor/client to move out of a "victim" role and to begin to take on a more active role in determining her choices in life and to develop a sense of agency in the world.

The client was eager to tell more details of her abuse history, and she was a quick study in terms of understanding that she was not responsible for the abusive relationship she had experienced with her father. However, the work became complicated for Susan during this phase. In the clinical process, she experienced a number of bodily reactions when Jane would describe that she was feeling better all the time. Susan was confused as she was experiencing intrusive thoughts during the therapy hour, often imagining that her client was harming herself in some way. The supervision hours also became somewhat confusing. Susan was getting more disorganized in her reporting about the clinical process, and I, as supervisor, also began to be aware of an intense feeling of dread when Susan talked about her client. In addition, in scanning my own physical reactions, I noticed that I was feeling anxious and somewhat nauseous when Susan discussed her client's progress—I was not convinced that the client was progressing, and I wondered what the client was hiding from herself and her therapist. Susan and I were conscious of the potential that Jane was acting out some part of the trauma triangle (victim/victimizer/bystander) through projective identification. Intellectually, we wondered if Susan was being positioned as a victimizer by her client; however, Susan kept insisting that her feelings during the interviews with Jane was that Jane was self-harming in some way. Susan reported that she felt more like a bystander but was unsure how to raise this with her client. Her client kept reporting that she was feeling better.

It was clear to me and Susan that all three of us were being dramatically affected by this treatment. Susan felt a dilemma as her client was reporting progress; however, Susan shared my sense of dread and also experienced some guilt for not believing her client's reports of progress. I was aware that I increasingly doubted the validity of Susan's reports to me and began to question what she and I were missing about her client's presentation. At one point, Jane missed a session with Susan—this was highly unusual, and I encouraged Susan to contact her client to assess her safety. Indeed, the client had gone on a destructive drinking binge and had essentially withdrawn from the world for 3 days, staying in an alcoholic stupor. Susan and I agreed that this was perhaps the self-destructive behavior that both of us had had some intuition about and had received some confirmation through our own bodily responses and intense feelings that something was going awry with the client. I encouraged Susan to assess Jane's stability in the next session; I suggested that Susan begin to gently share some of her bodily reactions, her imagery that Jane was harming herself and her confusion about this in the midst of the client saying she was "fine" and "doing better." I had already told Susan of my own reactions to this therapeutic dyad and that I thought her client was conveying information to her via nonconscious right-hemisphere communication. Susan agreed with this understanding of the impasse.

Jane appeared distraught in the following session—she was somewhat dissociated and having a hard time verbalizing her current status to Susan. The client was tearful, anxious, and disheveled in her appearance. She had missed work for four consecutive days. She was not drinking but said she was somewhat frozen in her own home and having a hard time getting out of bed. Susan had planned to share some of her own responses to Jane if she was more functional in the session. As noted above, Susan and I had wondered if deconstructing some of the implicit communication patterns between the two would assist Jane to feel more coherent and organized. In spite of Jane's apparent distress, Susan did tell her client that she had been worried about her and that she was having repeated images of Jane hurting herself. Jane seemed to crumble emotionally and began to sob saying, "yes, I have been carving myself for a number of weeks now." She acknowledged that it was a great relief to share this behavior with Susan.

Jane went on to describe that she deserved to be "punished" . . . Susan questioned why this was so and Jane revealed that she had been having a number of new and intrusive memories in which she was sexually abusing her young male nephew. Jane had been trying to ignore these images, but they had grown stronger. She admitted that she had used self-carving as an affective release in times of extreme distress and that she found the behavior to help her to calm down. Jane went on to report that she could no longer deny that she was a perpetrator as well. She imagined that Susan was disgusted with her. Susan felt a sense of empathy and also relief. She understood that Jane would need to work through this complex dynamic, but she also felt confident that Jane's disclosure was the beginning of another phase of her healing process. In her next supervision, Susan was focused again and was clearly able to map out what needed to happen in Jane's next phase of treatment. My own feelings of anxiety and dread also passed, and Susan and I were able to jointly anticipate the next phase of the clinical work with Jane.

Understanding the Vignette From a Neuroscience Perspective

This is a good example of how the three individuals influenced each other in powerful ways as they reverberated with each other in the nonconscious implicit communication of the right hemisphere interactions. The impasse in the treatment was first noted by the clinician and the supervisor when each had experiences of dread about the treatment process. The clinician, especially, picked up the implicit communication of the client when she had repeated images of her client harming herself. It is important to pay heed to these sorts of images—though disturbing, they offer real opportunity in the clinical situation to unearth an impasse. The supervisee and supervisor also experienced some "rupture" in their relationship as the supervisor began to distrust the veracity of the clinician's recounting of the clinical situation. It was important for the supervisor and client to rule out that the impasse in the treatment was not related to some aspect of projective identification of the victim/victimizer/bystander trauma triangle. Certainly, the nonconscious projective identification enactments of self-harm and secrets was conveyed between all three participants in the client/supervisee/supervisor triad. A deconstruction of the implicit messages paved the way for further development of insight and a more complex understanding of the client's identity as both a "victim" but also a "victimizer." Certainly the functions of the left-brain hemisphere could once again be accessed and utilized to move the therapy along once this impasse was uncovered and began to be worked through between the client and clinician and subsequently the supervisee and the supervisor.

CONCLUSION

It is clear that the neuroscience literature, in a broad sense, is exerting a major influence on clinical processes with a range of dyads. As noted above, neuroscience literature is expanding at a quick pace and is offering new insights about a range of psychodynamic psychotherapy treatment issues. This article furthered the literature on supervision theory by illustrating how concepts of neuroscience can be utilized to better understand supervisory dyads, especially at times of difficulty between the two. So often, clinicians are trained to rely on their cognitive and verbal capacities when they are engaged in psychotherapy. The development of these capacities is important; however, an increasing attention to right-hemisphere interactions that highlight implicit communication in dyads is illuminating novel ways to understand clinical process situations that would have been previously characterized as "stuck" or at an impasse. This is true in supervisory relationships as well.

Divino and Moore (2010) offered a number of suggestions about how to integrate neurobiological finds into psychodynamic psychotherapy training and practice. Their article elucidates their techniques in classroom teaching of psychotherapy practice. They explained that anyone's ability to practice reflexivity and with self-awareness is to a great extent dependent on the student's/clinician's interpersonal and environmental experiential history (p. 340). They suggested that students (and supervisees) need to be taught the art of observation. They suggest that "a combined focus on the content of a session, the patient's affect, the therapist's own affect, and any memories that may be kindled by the evoked affect is likely to reveal nonconscious aspects of the patient's communication" (p. 342). It is likely true that clinical intuition cannot be taught in a classroom or in supervision. However, encouraging our supervisees to continuously be aware of their bodily sensations, internal cues, and affective reactions while engaged with a client will open up many pathways for understanding clinical processes.

How we are practicing psychotherapy and supervision is currently changing; the influence of neuroscience literature is furthering our capacities to better respond to process issues at the implicit and explicit levels. We certainly will continue to value left-brain-hemisphere functions in psychotherapy and supervision. These are the executive functions of the prefrontal cortex that are necessary ingredients in any change process. However, a continued valuing of right-hemisphere communication will ensure that our therapeutic processes, including supervision, will honor the power and influence of all aspects of our complex interactions that we experienced during infancy and childhood. Many of these interactions, including right-hemisphere internalizing of implicit communication patterns between caretaker and child, set templates for who we become as individuals and clinical practitioners. These truly influence our responses in adult interpersonal experiences and thus need to be understood as we strive to become better clinicians and supervisors.

REFERENCES

Applegate, J., & Shapiro, J. (2005). *Neurobiology for clinical social work: Theory and practice.* New York, NY: W.W. Norton.

Basham, K., & Miehls, D. (2004). *Transforming the legacy: Couple therapy with survivors of childhood trauma.* New York, NY: Columbia University Press.

Bennett, S., & Holtz Deal, K. (2012). Supervision training: What we know and what we need to know. *Smith College Studies in Social Work, 82*(2/3), 195–215.

Binder, J. (1999). Issues in teaching and learning time-limited psychodynamic psychotherapy. *Clinical Psychology Review, 19*(6), 705–719.

Chapman, L. (2014). *Neurobiologically informed trauma therapy with children and adolescents: Understanding mechanisms of change.* New York, NY: W.W. Norton.

Cozolino, L. (2010). *The neuroscience of psychotherapy: Healing the social brain* (2nd ed.). New York: W.W. Norton.

Decety, J., & Chaminade, T. (2003). When the self represents the other: A new cognitive neuroscience view on psychological identification. *Consciousness and Cognition, 12*, 577–596.

DeKoven Fishbane, M. (2013). *Loving with the brain in mind: Neurobiology & couple therapy*. New York, NY: W.W. Norton.

Divino, C., & Moore, M. (2010). Integrating neurobiological findings into psychodynamic psychotherapy training and practice. *Psychoanalytic Dialogues: The International Journal of Relational Perspectives, 20*(3), 337–355.

Frawley-O'Dea, M. G. (1997). Who's doing what to whom? Supervision and sexual abuse. *Contemporary Psychoanalysis, 33*(1), 5–18.

Frawley-O'Dea, M. G. (2003). Supervision is a relationship too: A contemporary approach to psychoanalytic supervision. *Psychoanalytic Dialogues, 13*(3), 355–366.

Gallese, V. (2007). Before and below theory of mind: Embodied simulation and the neural correlates of social cognition. *Philosophical Transactions of the Royal Society, Biological Sciences, 362,* 659–669.

Ganzer, C., & Ornstein, E. (2004). Regression, self-disclosure, and the teach or treat dilemma: Implications of a relational approach for social work supervision. *Clinical Social Work Journal, 32*(4), 431–449.

Hahn, W. (2001). The experience of shame in psychotherapy supervision. *Psychotherapy, 38*(3), 272–282.

Lindy, J. (2012). Dynamics of the educational triad. *Smith College Studies in Social Work, 82*(2/3), 173–194.

Lyons-Ruth, K. (1998). Implicit relational knowing: Its role in development and psychoanalytic treatment. *Infant Mental Health Journal, 19,* 282–289.

Miehls, D. (2010). Contemporary trends in supervision theory: A shift from parallel process to relational and trauma theory. *Clinical Social Work Journal, 38,* 370–378.

Miehls, D. (2014). Neurobiology and clinical social work. In J. Brandell (Ed.), *Essentials of clinical social work* (pp. 84–102). Thousand Oaks, CA: Sage.

Montgomery, A. (2013). *Neurobiology essentials for clinicians: What every therapist needs to know*. New York, NY: W.W. Norton.

Sarnat, J. (2012). Supervising psychoanalytic psychotherapy: Present knowledge, pressing needs, future possibilities. *Journal of Contemporary Psychotherapy, 42,* 151–160.

Schamess, G. (2006a). Therapeutic processes in clinical supervision (Part II). *Clinical Social Work Journal, 34*(4), 427–445.

Schamess, G. (2006b). Transference enactments in clinical supervision. *Clinical Social Work Journal, 34*(4), 407–425.

Schamess, G. (2012). Mutual influence in psychodynamic supervision. *Smith College Studies in Social Work, 82*(2/3), 142–160.

Schore, A. N. (2012). *The science of the art of psychotherapy*. New York, NY: W.W. Norton.

Schore, J. R., & Schore, A. N. (2008). Modern attachment theory: The central role of affect-regulation in development and treatment. *Clinical Social Work Journal, 36,* 9–20.

Wilkinson, M. (2010). *Changing minds in therapy: Emotion, attachment, trauma & neurobiology*. New York, NY: W.W. Norton.

Biomania: Benefits, Risks, and Challenges

JON G. ALLEN

The Menninger Clinic, Houston, Texas, USA

As a tongue-in-cheek expression of protest, the author uses the term biomania *to characterize excessive enthusiasm for exclusively biological approaches to psychiatry, while fully appreciating the increasingly vital contributions of neuroscience to the profession. Advocating science-informed humanism, the article brings to bear psychological and philosophical thinking on age-old problems now informed by neuroscience, including free will, the mind–brain relation, and the nature of consciousness. All these problems are pertinent to understanding patients and to educating them and their family members in this age of biological psychiatry. Clinicians in all mental health disciplines must strive to balance science and humanism in their therapeutic endeavors without sacrificing either to the other. This article provides some guidance for that aspiration.*

I am grateful to Dennis Miehls and Jeffrey Applegate for providing me with the opportunity to express my reservations about what I have dubbed "biomania": enthrallment with exclusively neurobiological approaches to psychiatric disorders and treatment. These reservations are embedded in a broader concern about the potential eclipse of humanism in clinical practice by an overvaluation of science and related technological approaches to mental health care. Our language is evolving accordingly. What we formerly attributed to our "human nature," we now attribute to our "wiring" (Lieberman, 2013). To refine our practice of psychotherapy, we must identify *mechanisms* of change (Kazdin, 2007), and recent research is homing in on brain changes associated with psychotherapy—the neurobiological mechanisms.

In overview, my argument proceeds as follows: (1) Psychiatry must remain anchored in humanism but has become increasingly technological, with psychotherapy researchers promulgating a slew of evidence-based, manualized treatments. Neuroscience is further escalating technological thinking, which reinforces the need for balance in the form of science-informed humanism. (2) Reframing mental illnesses as brain disorders seems like a sympathetic and helpful approach to patients and families, but it is not without risk of abetting the stigma it aims to defuse. (3) Taking the brain seriously, as we now must do, confronts us with age-old philosophical conundrums, including free will, the mind–body relation, and the nature of consciousness. All these problems pertain to our sense of ourselves and other persons. With the ascendance of technology, we risk depersonalization, and we must strive to counter this trend. New thinking about consciousness has the potential to put some soul back into the brain. (4) How we clinicians think about the person–brain relation shapes the way we educate our patients and their family members about psychological problems, psychiatric disorders, and mental health treatment. Patients and families are at risk for becoming biomanics. We must learn to juggle contrasting scientific and humanistic perspectives on our complex human nature as we aspire to apply burgeoning scientific knowledge to understanding our patients and relating to them therapeutically. With scientific aspirations, psychology parted company with philosophy a century ago. With neuroscience now at the doorstep of psychology, it is time to welcome our philosophical colleagues back into our home. They have a strong voice in what follows.

SCIENCE-INFORMED HUMANISM

Prior to the recent enthusiasm for neurobiological explanations and psychopharmacological interventions, technology in psychotherapy gained ascendance in the proliferation of "evidence-based" specialized therapies, accompanied by a spate of acronyms. Are therapists at risk of becoming technicians? In protest, I declared myself a practitioner of plain old therapy (Allen, 2013d). This preference for plain old therapy is based on the abundant evidence for the contribution of the human relationship to the outcome of therapy (Castonguay & Beutler, 2006; Norcross, 2011), in contrast to the limited evidence for the general superiority of any brand-name therapy in relation to any other. I am not denying that specialized therapies have a place; it would make no sense to treat obsessive–compulsive disorder with plain old therapy when exposure and response prevention would be more effective. As in general medicine, generalists must know when to refer to specialists. Striving for balance and integration, I have argued that we need science-informed humanism as a basis for practice (Allen, 2013c).

This concern with humanistic aspects of care is hardly new. A few decades ago in the context of general medicine, Walter Menninger (1975) noted, "numerous examples of physicians who are absolutely superb technicians, with all the latest knowledge and skill, but who approach patients in such a cold manner as to prompt doubt and distress" (p. 837). His quotations from a 1927 publication by Francis Peabody underscore the truly longstanding nature of the science-humanism tension:

> The most common criticism made at present by older practitioners is that young graduates have been taught a great deal about the mechanism of disease, but little about the practice of medicine—or, to put it more bluntly, they are too 'scientific' and do not know how to take care of patients . . . . The good physician knows his patients through and through, and his knowledge is bought dearly. Time, sympathy and understanding must be lavishly dispensed, but the reward is to be found in the *personal bond* which forms the greatest satisfaction of the practice of medicine. One of the essential qualities of the clinician is interest in humanity, for *the secret of the care of the patient is in caring for the patient*. (pp. 836–837, emphasis added)

Bracken et al. (2012) recently echoed these sentiments in the context of mental health treatment, buttressing their arguments with research. These authors summarized research showing that "non-specific factors (client variables, extra-therapeutic events, relationship variables and expectancy and placebo effects) account for about 85% of the variance in therapeutic outcomes across the psychotherapy field," and they went on to note that "in a review of over 5000 cases treated in a variety of National Health Service settings in the UK, no significant variance in outcome could be attributed to the specific psychotherapeutic model use" (p. 431). Moreover, "many service users did not really value the technical expertise of the professionals. Instead, they were more concerned with the human aspects of their encounters such as being listened to, taken seriously, and treated with dignity, kindness and respect" (p. 432).

I am not minimizing the value of science in clinical practice; contra Peabody, I do not think we can be "too scientific." But we cannot rely exclusively on science, and I think we must take a broad view of the evidence base. The honorific label *evidence-based treatment* is based substantially on experimental trials that compare brand-name manualized therapies to control groups or to one another. As noted earlier, these ubiquitous horse-race comparisons of brands rarely yield winners. Yet, more than a half-century ago, Carl Rogers (1951, 1957) identified key relationship factors that contributed to treatment outcomes, each strongly buttressed by subsequent research: empathy (Elliott, Bohart, Watson, & Greenberg, 2011), positive regard (Farber & Doolin, 2011), and genuineness (Kolden, Klein, Wang, & Austin, 2011).

In addition, abundant research attests to the impact on treatment outcome of the therapeutic alliance (Horvath, Del Re, Fluckiger, & Symonds, 2011) and the process of repairing ruptures in the alliance (Safran, Muran, & Eubanks-Carter, 2011).

Equally impressive in its broad implications for psychotherapeutic treatment is research demonstrating the pervasive developmental benefits of secure attachment relationships as well as the developmentally pernicious impact of trauma in these relationships (Allen, 2013b). Peter Fonagy and his colleagues (Fonagy, 1989; Fonagy, Gergely, Jurist, & Target, 2002) made a major contribution in identifying the key process in the development of attachment security: mentalizing, that is, paying attention to mental states in self and others and interpreting behavior accordingly—holding mind in mind, for short. Fonagy and colleagues demonstrated an intergenerational process wherein parental attachment security is associated with parents' mentalizing of their early-attachment relationships; moreover, such security assessed prior to the birth of the child predicts the infant's security with the parent at age 1 year (Fonagy, Steele, & Steele, 1991; Steele, Steele, & Fonagy, 1996). Additional research shows that the relation between parental and infant security is mediated by parents' mentalizing of the infant during the first year of life (Arnott & Meins, 2007; Meins, Fernyhough, Fradley, & Tuckey, 2001; Slade, Grienenberger, Bernbach, Levy, & Locker, 2005). Furthermore, secure infants become better mentalizers in their childhood (Meins et al., 2002). In sum, mentalizing begets mentalizing, from generation to generation. Conversely, profoundly insecure parental attachment is associated with compromised mentalizing of the infant as well as insecurity in the infant; moreover, correspondingly compromised infant security is associated with impaired development of mentalizing in childhood as well as with developmental adversity that can extend into adulthood (Allen, 2013b; Fonagy, Gergely, & Target, 2007). Accordingly, parent–child interventions that promote psychological attunement are yielding promise for interrupting a potential course of developmental adversity (Berlin, Zeanah, & Lieberman, 2008; Sadler, Slade, & Mayes, 2006).

In humans, mentalizing is the psychological glue of attachment, and an exceptional capacity for mentalizing distinguishes us from other species. Indeed, emerging consensus suggests that the escalating demand for social cognition played a major role in driving the evolution of the human neocortex (Bogdan, 1997; Humphrey, 1988; Lieberman, 2013). In light of the developmental principle that mentalizing begets mentalizing and the evidence that skilled mentalizing promotes attachment security, we have argued that promoting mentalizing in the context of a secure attachment relationship is the most fundamental common factor that contributes to the effectiveness of a wide variety of psychotherapeutic approaches (Allen, Fonagy, & Bateman, 2008). We also have acknowledged that, given its fundamental and ubiquitous role, mentalizing is the least novel approach to therapy imaginable (Allen & Fonagy, 2006). Thus, if mentalizing is our uniquely human skill, our effectiveness as psychotherapists boils down to our skill in being human (Allen, 2013d). This reasoning was my pathway to advocating plain old therapy anchored in attachment research and to regarding this approach as exemplifying science-informed humanism.

Biomania knows no bounds; neuroscience has established a strong foothold in research on attachment (Allen, 2013b), and social-cognitive neuroscience is refining our understanding of the complexities of mentalizing (Adolphs, 2003; Amodio & Frith, 2006; Frith & Frith, 2006; Lieberman, 2013). Developmental neuroscience also is underscoring the potentially enduring adversities associated with early-attachment trauma (Alter & Hen, 2009; Polan & Hofer, 2008; Suomi, 2008; Weaver et al., 2004). Hence neuroscience potentially has much to contribute to the fundamentally humanistic agenda of treating trauma with plain old therapy.

In expressing reservations about biomania, I do not intend to give short shrift to its benefits. Although we could be heading toward a plateau in the effectiveness of psychotherapy (as the horse races might imply), I believe that major advances in understanding and treating psychopathology will come from neuroscience. Nonetheless, it is hard for me to imagine that such advances will obviate the need for psychotherapy as a humanistic and ethical endeavor (Allen, 2008, 2013c). Notwithstanding the controversy that Thomas Szasz (1974) evoked with the tendentious title of his book, *The Myth of Mental Illness*, I am sympathetic with his focus on problems in living and with his conclusion that "Psychologists and psychiatrists deal with moral problems which, I believe, they cannot solve by medical methods" (p. 9). Yet, in the context of severe psychopathology, medical methods must be part of the solution—not infrequently, a critical part. For example, I have worked with a number of patients who were so profoundly depressed or psychotic that they were beyond the reach of psychotherapy. They needed medical intervention (e.g., medication, electroconvulsive therapy) to make any use of psychotherapy. The use of technology is not borne solely of technological zeal; relief of suffering by medical methods also is science-informed humanism at its best.

DOES FOCUSING ON THE BRAIN DECREASE STIGMA?

Whatever reservations one might have about the ascendance of neuroscience in the field of mental health, one potential benefit would seem obvious: reframing mental illnesses as "brain disorders" should reduce social stigma. The reasoning for this premise is straightforward: physical illnesses are generally less stigmatizing than mental illnesses, such that shifting the focus from the person to the brain should alleviate stigma.

We now have a corpus of research evidence to test this hypothesis. Erlend Kvaale and colleagues (Kvaale, Haslam, & Gottdiener, 2013) combined data from all pertinent research studies bearing on whether characterizing psychological problems as diseases with biogenetic causes reduces stigma. They refined this question by distinguishing four different facets of stigma: blame of the individual for problems, pessimism about prognosis for recovery, perceived dangerousness, and desire to maintain social distance. Aggregating data across studies yielded large samples for each of the four facets, ranging from 1,207 to 3,469 participants.

Surprisingly, shifting the focus from the person to the brain does not consistently reduce stigma and might even increase it in some respects. On the positive side, the disease perspective is associated with less blaming attitudes; on the negative side, it is associated with greater pessimism about prognosis. Moreover, there was suggestive but inconclusive evidence that the disease model is associated with higher perceived dangerousness. Notably, there is no evidence that the disease model affected social distancing.

Plainly, focusing on brain disorders is a problematic approach to alleviating stigma. As Kvaale et al. (2013) point out, the disease model decreases blame, but this shift comes with a cost: it increases pessimism about recovery and might also contribute to perceived dangerousness. The matter of perceived dangerousness is of great current concern, given the burgeoning alarm about the role of mental illness in mass shootings. The finding that construing mental illnesses as brain disorders does not reduce social distancing is noteworthy, given that rejection and discrimination are key consequences of stigma; these most pernicious social attitudes are not ameliorated by the disease model. The authors' conclusion is worth heeding: "Explanations that invoke biogenetic factors may reduce blame but they may have unfortunate side-effects, and they should not be promoted at the expense of psychosocial explanations, which appear to have more optimistic implications" (Kvaale et al., 2013, p. 790). We cannot take the person out of the problem.

BEING A PERSON IN A BRAIN

Over the course of recent centuries, scientists have progressively dethroned us humans. With Copernicus, we lost our place as the center of the universe. With Darwin, we learned that we are the current products of gradual evolution; moreover, evolution is no guarantor of progress—much less perfection—inasmuch as the vast majority of species that existed have become extinct. With Freud, we came to understand the limitations of our rationality in light of the pervasive influence of unconscious processes on our thoughts, feelings, actions, and relationships. With the burgeoning of neuroscience, we are now in a position to appreciate the impact of genetic influences not only on our physical characteristics but also on our personality as well as our vulnerability to various psychiatric disorders. Moreover, with the advent of functional neuroimaging, we are unearthing myriad relationships between patterns of brain activity and our cognitive and emotional functioning. By means of this activity, our brains are conscious. With this latest potential dethroning, we are at risk for losing our minds and sense of self, ceding all the power to our brains. There are two age-old philosophical problems that bear addressing insofar as they might threaten our sense of personhood: free will and the neurobiological basis of consciousness. Although giving the brain its due, it might be possible to arrive at an understanding that enhances rather than diminishes our personhood.

Free Will

Neuroimaging is enabling us to become much more intimately acquainted with our brains insofar as brain activity and mental activity can be correlated directly. These scientific observations are consistent with a long-held (but much debated) philosophical view that mental activity is entirely dependent on brain activity—no mind apart from brain. Moreover, given that the brain is a material object and hence subject to all the laws of chemistry and physics, we can conclude that the mind is subject to these laws. This chain of reasoning raises the specter of determinism which, by some accounts, is incompatible with free will. If ever there were a neurobiological threat to our sense of ourselves as persons, this is it: My feeling of control over my thoughts and actions is an illusion; not only am I along for the ride in my brain but also my fate is cast in stone.

As philosopher John Searle (2007) wrote, "The problem of free will is unusual among contemporary philosophical issues in that we are nowhere remotely near to having a solution" (p. 11). The problems of free will and determinism are enormously complex and subtle; debate is endless (Kane, 2011), but research might yield progress (Baumeister, Mele, & Vohs, 2010). Although we can entertain all kinds of ideas about ourselves, in practice we cannot feel that we are the passive pawns of our determinism-governed brains. Consider this from Searle:

> Suppose you are given a choice in a restaurant between steak and veal. The waiter asks you "And sir, which would you prefer, the steak or the veal?" You cannot say to the waiter, "Look, I am a determinist. I will just wait and see what I order because I know that my order is determined." (p. 11)

My hunch is this: When we discover how the process of making choices relates to brain activity, we will find some counterpart to our experience of free will (genuine choice). But I also consider our choices to be profoundly constrained by much that is out of our control (Ayer, 1982), such that free will always corresponds to limited "elbowroom" (Dennett, 1984)—choice within constraints. Thus I believe that neuroscience also will inform us about the biological constraints on choice. Meanwhile, I am partial to neurophilosopher Patricia Churchland's (2013) commonsensical approach to free will:

> If you are *intending* your action, *knowing* what you are doing, and are of sound mind, and if the decision is not coerced (no gun is pointed at your head), then you are exhibiting free will. This is about as good as it gets (p. 180) . . . [T]he fuzzy boundaries of concepts such as *self-control* and *voluntary* and *free will* explain why intelligent, conscientious people might disagree about how to judge problematic cases. (p. 183)

The problem of free will is not mere philosophical hairsplitting; I encounter it on a daily basis in my clinical work. The clinical problem takes the form of judgments about the extent to which patients "can't" or "won't" do as we think they must do to recover. Consider the profoundly depressed patient who does not get out of bed and thus does not do what is necessary for recovery. Can't or won't get going? I find it difficult to judge the balance of can't and won't, and I confess a belief that brain imaging data would render us more sympathetic to the patient's experience of "can't." We therapists are better equipped to deal with the "won't" (e.g., in addressing the thoughts and feelings that stand in the way of adaptive action). In striving to judge the balance of can't and won't, we should keep in mind Churchland's (2013) point that intelligent people will disagree. Thus, in navigating this routine challenge, we must not be caught in a forced-choice way of thinking: can't and won't intermingle in the context of limited elbowroom.

Consciousness

The relation of consciousness to brain activity takes us into another age-old philosophical conundrum, the mind–body problem. How can a material object—the brain—be conscious and have a mind? This problem now comprises the bedrock of the nature of human nature, and contemporary neuroscience brings it to the fore. To me, the study of the neural correlates of consciousness is the most fascinating domain of neuroscience, and researchers are making considerable headway in identifying unique patterns of brain activity associated with conscious experience (Damasio, 2010; Dehaene, Changeux, Naccache, Sackur, & Sergent, 2006; Edelman, 2004; Shallice & Cooper, 2011). Concomitantly, research is demonstrating the brain's enormous capacity for unconscious processing and its pervasive impact on our functioning, including on our conscious experience (Churchland, 2013). By any account, consciousness is a narrow window on brain activity, albeit a profoundly important one that comprises the core of our personhood.

Correlating brain activity with conscious experience does not answer the fundamental question: How does a physical object create a mental world? How does the brain create visual sensations from light waves? How can a person inhabit a brain without being separate from the brain? Beware: striving to fathom the answers to these questions can shake up your sense of self. Merely taking seriously the idea that you are your brain's continuous creation can be mindboggling.

No one claims to have solved the mind–body problem, but there is some convergence among current scholars on an idea I will merely sketch here, at the risk of gross oversimplification (Baars, 1997; Graziano, 2013; Humphrey, 2006, 2011). In interaction with the material world, the material brain constructs the mind as an illusion akin to a theater. How the brain accomplishes this feat remains to be understood, but we are now in a better position to appreciate the problems to be solved (Humphrey, 2006). The "stuff" of the mind is vastly different from the "stuff" of chemistry and physics: mental experience is comparatively ghostly, immaterial, and spiritual. And we not only experience ourselves and the world in this illusory (i.e., mental) way but also perceive other persons (and animals) as doing likewise. We inhabit a world of persons and theaters, which our highly evolved brains created to enable us to live and thrive in their world of chemicals and atoms.

Given the ways of evolution, it seems highly unlikely that consciousness came into being without purpose—as if consciousness is merely along for the ride in the brain, which does all the real work. Mainstream thinking has it thus: we need consciousness when automatic and habitual (nonconscious) behavior is insufficient—typically, when we engage with novel and complex situations that require flexibility and deliberation (Damasio, 2010; Shallice & Cooper, 2011). Social interactions are a prime example of complex situations that call for conscious deliberation. Our elaborate consciousness evolved in concert with our expanding prefrontal cortex in relation to the cognitive challenges of complex social problem solving related to the adaptive need for social cooperation and competition (Lieberman, 2013). But this view leaves out the profound emotional value of consciousness.

Countering the risk of our feeling diminished by linking our most prized possession—consciousness—to the brain, Nicholas Humphrey (2011) conceived the mind–brain relation in a way that dramatically enhances our sense of self and personhood while keeping us true to emerging scientific knowledge. Humphrey gave us science-informed humanism at its very best. He does so eloquently, and I will take the liberty of letting him speak for himself. My enthusiasm for Humphrey's thinking takes me on a bit of a tangent, but this excursion provides a strong antidote to the technological cast of biomania.

Boldly titling his book *Soul Dust*, Humphrey (2011) puts soul back into psychology: "Though I have no belief whatever in the supernatural, I make no apology for putting the human soul back where I am sure it belongs: at the center of consciousness studies" (p. xi). Humphrey bucks the scientific tide, quoting his equally philosophical scientific forbear, William James: "Like it or not, you see yourself, in James's words, as a 'simple spiritual substance in which the various psychic faculties, operations, and affections inhere.' If that is not to have a soul, I do not know what is" (p. 158).

As Humphrey (2011) sees it, the adaptive value of consciousness goes beyond problem solving by infusing conscious life with emotional value and a feeling of vitality:

> natural history reveals . . . that consciousness—on several levels—*makes life more worth living*. Conscious creatures enjoy being phenomenally conscious . . . they *revel in being* phenomenally conscious . . . there is real biological value in all this. The added *joie de vivre* . . . dramatically increased the investment individuals make in their own survival. (p. 75)

But Humphrey (2011) does not stop with our personal experience; consciousness infuses the world with the same spirit: "The material world has given human beings magical souls. Human souls have returned the favor and put a magical spell upon the world" (p. xii). He elaborated, "It is as if, when you see and hear and touch and taste things, some of the magic of your phenomenal sensation is rubbing off onto the things as such" (p. 111). And further, "it is indeed *you* who are the enchanter, *you* who are, as it were, coloring things with the fairy dust of your own consciousness" (p. 117). This line of thought leads into the import of his book's title, *Soul Dust*:

> you are responsible at the very deepest level for *what it feels like to be you*. But then, for your next trick, well, how about spreading some of that soul dust onto the things around you? Remember, too, that it is your mind that projects phenomenal qualities onto external objects. If you only knew it, you yourself are responsible for *the feel of the world*. (Humphrey, 2011, p. 134)

Crucially, we spread the soul dust onto each other in a way that enhances the evolutionary value of our sociality in tandem with our individual survival value:

> What human beings wake up to is that they are indeed a part of a *society of selves*. The idea is extraordinarily potent—on psychological, ethical, and political levels. And there can be no question that from the moment it took off among our ancestors, it must have been highly adaptive. For from the beginning it would have transformed human relationships,

encouraging new levels of mutual respect, and greatly increasing the value individuals placed on their own and others' lives. (Humphrey, 2011, p. 152)

Here is how Humphrey sums it all up:

> Consciousness is a magical mystery show that you lay on for yourself. You respond to sensory input by creating, as a personal response, a seemingly otherworldly object . . . which you present to yourself in your inner theater. Watching from the royal box, as it were, you find yourself transported to that other world. (Humphrey, 2011, p. 40)

Some readers might bristle at Humphrey's (2011) unabashed dualism—seemingly the same sort of dualism for which Descartes (1637/1968) has been much maligned. But Humphrey (2011) is no lone anachronistic dualist; we all are: "all my arguments about the magical mystery show would fall flat if human beings were *not* dualists. It would mean the show had failed" (p. 195, *emphasis in original*). Matthew Lieberman (2013) instructively summed up the brain basis of our entrenched dualism:

> the neural separation of representing our own bodies and representing our own minds explains why we can't get away from Descartes' mind-body dualism. All signs point toward mind-body dualism being a bad explanation of what we are, and yet most of us operate like card-carrying dualists. We can't help it because it is literally wired into our operating system to see the world in terms of minds and bodies that are separated from one another. We have one system for thinking about our own minds and another one for recognizing our own bodies, and these systems are separated in the brain. (p. 186)

Yet in our exuberance for this great evolutionary gift that we cannot return to our brains, we should not give short shrift to the downsides of consciousness; these downsides—exemplified in suffering—make up the basis of our clinical work. Being self-conscious creatures, we face existential concerns. At the core of these concerns is our awareness of our inevitable death—the termination of consciousness. Moreover, this recognition opens up the possibility of suicide; as Humphrey (2011) stated (quoting another author): "At some stage of evolution man must have discovered that he can kill not only animals and fellow-men but also himself. It can be assumed that life has never since been the same to him" (p. 173). Furthermore, being meaning-making creatures, we are liable to grapple with the potential loss of meaning and purpose—at worst leading to nihilism. And the imaginative theater we create can be replete with tragic or nightmarish dramas that we author to our detriment. Moreover, depression as well as dissociative detachment can rob consciousness of its inherent adaptive vitality. Hence, adaptive and glorious as it might be in general, consciousness is a double-edged sword out of which psychiatric disorders and existential despair are forged.

In agreeing with current thinking that our subjective experience is an illusion in theater created by the brain, I do not imply that the world as we live it is not "real." Nothing could be more "real" to us than our direct experience. But coming to grips with the fact (in my mind) that this world as we live it is a creation in a material object that is best described by science (biology, chemistry, and physics) is no small feat. I speculate that we will become increasingly amazed by our brains' mental creations as we learn more from neuroscience. Doubtlessly, we will be humbled. But we need not feel further dethroned, and we certainly should feel grateful for the evolution of the brain and its creation of the mind that enables us to thrive in the social world—barring the psychiatric and existential threats to our well-being.

BALANCING PERSPECTIVES IN CLINICAL PRACTICE

I view the mental health professions as being fundamentally humanistic in their grounding in psychological attunement in attachment relationships—caring, in short. My protesting "biomania" is borne of concern that we risk insidiously morphing our clinical practice into a technological enterprise. Manualizing therapies in relation to psychiatric diagnosis is one step; objectifying persons as brains in action could take technological thinking to new heights. Economic constraints on health care—including limited personal contact with patients—could abet this transition. We are heading down a path to employing genetic testing and brain scans to guide medical interventions. This progression promises to be a great boon to our patients and to our work as therapists. But not if it comes at the expense of addressing problems in living, as Szasz (1974) warned in his provocative way. Creation of the brain though it may be, we live in the theater and must work out our dramas there.

To reiterate, I am on board with learning all we can about neuroscience and using this knowledge to develop more effective neurobiological treatments: relief of suffering by any means is a fundamentally humanitarian project, and neuroscience will make an increasingly essential contribution to this enterprise. But we must remain mindful of our humanity as we juggle these dramatically contrasting perspectives on who we are—persons in brains.

I have devoted considerable effort—in writing and in psychoeducational groups—to educating patients and their family members about the biological basis of trauma (Allen, 2005) and depression (Allen, 2006). Contra Szasz (1974), I include the illness perspective to help patients be more compassionate toward themselves in relation to the daunting challenges of recovering from these potentially disabling conditions. In taking responsibility for their recovery, patients must face the reality of the seriousness of their illness; as contrasted with wishful thinking, hope is based on reasonable expectations (Allen, 2013a; K. A. Menninger, 1959/1987; Pruyser, 1987). In taking this biological approach, however, we must be mindful of the dangers of increasing stigma by implying a pessimistic prognosis (Kvaale et al., 2013). In particular, we must emphasize brain plasticity and the capacity for restoration of normal brain function, without which recovery would be impossible.

Perhaps more problematic than professional biomania is the prospect for patients to become biomanics in adopting a reductionistic biological view of their illness. I remember vividly reviewing with a group of patients the "stress pileup" model of vulnerability to depression, which encompasses a developmental perspective (Allen, 2006). After listening attentively, one patient protested, "But my doctor said I have a *biochemical* depression!" I responded that, of course, her depression has a biochemical basis, but I was outlining the kinds of developmental experiences that contribute to biochemical changes and associated alterations in patterns of brain functioning.

One obvious problem with patients' adoption of the biological view is their fixation on solely biological treatments. I encourage patients to get all the help they can from medication and other biological interventions, but I emphasize that illnesses of all sorts stem partly from problems in living and that recovery and health is based on behavior and relationships—putting attachment relationships at the forefront. I am most disconcerted by patients who have been told that their depression is "treatment resistant," such that they feel utterly hopeless. Having adopted biomania, they do not realize that, though they may not have responded to medication, they can benefit from behavioral, psychological, interpersonal, and family interventions. Moreover, as my colleague, psychiatrist David Console emphasized to me years ago, benefit from psychological interventions is likely to render patients more responsive to medication, just as medication can render patients more responsive to psychotherapy.

We have lived for a long time with the knowledge that the earth is not the center of the universe, that we evolved over eons, and that we are unaware of our mental activity to a considerable degree. Of course, the sheer availability of knowledge does not translate automatically into learning or acceptance of the knowledge (evolution being a prime example). Although we have long known—in principle—that the mind relates to the brain, we are only recently becoming aware of the neurobiological details that make this principle increasingly real—disconcertingly so. How this dawning awareness will shape our view of ourselves will only be seen over the decades (perhaps centuries) to come. At this point, we remain on the cusp of understanding the biological basis of our humanity—our consciousness, attachment relationships, mentalizing capacity, and moral proclivities. We mental health professionals are likely to be more aware of this research than laypersons insofar as biomania is infusing our work. This special issue of *Smith Studies* exemplifies our need to educate ourselves, if only to develop a balanced perspective that we can use to educate our patients and their family members who are liable to be misled by the latest "discovery" of the gene that causes *x* or the brain region responsible for *y*— or worse, those who despair because the have not responded to a plethora of medications but have not appreciated the value of psychotherapies and family interventions.

If we are to help our patients and their family members navigate the mental health care system in this dawning age of biomania, we must come to grips with the brain–mind relation in our own minds. For the foreseeable future, dualists as we will remain, we will necessarily juggle two perspectives. Philosopher Peter Strawson's (1962/1982) seminal chapter, "Freedom and Resentment," published long before the ascendance of neuroscience, continues to shape the way I think about my clinical work. I conclude this article with a précis of Strawson's clear thinking, now more needed than ever.

Strawson (1985) helpfully distinguished two contrasting attitudes toward others' actions: The emotionally detached attitude is objective, employing scientific thinking to construe behavior as based on causes. The emotionally reactive attitude is subjective, based on moral reasoning that views individuals as responsible for choices. We must accommodate both attitudes in the field of mental health and in our relationships more generally. Strawson characterized the detached, scientific-deterministic view as follows:

> To see human beings and human actions in this light is to see them simply as objects and events in nature, natural objects and natural events, to be described, analyzed, and causally explained in terms in which moral evaluation has no place; in terms, roughly speaking, of an observational and theoretical vocabulary recognized in the natural and social sciences, including psychology. (p. 40)

From this perspective, treatments for psychiatric disorders, based on scientific research, constitute an additional set of intervening causes, changing patients' thoughts, feelings, and behavior in the grand causal chain of determinism. As Strawson (1962/1982) put it, from the standpoint of treatment, the person is to be "managed or handled or cured or trained" (p. 66). As described earlier, this emotionally detached approach has the potential advantage of ameliorating blame. With alcoholism in mind, consider Strawson's (1985) point:

> What from one [reactive] point of view is rightly seen as a piece of disgraceful turpitude, an appropriate object of a reaction of moral disgust, is,

from the other [detached] point of view, rightly seen as merely the natural outcome of a complex collocation of factors, an appropriate object of scientific, psychological, and sociological analysis and study. (pp. 41–42)

Not so fast! Consistent with our dualistic thinking, Strawson (1962/1982) made the compelling argument that we can temporarily suspend our moral reactive attitudes, but we cannot and should not strive to eliminate them: "A sustained objectivity of inter-personal attitude, and the human isolation which that would entail, does not seem to be something of which human beings would be capable, even if some general truth were a theoretical ground for it" (p. 68). Furthermore, "it is useless to ask whether it would not be rational for us to do what it is not in our nature to (be able to) do" (p. 74). As therapists and in our other relationships, we naturally respond emotionally to others as persons with intentions who are free agents, make choices, and are responsible for their actions. Hence Strawson proposed that we cannot altogether avoid the emotionally reactive attitude. Indeed, detached and reflective moral reasoning typically is preceded and influenced by relatively fast, automatic, and emotional moral intuition (Haidt, 2007). This is the proper junction to acknowledge that I have set up a straw man in this article because, in our clinical work, we are incapable of being full-blown biomanics—technicians devoid of humanity. But we certainly are capable of tilting too far in that direction.

Advocating detachment, Strawson (1962/1982) also made clear that, in our unavoidable feelings and judgments, we take into account the possibility of accidents and unwitting actions—it makes a big difference if someone steps on your foot on purpose or not. And he also allowed for factors that limit the capacity for freedom of action, including compulsions and psychiatric disorders; in such situations, we might "suspend our ordinary reactive attitudes toward the agent, either at the time of his action or all the time" (p. 65). Moreover, he allowed for degrees of mitigation; in suspending the ordinary reactive attitudes, we might feel less perturbed rather than not at all perturbed about offensive actions. This point is consistent with Churchland's (2013) acknowledgment of the fuzzy boundaries between voluntary and involuntary action and with my emphasis on our limited elbowroom (Allen, 2006).

To summarize: In contrast with our scientific detachment, our reactive attitudes are embedded in our emotional engagement with each other. Such engagement is based on our natural proclivity to mentalize, that is, to respond emotionally and to interpret others' actions as based on intentions, desires, feelings, and beliefs—with the implicit assumption that their actions reflect at least some degree of free agency and choice. Freedom of choice always comes in degrees; our choices always take place in the context of constraints—we are constrained by external circumstances and by personal limitations. Plainly, psychiatric conditions such as alcoholism and depression limit the individual's elbowroom, and we professionals are in the best position to mentalize these limitations and to help our patients and their family members appreciate them. Yet psychiatric disorders do not entirely eliminate elbowroom—certainly not at every moment. Hence, as Strawson maintained, we must be able to straddle the detached and reactive attitudes. Strawson (1962/1982) took the psychoanalyst as an example of such straddling; he pointed out, ironically, that the psychoanalytic aim of adopting the detached attitude and suspending morally reactive attitudes is to "make such suspension unnecessary or less necessary" by virtue of "restoring the agent's freedom" (p. 75).

Strawson (1962/1982) provided us clinicians with a philosophical platform for maintaining balance that will support science-informed humanism. This platform is the basis of my conviction that our psychotherapeutic work with individuals, groups, and families is an ethical endeavor (Allen, 2013c). This ethical endeavor has been intermingled with scientific aspirations since Freud pioneered psychoanalytic treatment a century ago (Tauber, 2010). This intermingling is becoming increasingly challenging as we grapple with the discoveries of neuroscience. Now Humphrey (2011) has charted a path for putting soul back into the brain—the epitome of science-informed humanism. For one, I am glad to live in my brain's theater of consciousness, enjoying the contemporary version of the age-old quest to understand our place in the world.

REFERENCES

Adolphs, R. (2003). Cognitive neuroscience of human social behavior. *Nature Reviews Neuroscience, 4*, 165–178.

Allen, J. G. (2005). *Coping with trauma: Hope through understanding* (2nd ed.). Washington, DC: American Psychiatric Publishing.

Allen, J. G. (2006). *Coping with depression: From catch-22 to hope.* Washington, DC: American Psychiatric Publishing.

Allen, J. G. (2008). Psychotherapy: The artful use of science. *Smith College Studies in Social Work, 78*, 159–187.

Allen, J. G. (2013a). Hope in human attachment and spiritual connection. *Bulletin of the Menninger Clinic, 77*, 302–331.

Allen, J. G. (2013b). *Mentalizing in the development and treatment of attachment trauma.* London, UK: Karnac.

Allen, J. G. (2013c). Psychotherapy is an ethical endeavor: Balancing humanism and science in clinical practice. *Bulletin of the Menninger Clinic, 77*, 103–131.

Allen, J. G. (2013d). *Restoring mentalizing in attachment relationships: Treating trauma with plain old therapy.* Washington, DC: American Psychiatric Publishing.

Allen, J. G., & Fonagy, P. (2006). Preface. In J. G. Allen & P. Fonagy (Eds.), *Handbook of mentalization-based treatment* (pp. ix–xxi). Chichester, UK: Wiley.

Allen, J. G., Fonagy, P., & Bateman, A. (2008). *Mentalizing in clinical practice*. Washington, DC: American Psychiatric Publishing.

Alter, M. D., & Hen, R. (2009). Serotonin, sensitive periods, and anxiety. In G. Andrews, D. S. Charney, P. J. Sirovatka, & D. A. Reiger (Eds.), *Stress-induced and fear circuitry disorders: Refining the research agenda for DSM-V* (pp. 159–173). Arlington, VA: American Psychiatric Publishing.

Amodio, D. M., & Frith, C. D. (2006). Meeting of minds: The medial frontal cortex and social cognition. *Nature Reviews Neuroscience, 7,* 268–277.

Arnott, B., & Meins, E. (2007). Links between antenatal attachment representations, postnatal mind-mindedness, and infant attachment security: A preliminary study of mothers and fathers. *Bulletin of the Menninger Clinic, 71,* 132–149.

Ayer, A. J. (1982). Freedom and necessity. In G. Watson (Ed.), *Free will* (pp. 15–23). New York, NY: Oxford University Press.

Baars, B. J. (1997). *In the theater of consciousness: The workspace of the mind*. New York, NY: Oxford University Press.

Baumeister, R. F., Mele, A. R., & Vohs, K. D. (Eds.). (2010). *Free will and consciousness: How do they work?* New York, NY: Oxford University Press.

Berlin, L. J., Zeanah, C. H., & Lieberman, A. F. (2008). Prevention and intervention programs for supporting early attachment security. In J. Cassidy & P. R. Shaver (Eds.), *Handbook of attachment: Theory, research, and clinical applications* (2nd ed., pp. 745–761). New York, NY: Guilford.

Bogdan, R. J. (1997). *Interpreting minds: The evolution of a practice*. Cambridge, MA: MIT Press.

Bracken, P., Thomas, P., Timimi, S., Asen, E., Behr, G., Beuster, C., . . . Yeomans, D. (2012). Psychiatry beyond the current paradigm. *British Journal of Psychiatry, 201,* 430–434.

Castonguay, L. G., & Beutler, L. E. (Eds.). (2006). *Principles of therapeutic change that work*. New York, NY: Oxford University Press.

Churchland, P. S. (2013). *Touching a nerve: The self as brain*. New York, NY: Norton.

Damasio, A. (2010). *Self comes to mind: Constructing the conscious brain*. New York, NY: Pantheon.

Dehaene, S., Changeux, J.-P., Naccache, L., Sackur, J., & Sergent, C. (2006). Conscious, preconscious, and subliminal processing: A testable taxonomy. *Trends in Cognitive Sciences, 10,* 204–211.

Dennett, D. C. (1984). *Elbow room: The varieties of free will worth wanting*. Cambridge, MA: MIT Press.

Descartes, R. (1968). *Discourse on method and the meditations* (F. E. Sutcliffe, Trans.). New York, NY: Penguin. (Original work published 1637)

Edelman, G. M. (2004). *Wider than the sky: The phenomenal gift of consciousness*. New Haven, CT: Yale University Press.

Elliott, R., Bohart, A. C., Watson, J. C., & Greenberg, L. S. (2011). Empathy. In J. C. Norcross (Ed.), *Psychotherapy relationships that work: Evidence-based responsiveness* (2nd ed., pp. 132–152). New York, NY: Oxford University Press.

Farber, B. A., & Doolin, E. M. (2011). Positive regard and affirmation. In J. C. Norcross (Ed.), *Psychotherapy relationships that work: Evidence-based responsiveness* (2nd ed., pp. 168–186). New York, NY: Oxford University Press.

Fonagy, P. (1989). A child's understanding of others. *Bulletin of the Anna Freud Centre, 12,* 91–115.

Fonagy, P., Gergely, G., Jurist, E. L., & Target, M. (2002). *Affect regulation, mentalization, and the development of the self.* New York, NY: Other Press.

Fonagy, P., Gergely, G., & Target, M. (2007). The parent-infant dyad and the construction of the subjective self. *Journal of Child Psychology and Psychiatry, 48,* 288–328.

Fonagy, P., Steele, H., & Steele, M. (1991). Maternal representations of attachment during pregnancy predict the organization of infant-mother attachment at one year of age. *Child Development, 62,* 891–905.

Frith, C. D., & Frith, U. (2006). The neural basis of mentalizing. *Neuron, 50,* 531–534.

Graziano, M. S. A. (2013). *Consciousness and the social brain.* New York, NY: Oxford University Press.

Haidt, J. (2007). The new synthesis in moral psychology. *Science, 316,* 998–1002.

Horvath, A. O., Del Re, A. C., Fluckiger, C., & Symonds, D. (2011). Alliance in individual psychotherapy. In J. C. Norcross (Ed.), *Psychotherapy relationships that work: Evidence-based responsiveness* (2nd ed., pp. 25–69). New York, NY: Oxford University Press.

Humphrey, N. K. (1988). The social function of intellect. In R. W. Byrne & A. Whiten (Eds.), *Machiavellian intelligence: Social expertise and the evolution of intellect in monkeys, apes, and humans* (pp. 13–26). New York, NY: Oxford University Press.

Humphrey, N. K. (2006). *Seeing red: A study in consciousness.* Cambridge, MA: Harvard University Press.

Humphrey, N. K. (2011). *Soul dust: The magic of consciousness.* Princeton, NJ: Princeton University Press.

Kane, R. (Ed.). (2011). *The Oxford handbook of free will* (2nd ed.). New York, NY: Oxford University Press.

Kazdin, A. E. (2007). Mediators and mechanisms of change in psychotherapy research. *Annual Review of Clinical Psychology, 3,* 1–27.

Kolden, G. G., Klein, M. H., Wang, C.-C., & Austin, S. B. (2011). Congruence/genuineness. In J. C. Norcross (Ed.), *Psychotherapy relationships that work: Evidence-based responsiveness* (2nd ed., pp. 187–202). New York, NY: Oxford University Press.

Kvaale, E. P., Haslam, N., & Gottdiener, W. H. (2013). The 'side effects' of medicalization: A meta-analytic review of how biogenetic explanations affect stigma. *Clinical Psychology Review, 33,* 782–794.

Lieberman, M. D. (2013). *Social: Why our brains are wired to connect.* New York, NY: Random House.

Meins, E., Fernyhough, C., Fradley, E., & Tuckey, M. (2001). Rethinking maternal sensitivity: Mothers' commments on infants' mental processes predict security of attachment at 12 months. *Journal of Child Psychology and Psychiatry, 42,* 637–648.

Meins, E., Fernyhough, C., Wainwright, R., Das Gupta, M., Fradley, E., & Tuckey, M. (2002). Maternal mind-mindedness and attachment security as predictors of theory of mind understanding. *Child Development, 73,* 1715–1726.

Menninger, K. A. (1987). Hope. *Bulletin of the Menninger Clinic, 51,* 447–462. (Original work published 1959)

Menninger, W. W. (1975). "Caring" as part of health care quality. *Journal of the American Medical Association, 234,* 836–837.

Norcross, J. C. (Ed.). (2011). *Psychotherapy relationships that work: Evidence-based responsiveness* (2nd ed.). New York, NY: Oxford University Press.

Polan, H. J., & Hofer, M. A. (2008). Psychobiological origins of infant attachment and its role in development. In J. Cassidy & P. R. Shaver (Eds.), *Handbook of attachment: Theory, research, and clinical applications* (2nd ed., pp. 158–172). New York, NY: Guilford.

Pruyser, P. W. (1987). Maintaining hope in adversity. *Bulletin of the Menninger Clinic, 51*, 463–474.

Rogers, C. R. (1951). *Client-centered therapy: Its current practice, implications, and theory*. Boston, MA: Houghton Mifflin.

Rogers, C. R. (1957). The necessary and sufficient conditions of therapeutic personality change. *Journal of Consulting Psychology, 21*, 95–103.

Sadler, L. S., Slade, A., & Mayes, L. C. (2006). Minding the baby: A mentalization-based parenting program. In J. G. Allen & P. Fonagy (Eds.), *Handbook of mentalization-based treatment* (pp. 271–288). Chichester, UK: Wiley.

Safran, J. D., Muran, J. C., & Eubanks-Carter, C. (2011). Repairing alliance ruptures. In J. C. Norcross (Ed.), *Psychotherapy relationships that work: Evidence-based responsiveness* (2nd ed., pp. 224–238). New York, NY: Oxford University Press.

Searle, J. R. (2007). *Freedom and neurobiology*. New York, NY: Columbia University Press.

Shallice, T., & Cooper, R. P. (2011). *The organisation of mind*. New York, NY: Oxford University Press.

Slade, A., Grienenberger, J., Bernbach, E., Levy, D., & Locker, A. (2005). Maternal reflective functioning, attachment, and the transmission gap: A preliminary study. *Attachment and Human Development, 7*, 283–298.

Steele, H., Steele, M., & Fonagy, P. (1996). Associations among attachment classificaitons of mothers, fathers, and their infants. *Child Development, 67*, 541–555.

Strawson, P. F. (1982). Freedom and resentment. In G. Watson (Ed.), *Free will* (pp. 59–80). New York, NY: Oxford University Press. (Original work published 1962)

Strawson, P. F. (1985). *Skepticism and naturalism: Some varieties*. New York, NY: Columbia University Press.

Suomi, S. J. (2008). Attachment in rhesus monkeys. In J. Cassidy & P. R. Shaver (Eds.), *Handbook of attachment: Theory, research, and clinical applications* (2nd ed., pp. 173–191). New York, NY: Guilford.

Szasz, T. S. (1974). *The myth of mental illness: Foundations of a theory of personal conduct* (Rev. ed.). New York, NY: Harper and Row.

Tauber, A. I. (2010). *Freud: The reluctant philosopher*. Princeton, NJ: Princeton University Press.

Weaver, I. C. G., Cervoni, N., Champagne, F. A., D'Alessio, A. C., Sharma, S., Seckl, J. R., . . . Meaney, M. J. (2004). Epigenetic programming by maternal behavior. *Nature Neuroscience, 7*, 847–854.

Index

Printed and bound by CPI Group (UK) Ltd, Croydon, CR0 4YY

18/10/2024

01776204-0005